# History, Philosophy and Theory of the Life Sciences

## Volume 15

**Editors**
Charles T. Wolfe, Ghent University, Ghent, Oost-Vlaanderen Belgium
Philippe Huneman, IHPST (CNRS/Université Paris I Panthéon-Sorbonne), France
Thomas A.C.Reydon, Leibniz Universität, Hannover, Germany

More information about this series at http://www.springer.com/series/8916

Jerome C. Wakefield • Steeves Demazeux
Editors

# Sadness or Depression?

International Perspectives on the Depression
Epidemic and Its Meaning

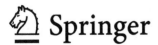 Springer

*Editors*
Jerome C. Wakefield
Silver School of Social Work
  and Department of Psychiatry
New York University
New York, NY, USA

Steeves Demazeux
Department of Philosophy, SPH Laboratory
Université Bordeaux Montaigne
Pessac, France

ISSN 2211-1948          ISSN 2211-1956   (electronic)
History, Philosophy and Theory of the Life Sciences
ISBN 978-94-017-7421-5          ISBN 978-94-017-7423-9   (eBook)
DOI 10.1007/978-94-017-7423-9

Library of Congress Control Number: 2015959694

Springer Dordrecht Heidelberg New York London

Printed on acid-free paper

Springer Science+Business Media B.V. Dordrecht is part of Springer Science+Business Media (www.springer.com)

# Contents

# Contributors

**Xavier Briffault** is a social scientist and epistemologist working on mental health at the French National Centre for Scientific Research and in one of the main French social sciences research centre, Cermes3 (Centre de recherche, médecine, sciences, santé, santé mentale, société). His main research interests are depression, obsessive-compulsive disorders, psychotherapy and mental health prevention programmes, as well as public health interventions in those areas. He conducts on these issues a sociologically and epistemologically informed analysis of the effectiveness of interventions, particularly in the context of the extension of the evidence-based medicine paradigm (EBM) to mental medicine. He also operates as an expert for several public health institutions.

**Pierre-Henri Castel** PhD in Philosophy, PhD in Psychology, 52, is French. He is a senior research fellow at the Centre National de la Recherche Scientifique (CNRS) at the Ecole des Hautes Etudes en Sciences Sociales (EHESS) in Paris. He has worked as a clinician for 20 years in various psychiatric hospitals. He also is a psychoanalyst in private practice. His scholarly specialty is the history and philosophy of mental medicine, from psychoanalysis to psychiatric neuroscience. He has written nine books, on hysteria and neurology in Charcot's circle, a detailed analysis of Freud's *Traumdeutung*, a history of transsexualism focusing on personal identity, a collection of essays on contemporary psychiatry from the point of view of a neo-Wittgensteinian philosophy of mind and, recently, a two-volume critical history of obsessions and compulsions from antiquity to present-day neuroscience and CBT: *Âmes scrupuleuses, vies d'angoisse, tristes obsédés. Obsessions et compulsions de l'Antiquité à Freud* (2011) and *La Fin des coupables, suivi du cas Paramord. Obsessions et compulsions de la psychanalyse aux neurosciences* (2012). His work can be seen as a form of philosophical anthropology based on the history of major mental disorders (along with their cures), but he has also worked extensively to try to bridge the gap between the main philosophical currents, the analytic and the 'continental', underlying many recent developments in the philosophy of psychopathology (personal website: http://pierrehenri.castel.free.fr).

**Steeves Demazeux** is an associate professor of philosophy at the Université Bordeaux Montaigne (France). He received his doctoral degree at Paris Sorbonne University (IHPST laboratory) and spent 2 years as a postdoctoral fellow at CERMES Institute (Paris Descartes University). His research interests include history and philosophy of psychiatry, philosophy of medicine and philosophy of science. He is the author of *Qu'est-ce que le DSM? Genèse et transformations de la bible américaine de la psychiatrie* (Ithaque 2013); the co-author, with Françoise Parot and Lionel Fouré, of *Psychothérapie, fondements et pratiques* (Belin 2011); and the co-editor, with Patrick Singy, of the collective volume, *The DSM-5 in Perspective. Philosophical Reflections on the Psychiatric Babel* (Springer 2015).

**Christopher Dowrick, M.D., FRCGP** is professor of primary medical care in the University of Liverpool and a general practitioner in north Liverpool, England. He is also board advisor for Mersey Care NHS Trust, senior investigator emeritus for the National Institute for Health Research in England and professorial research fellow in the University of Melbourne in Australia. He is a member of the World Organization of Family Doctors' working party on mental health and a technical expert for the World Health Organization's mhGAP programme.

His research portfolio covers common mental health problems in primary care, with a focus on depression and medically unexplained symptoms. He critiques contemporary emphases on unitary diagnostic categories and medically oriented interventions and highlights the need for socially oriented perspectives. He is currently exploring the role of placebo and contextual effects in antidepressant drug prescribing and investigating ways to reduce inequity of access to primary mental health care for people from marginalised and disadvantaged communities. He has over 200 academic publications. The second edition of his book *Beyond Depression* was published by Oxford University Press in 2009. With Allen Frances, he has contributed to the *British Medical Journal*'s 'Too Much Medicine' series on the over-medicalisation of depression (http://bmj.com/cgi/content/full/bmj.f7140).

**Alain Ehrenberg** is a sociologist and director of research at the CNRS (Centre National de la Recherche Scientifique). He has developed research programmes and research units on mental health issues. His main books are about transformations of individualism and autonomy, mainly through the area of mental health: *Le Culte de la performance* (Calmann-Lévy 1991), *L'Individu incertain* (Calmann-Lévy 1995), *La Fatigue d'être soi* (Odile Jacob 1998, translated into six languages including in English: *The Weariness of the Self. Diagnosing the History of Depression in the Contemporary Age*, McGill UP, 2010, with an original foreword) and *La Société du Malaise* (translated in German and Italian).

**Luc Faucher** is full professor in philosophy at the Université du Québec à Montréal (UQAM, Canada). After a PhD in Montréal, he has been postdoctoral fellow at Rutgers University under the direction of Stephen Stich. His research interests cover philosophy of cognitive sciences, philosophy of race, philosophy of emotions and philosophy of psychiatry. He is the co-editor (with Christine Tappolet) of *The*

*Modularity of Emotions* (2008) and the editor of *Philosophie et psychopathologies* (2006). He published papers in *Philosophy of Science, Philosophy of the Social Sciences, Emotion Review, Journal of Social Philosophy, Synthese* and *The Monist*. A former student of the Ecole Normale Supérieure, Paris.

**Denis Forest** is professor of philosophy at the University Paris Ouest Nanterre and an associate member of the Institut d'Histoire et de Philosophie des sciences et des techniques (IHPST, Paris). His main areas of research are philosophy of neuroscience and philosophy of mind. He has recently collaborated to the volume *Brain Theory: Essays in Critical Neurophilosophy* edited by Charles Wolfe (Palgrave Macmillan 2014). His second book, *Neuroscepticisme: les sciences du cerveau sous le scalpel de l'épistémologue*, has been published by Ithaque (Paris 2014).

**David Goldberg** has devoted his professional life to improving the teaching of psychological skills to doctors of all kinds and to improving the quality of services for those with severe mental illnesses. He has advised the Department of Health over the years about service developments and has been extensively used by the World Health Organization as a mental health consultant. He completed his psychiatric training at the Maudsley Hospital. He went to Manchester, where for over 20 years he was head of the Department of Psychiatry and Behavioural Science. In 1993 he returned to Maudsley as professor of psychiatry and director of research and development. His interests are in vulnerability factors which predispose people to develop depression and in teaching general practitioners to give a better service to psychologically distressed patients. His research over many years has been concentrated on the details of communication between GPs and their patients, and he has applied these principles to his teaching of mental health workers in developing countries. He has a major interest in the best way primary care and specialist mental health services should relate to one another. For the past 25 years, his interests have extended away from doctors to the people who are in states of distress with particular attention to the factors that make people vulnerable to stressful life events. His first book on this subject dealt with both GPs and their patients (*Mental Illness in the Community, the Pathway to Psychiatric Care* with Peter Huxley), and his most recent book takes a thorough, developmental look at the determinants of this vulnerability (*The Course and Origin of Common Mental Disorders* with Ian Goodyer). He has been chairman of two NICE Guideline Development Groups, the first for depression and more recently for the guideline for depression among those with physical illnesses. He is a fellow of Hertford College, Oxford; King's College, London; and the Academy of Medical Sciences. He retired in 1999 and now works part time at the institute. He is currently chairman of the Psychiatry Research Trust at the Institute Of Psychiatry, London.

**Allan V. Horwitz** is board of governors professor in the Department of Sociology and interim director of the Institute for Health, Health Care Policy and Aging Research at Rutgers University. He has published over 100 articles and chapters about various aspects of mental health and illness and eight books including

*Creating Mental Illness* (University of Chicago Press 2002), *The Loss of Sadness: How Psychiatry Transformed Normal Misery into Depressive Disorder* (Oxford University Press 2007 with Jerome Wakefield), *All We Have to Fear* (Oxford University Press 2012 with Jerome Wakefield) and *A Short History of Anxiety* (Johns Hopkins University Press 2013). He was also the co-editor, with Teresa Scheid, of *A Handbook for the Study of Mental Health: Social Contexts, Theories, and Systems* (Cambridge University Press 1999). He also served as dean of social and behavioral sciences at Rutgers. Since 1980 he has been the co-director (with David Mechanic) of the NIMH-funded Rutgers' Postdoctoral Program in Mental Health. Professor Horwitz is the current chair of the Medical Sociology Section of the American Sociological Association and is a past chair of the Mental Health Section of the ASA. In 2006 he received the Leonard Pearlin Award for Distinguished Lifetime Contributions to the Sociology of Mental Health. He has been a fellow-in-residence at the Netherlands Institute for Advanced Study (2007–2008) and at the Center for Advanced Study in the Behavioral Sciences at Stanford (2012–2013).

**Junko Kitanaka, Ph.D.** is a medical anthropologist and associate professor in the Department of Human Sciences, Keio University, Tokyo. For her McGill University doctoral dissertation on depression, she received a number of awards including the 2007 Dissertation Award from the American Anthropological Association's Society for Medical Anthropology. This has since been published by Princeton University Press as a book titled *Depression in Japan: Psychiatric Cures for a Society in Distress*, which won the American Anthropological Association's Francis Hsu Prize for Best Book in East Asian Anthropology in 2013. The book has been translated by Dr. Pierre-Henri Castel at Paris Descartes University and published by Ithaque as *De la mort volontaire au suicide au travail: Histoire et anthropologie de la depression au Japon* (2014). She is currently working on a new project on dementia, old age and the psychiatrisation of the life cycle.

**Maël Lemoine** is an associate professor in the philosophy of biomedical science in Tours (France) and at the Institut d'Histoire des Sciences et des Techniques (Paris). In 2011, he published a book on explanations in medicine. He has since been working on the 'naturalisation' of mental disorders, on model organisms in biomedicine and on the concept of disease. He published half a dozen papers in English on these questions. He is currently preparing a book entitled *The Naturalization of Depression*.

**Mario Maj** is professor of psychiatry and chairman at the University of Naples SUN, Naples, Italy, and director of the Italian WHO Collaborating Center for Research and Training in Mental Health. He has been president of the World Psychiatric Association, the European Psychiatric Association and the Italian Psychiatric Association. He is editor of *World Psychiatry*, official journal of the World Psychiatric Association (impact factor 2014: 12.896).

He is member of the advisory board for the Chapter on Mental and Behavioural Disorders of the ICD-11 and chairperson of the Work Group on Mood and Anxiety

Disorders for that chapter. He has been member of the Work Group for Mood Disorders of the DSM-5.

He is honorary fellow of the Royal College of Psychiatrists, UK, and the American College of Psychiatrists and doctor honoris causa at the University of Craiova.

He has been active as a researcher and an educator on behalf of the WHO in sub-Saharan Africa, South East Asia and Latin America. He has been chairman of the Section on Neuropsychiatry of the Global Programme on AIDS at the WHO Headquarters in Geneva.

He is member of the editorial board of several international journals. He has been author of more than 450 scientific papers indexed in Scopus, mostly in the area of mood, psychotic and eating disorders. His H-index is 50.

**Jerome C. Wakefield** is university professor, professor of social work and professor of the conceptual foundations of psychiatry at New York University. He is also an affiliate faculty in bioethics and an honorary faculty member of the Institute for Psychoanalytic Education at NYU. He holds a PhD in philosophy, a DSW in clinical social work and an MA in mathematics (logic and methodology of science), all from the University of California, Berkeley. After post-doctoral fellowships in women's studies (Brown University), cognitive science (University of California, Berkeley) and mental health services research (Rutgers University), he held faculty positions at the University of Chicago, Columbia University and Rutgers University, before coming to NYU in 2003. He has published over 250 scholarly articles on the conceptual foundations of diagnosis and clinical theory, with recent publications focusing on controversies over proposed changes to DSM-5, especially issues concerning the relationship between depression and grief and the boundary between normal distress and mental disorder. He is the co-author (with Allan Horwitz) of *The Loss of Sadness: How Psychiatry Transformed Normal Sorrow into Depressive Disorder* (Oxford 2007), named the best psychology book of 2007 by the Association of Professional and Scholarly Publishers, and *All We Have to Fear: How Psychiatry Transforms Natural Fear into Mental Disorder* (Oxford 2012), named best book of the year by the American Sociological Association, Section on Evolution, Biology, and Society. He is currently completing a book on Freud's case history of Little Hans and its significance in the history of psychoanalysis, to be published by Routledge.

# Introduction: Depression, One and Many

Jerome C. Wakefield and Steeves Demazeux

This collective volume takes a fresh look at the psychiatric diagnosis of "major depressive disorder", the disorder's nature and its social meaning today. The heterogeneity of the conditions we call "depression" is so great that it raises difficult questions of individuation and identity. Major depression is one category of disorder in the DSM-5 and ICD-10, yet it is virtually universally agreed that the conditions that fall under that category constitute several different disorders caused by quite different etiologies. Similarly, depression varies across cultures in the way it presents, the way it is experienced, and the way it is valued or disvalued, so if it is so different, what makes it the same condition of "depression" that is being studied across cultures? Depression is the category of mental disorder most clearly recognized continuously since antiquity, yet it is also a category that has transformed and dramatically expanded during the twentieth century, so what makes it the same category over time? This is both a major intellectual challenge and a more immediate editorial challenge of explaining how the many diverse contributions to this volume could possibly be talking about a common topic. In attempting to provide an encompassing perspective, we acknowledge that some of the contributors to this volume may well disagree (and that at times we two disagree), and put forward the following thoughts in the spirit of offering one possible perspective among many.

J.C. Wakefield (✉)
Silver School of Social Work and Department of Psychiatry,
New York University, New York, NY, USA
e-mail: jw111@nyu.edu

S. Demazeux
Department of Philosophy, SPH Laboratory, Université Bordeaux Montaigne, Pessac, France
e-mail: steeves.demazeux@u-bordeaux-montaigne.fr

© Springer Science+Business Media Dordrecht 2016
J.C. Wakefield, S. Demazeux (eds.), *Sadness or Depression?*
History, Philosophy and Theory of the Life Sciences 15,
DOI 10.1007/978-94-017-7423-9_1

# A Short or a Long History?

The historiography on depression indicates the profound difficulty of finding the right balance for addressing in a unified way depression's anthropological, social and biological components. First of all, should depression be considered the result of a short or a long history? If we rely merely on terminology, we should recall that the medical use of the term "depression" as opposed to "melancholia" is rather recent. Following scattered references to sadness as "depressed spirits" in the prior centuries – including in Samuel Johnson's *Dictionary* (Johnson 1755, 21) – Jean-Etienne Esquirol characterized the condition of lypemania in 1838 as a "sad and *depressed* passion" (our emphasis), becoming one of the first alienists to use this metaphor inside a medical treatise. By the middle of the nineteenth century, the substantive "depression" spread in the writings of many European psychiatrists, such as French psychiatrist Jules Séglas who aimed at characterizing by this term a new specific form of moral suffering with all the clinical features of melancholia but without its component of delirium (see Lantéri-Laura 2003).

The history of melancholia seems easiest to trace back. It goes back to ancient times (around fifth century BC) and to the theory of humors ("melancholia" means "black bile disease"). In antiquity and until relatively recently, "melancholia" often referred to conditions that involved delusions ("delirium") and would likely be labeled as schizophrenia today, such as a melancholic patient described by Pinel who believed that he was actually dead and thus could not eat anymore (Starobinski 2012, 90). Today, melancholia is generally considered a severe form of depression, but there is still controversy about whether the two clinical entities really overlap with each other or should be distinguished. Despite a wave of studies some decades ago that argued that no such distinction had been scientifically confirmed (Kendell 1976; Lewis 1934), many in psychiatry continue to argue that the distinction is real and the histories divergent (Fink and Taylor 2007; Fink et al. 2007; Parker et al. 2010; Shorter 2007).

# Some Arguments in Favor of the Long History View

Whereas some medical historians have documented the swarming multiplicity of uses, theoretical assumptions, moral implications and treatment indications behind the terms "depression" and "melancholia" (Starobinski 2012), other medical historians have insisted to the contrary on the "remarkable consistency" of the medical condition that we now call depression (Jackson 1986, ix). The latter historians claim that, notwithstanding the many changes in concepts, theories and treatments through two and a half millennia, we can recognize in medical descriptions something like a stable medical condition tantamount to our modern conception of major depressive disorder, with a strikingly stable clinical picture. The individual is sad most of the day, he cries a lot and has lost his appetite, his energy, his sleep and most of his social interests, and often the individual cannot explain to himself and to others why he is in such a state of low mood. An intense episode of sadness, combined with the lack of a rational explanation for it in the circumstances of a person's life, are the two most traditionally mentioned characteristics from Aristotle (Jackson 1986, 32) and Galen (1929) through Burton (2001) to Kraepelin (1915), and they remain tempting reasons to speak of a common phenomenon of depressive episodes both retrospectively and in our present time.

Some medical historians emphasize the dangers of retrospective diagnosis. As Strarobinski observes, there is always something missing in the short clinical accounts that we find in old books, most importantly the presence of the patient (Starobinski 2012, 15). But is this a sufficient reason to condemn any retrospective diagnosis? To take one historical example of many, when the philosopher David Hume told the Comtesse de Boufflers about the "strange condition" of Lord Chatham that rendered him incapable of making decisions, Hume surely was describing something close to our modern concept of depression:

> You ask the present state of our politics....[W]e are in greater confusion than usual; because of the strange condition of Lord Chatham, who was regarded as our first minister. The public here, as well as with you, believe him wholly mad; but I am assured it is not so. He is only fallen into extreme low spirits and into nervous disorders, which render him totally unfit for business, make him shun all company, and, as I am told, set him weeping like a child, upon the least accident. Is not this a melancholy situation for so lofty and vehement a spirit as his? And is it not even an addition to his unhappiness that he retains his senses?... Meanwhile, the public suffers extremely by his present imbecility: no affairs advance: the ministers fall in variance: and the King entertains thoughts of forming a new administration. (Hume 1767)

The mysterious illness that gnawed at Lord Chatham intrigued many political commentators of his time. How to explain that, as Lady Chatham reported to the King, he suddenly became unable to make a decision about anything? Was he affected by a real illness, as invoked in his Resignation Letter addressed to the King in 1768? Or should we suspect political cowardice, as did some of his opponents? Resolving this question requires an investigation of the complex nexus of *causes* and/or *reasons* that can explain his behavior at a particular time and in a particular historical context, challenging us with endless ambiguities. The best explanation could be moral or sociological rather than psychological or medical. Yet even Hume identified "extreme low spirits" that are "nervous disorders" as a possible explanation, distinguishing it from rank "madness" and thus from psychotic conditions. Granting that basing our view of the history of depression on patchy stories from the past has its methodological dangers, why should we deny that many of our ancestors were affected by a condition that appears so common nowadays? Should we refuse to allow individuals of the past the intuitive demarcation that even they seem to have made between a normal episode of sadness and pathological sorrow?

Those who consequently opt for a long history of depression would see the use of the term 'depression' as simply a recent stylistic variant that refers to a condition recognized since antiquity. It is true that in antiquity it was often what we would now classify as "psychotic depression" – overlapping with what we now might classify as schizophrenia – that fell under "melancholia." And it is quite possible that milder forms have gradually been coopted by this category with the advent of "simple depression" and like states. Yet, many historical considerations support a continuity within the changes.

While theories of depressive disorder have changed, the symptoms that indicate the disorder have not. Writing in the fifth century B.C., Hippocrates provided the first known definition of melancholia as a distinct disorder: "If fear or sadness last for a long time it is melancholia" (Hippocrates 1931, 185). In addition to fear and sadness, Hippocrates mentioned as symptoms "aversion to food, despondency, sleeplessness, irritability, restlessness," much like today's criteria (Hippocrates 1923, 263). In another case, Hippocrates describes a woman who became morose during grief as not taking to her bed but suffering from insomnia, anorexia, anxiety, and somatic symptoms (Hippocrates 1923). Moreover, Hippocrates's definition indicated that it is not such symptoms alone but only symptoms of unexpected duration that indicate disorder. Hippocrates's insistence that the sadness or fear must be prolonged can be interpreted as a first attempt to capture the notion that disproportion to circumstances and thus lack of an explanation in terms of circumstances is an essential aspect of depressive disorder.

A century after Hippocrates, Aristotle (or one of his students) in the *Problemata* elaborated the distinction between a variety of normal mood states of sadness, on the one hand, and pathological disease states, on the other. Aristotle clearly expressed the idea that disordered sadness is disproportionate to events. He noted that, if the black bile "be cold beyond due measure, it produces groundless despondency" (Aristotle 1927, 165). Here "beyond due measure" refers to what is disproportionate to the circumstances, making the resultant sadness "groundless." Such despondency, for example, "accounts for the prevalence of suicide by hanging amongst the young and sometimes amongst older men too" (Aristotle 2000, 59). Aristotle also inaugurated the tradition that has lasted to our own day of associating depressive temperament or even depressive disorder with exceptional artistic and intellectual ability, asking: "Why is it that all men who have become outstanding in philosophy, statesmanship, poetry or the arts are melancholic, and some to such an extent that they are infected by the diseases arising from black bile…They are all, as has been said, naturally of this character" (Aristotle 2000, 57).

Further supporting a continuity of conception of depression, the ancients clearly distinguished between melancholic disordered sadness and intense but normal sadness with similar symptoms due to events in a person's life. This distinction was often illustrated with stories of a famous diagnostic triumph by Erasistratus (304–250 B.C.), physician to King Seleucus of Syria, in which Erasistratus discovered through shrewd observation that the King's son, Antiochus, was not suffering from melancholia as his symptoms suggested, but was instead suffering from unrequited (and unexpressable) love – for his father's young wife! As Aretaeus tells it:

> A story is told, that a certain person, incurably affected, fell in love with a girl; and when the physician could bring him no relief, love cured him. But I think that he was originally in love, and that he was dejected and spiritless from being unsuccessful with the girl, and

appeared to the common people to be melancholic. He then did not know that it was love; but when he imparted the love to the girl, he ceased from his dejection, and dispelled his passion and sorrow; and with joy he awoke from his lowness of spirits, and he became restored to understanding, love being his physician (Jackson 1986, 40).

Similarly, Galen (1929) describes a case in which he is unsure whether the problem lies in normal despair over some loss that is being hidden from the physician or the development of a depressive medical disorder:

> I was called in to see a woman who was stated to be sleepless at night and to lie tossing about from one position into another. Finding she had no fever, I made a detailed inquiry into everything that had happened to her, especially considering such factors as we know to cause insomnia. But she either answered little or nothing at all, as if to show that it was useless to question her. Finally, she turned away, hiding herself completely by throwing the bedclothes over her whole body, and laying her head on another small pillow, as if desiring sleep. After leaving I came to the conclusion that she was suffering from one of two things: either from a melancholy dependent on black bile, or else trouble about something she was unwilling to confess. I therefore deferred till the next day a closer investigation of this. (Galen 1929, 213)

DSM-5 contains a note stating that the clinician must use judgment when diagnosing depression because intense normal responses of sadness to various losses and stresses may resemble depressive disorder symptomatically. We may thus presume that many modern psychiatrists continue to be confronted by the same dilemma facing Galen that challenges the symptom-based core of the modern definition of a depressive disorder.

## What Is the Meaning of the Depression Epidemic in the Twentieth Century?

Whatever the historical perspective we should embrace (the short or the long view), one of the most intriguing and distinctive modern phenomena about depression is its epidemic character. This supposedly devastating and recurrent psychiatric disorder just a few decades ago was estimated to afflict perhaps 2–3 % of the population of the United States over a lifetime (Klein and Thase 1997), whereas the latest and most methodologically sophisticated studies indicate that the disorder occurs in more than half of the U.S. population (Moffitt et al. 2010; Rohde et al. 2013). The World health Organization (WHO) predicts that the situation will even get worse by 2020, with depression becoming the second major cause of worldwide disability.

How to explain such an epidemic expansion in prevalence and the corresponding treatment and prevention efforts regarding the disorder that has come to be known as "major depression"? In a huge literature devoted to this specific subject, one can discern two basic hypotheses. The first hypothesis accepts the growth of depression during the twentieth century as in some sense "real" and attempts to identify the cause. Some researchers, for instance, have speculated that some novel toxic or infectious agents or the influence of dietary changes may explain the epidemic of depression. Others researchers have focused on changes in lifestyle, such as our relationship with nature or lack of exposure to external light. Still others have considered such social changes as the rise of individualism, the development of neoliberalism, the culture of narcissism, social mobility, constant exposure to imagies of those with greater beauty or wealth through the media, and the effects of these phenomena on our psyches as possible causes of the epidemic of depressions. On the other hand, it is pointed out that major traditional sources of dejection, such as loss of children, poverty, and early death due to disease, have receded markedly in the developed societies that nonetheless report high rates of depression.

The second hypothesis is that the overwhelming increase in the prevalence of depression during the past century is mostly in some sense *artificial*. Epidemiological data in psychiatry have never been very reliable, especially in community populations. Few studies exist before the 1970s, and they were rarely replicated and were lacking a careful delineation between disorder and social distress (Horwitz and Wakefield 2007, 205). The widely used diagnostic criteria for depression provided in the American Psychiatric Association's *Diagnostic and Statistical Manual of Mental Disorders* (APA 2013) is clinically fuzzy, its boundaries have broadened over time, and it is based on symptoms that can easily occur in normal sadness, so that the mistaken "false positive" diagnoses of normal sadness as depressive disorder is possible. For example, recent changes in which a "bereavement exclusion" from diagnosis with major depression was removed from the diagnostic criteria implies that even intense sadness when mourning a relative can qualify as depressive disorder. A positive aspect of this artificial expansion is that it makes depression more visible and thereby creates better support and social acceptance for a disease that has long been considered shameful. A less optimistic perspective is that the modern expansion of depression is a pathologization process that progressively blurs the traditional and intuitive demarcation between normal sadness and pathological sorrow and yields the medicalization of the normal emotions of ordinary life (Horwitz and Wakefield 2007). This perspective raises concerns about the strategies employed by the pharmaceutical industries over the past 40 years, resulting in very high rates of consumption of antidepressants. The fact that in 1994, a selective serotonine reuptake inhibitor called "Prozac" became the second top-selling drug in the world is indicative of the scope of the social phenomena of depression using our contemporary DSM-based definitions.

Depression is closely associated symptomatically not only with normal intense sadness, but also with culpability and guilt, feeling stressed at work, excessive fatigue, deep sorrow, general lassitude, and diffuse unhappiness. Because of its medical nature, depression is the only one in this list that has a chance to get socially accepted as an excuse for impaired role functioning. However, it will be accepted as a social excuse only if, as the "sick role" demands, you show no complacency and demonstrate a willingness to get better rather than accepting your condition (Wakefield 2009, 2010). By contrast, lassitude (*lassitude*), tiredness (*fatigatio*) – two terms that carry in old Latin, exactly like the word *depressio*, the same image of exhaustion, of weariness, of a progressive slide down, of something being deflated –

have no positive place in society as justifiable, excusable phenomena that relieve you from your social obligations. Indeed, the French philosopher Roland Barthes, in one of his lectures at the College de France in 1978, wondered why tiredness is so negatively connoted is our societies and undertook the philosophical rehabilitation of tiredness as one of his figures of the "neutral" (Barthes 2005).

The same could largely be said of bereavement, except that for a long time in human history there has been a strict social codification of the process of bereavement. When an intimate dies, you are relieved of your social obligations for a certain time, after which society reasserts itself. Barthes noted in his diary a few days after the death of his mother: "The *measurement* of mourning. (Dictionary, Memorandum): eighteen months for mourning a father, a mother" (Barthes 2010, 28). According to the old dictionary that Barthes quotes, this measure was seen as the normal expected duration of bereavement. Eighteen months is also approximately the duration of Barthes' diary. The acceptable period of mourning today, before it is reclassified as pathology, can be considerably shorter. The pathological threshold was two months in DSM-IV, but even this threshold was removed in the DSM-5, making it possible to diagnose the bereaved as disordered after just two weeks of intense sadness. Barthes deplores the fact that our society today denies mourning, leaving to the individual the moral duty to internalize his or her suffering (Barthes 2010, 163). Whatever the intensity of his sorrow, Barthes categorically refused the medical term of depression for describing his condition. He intentionally distorted the term's meaning by inferring, for example, from the observation, "I resist the world, I suffer from what it demands of me, from its demands," to the conclusion that "The world depresses me" (Barthes 2010, 135). Barthes refused to consider himself to be suffering from a depression because admitting (in the passive form) "I'm depressed" appeared to him as a kind of surrender that commands you to clinically behave like a depressed person. That is, depression is a medical label that carries contradictory meanings in the eyes of the patient. On the one hand, it commonly functions as a welcome legitimate medical social excuse. On the other hand, social or familial pressure that demands a medical definition of the sadness may obscure its existential meaning to the individual.

## "Diagnosis Creep" and the Philosophical Sociology of Concept Deployment

The dramatic changes in estimated prevalence concerning depression raise another question: Why is it so easy to expand diagnostic categories beyond the strict bounds of mental disorder? There is of course the simple ambiguity that the term can be used to refer to both pathological and normal emotions. Beyond that, there is a missing discipline of the "sociology of concept deployment" that would explore the techniques, ambiguities, and fallacies by which concepts are expanded beyond their previous bounds to encompass a larger domain with the acquiescence of those using the concept. Perhaps part of this puzzle in the case of depression is not so much conceptual but has to do with a sense of compassion, that people who are suffering are in need and deserving of help and should be able to receive the help they need, even if the source of their suffering is not a genuine medical disorder.

One important piece of the "concept deployment" puzzle has to do with psychological essentialism (Medin and Ortony 1989). Many concepts apply not only to things that share apparent properties but to anything that shares some inferred underlying essential nature with an initially identified class of prototypical cases. Because we do not know the underlying essential processes that constitute the dysfunctions that occur in depressive disorder, it is possible to argue without fear of being conclusively refuted that further processes that are considered normal sadness might share that underlying essence and be disorders. Such essentialist extensions of concepts can also be supported by a theory. For example, if one claims that mild depression tends to lead to severe depression and thus tends to be prodromal for a full-blown disorder, then one may tend to categorize milder states of sadness as likely depressive disorders; and, if one theorizes about depression as lack of serotonin, one may extend the concept to milder cases based on lowered serotonin.

Another reason it is easy to extend the concept of depression might be called the "fallacy of prototype extension." When trying to define the domain of application of a concept, people commonly tend to focus on central, prototypical examples but not to systematically address potential counterexamples, thus emphasizing necessary conditions over sufficient conditions. If one tries to define the notion of a depressive disorder, one will naturally be drawn to the idea that it is a matter of extraordinarily high levels of sadness. The problem is that the definitional process includes no systematic counterexample formulation of cases of intense sadness that are not disorders to ensure that the proposed definition is not only necessary but a sufficient condition. The "dimensional" approach to diagnosis combined with such essentialist thinking leads to the classic "slippery slope fallacy" – the fallacy of thinking that just because there is lack of any sharp dividing line between mild and severe depression, therefore there is no essential difference between the extremes. This leads to the conclusion that sadness must be disorder "all the way down" to the mildest cases. Thus, in some diagnostic formulations, even one or two depressive symptoms can constitute "subthreshold" or "subsyndromal" depressive disorder.

Additionally, mental health professionals are heavily biased towards not missing genuine cases and less concerned about false-positive diagnoses in which a normal individual is mistakenly diagnosed as disordered. Professionals are apt to err on the side of seeing pathology to avoid making a mistake that could lead to terrible consequences for the misdiagnosed individual, whereas the impact of unneeded treatment is not seen as so worrisome. The attempt to understand the concept of depression and its extensive deployment within the mental health professions requires cross-disciplinary perspectives from at least psychiatry, philosophy, and sociology to understand our transformed application of this concept.

## Integrating Biological and Social Views of Depressive Disorder

One opposition firmly embraced by most scholars is that between biological and social-constructivist approaches to depression. Many of the authors in this volume, while no doubt wanting to escape any such dichotomy, do tend to focus their attention on one or the other of these poles. Yet it is obvious both that there is a species-typical biological substrate that forms the foundation for social constructions of depression, and that human sociocultural malleability allows great scope to social formulations. A "hybrid" conception attempts to encompass both truths by acknowledging a biologically based etiology for mental disorder while affirming the role of social construction in cultural manifestations of disorder (Wakefield 1992; Hacking 1999). Even if a mental disorder has a biological essence that is a real malfunction of mental processes in the medical sense, its superficial features might vary with social circumstances because underlying biological conditions may express themselves in a context-sensitive way.

If one assumes that sociocultural shaping involves alteration of brain tissue functioning, then novel social constructions can yield genuinely novel dysfunctions (i.e., novel breakdowns in biologically designed capacities) as side effects. For example, as technology advances, we are forced to make deliberative decisions about learning, eating, sex, reproduction, aggression, and play that were not needed in earlier epochs in which natural motivational systems would have held sway. The tension created by the provocation and exploitation of desire in market-driven economies even while demanding extraordinary levels of control over these desires can yield genuinely new pathologies.

When do the results of the interaction of biology and society become disorders? The result of cultural sculpting of human beings in socially desired ways, from stretching lips to developing autonomy to exploiting differences in mathematical talent to create a technical elite, is not a disorder if there is no socially defined harm. However, in the process of reshaping human beings as social artifacts, disorder attributions do commonly arise in three ways.

First, the construction process can be pursued so relentlessly that damaging side effects occur that constitute true disorders. For example, the chronic stress of contemporary competitive educational and occupational environments that wring as much productivity as possible from the naturally talented can cause anxiety disorders in the vulnerable.

Second, when novel social practices are embraced, dysfunctions that have existed all along but been considered only minor anomalies because they have not caused sufficient harm may be reevaluated, and their harm may now be deemed sufficient to constitute a disorder. For example, minor dysfunctions in corpus collosum growth caused no harm and thus were not disorders until cultures exploited human capacities to invent reading, which demands high brain-hemispheric information transfer for which the corpus collosum is responsible. Consequently, those minor dysfunctions have emerged as major obstacles to social participation and constitute the genuine disorder of "dyslexia."

Third, due to normal variations unfavorable to the social resculpting process, some individuals may fail to adequately reach a constructed ideal. These individuals are sometimes claimed to be defective and classified as disordered. However, such judgments are conceptually questionable. When normal biological variation resists conformity to social construction, that is best not considered a disorder no matter how tempting it is for societies to use the "disorder" label as a cudgel to enforce socially preferred change, because otherwise psychiatry becomes an oppressive social control profession. The fallacy underlying such mislabeling is that cultural ideology falsely declares the constructed ideal as "natural" so that when individuals who are in fact quite normal do not match it, they are judged disordered.

Incorrectly labeling socially valued outcomes as natural and therefore classifying normal variations that fail to manifest the socially desirable features as disorders is not only incorrect but oppressive at its core. It encompasses such historical episodes as classifying runaway slaves as suffering from "drapetomania," and classifying men who masturbated and women who experienced clitoral orgasms as disordered during the Victorian era. In our own day, this fallacy encompasses labeling normal-range anxiety about public performances demanded by many of today's occupations as "social phobia," labeling normal-range rambunctiousness in children who have difficulty satisfying demands to sit quietly at their desks in school as ADHD, and labeling those who are sad and therefore inefficient in their social role performances as depressively disordered.

## Overview of the Contributions

Always too close or too far: the phenomenon of depression is an object that seems to accept no good focal length. This volume's aim is to bring depression more into focus by bringing together psychiatrists, philosophers, sociologists and anthropologists to create a multidisciplinary composite of depression and shed light on depression's multifaceted nature. A second goal is to present a truly international perspective on depression. It seemed important to encompass the experiences of psychiatrists from different cultural contexts, but also to include scholars with different theoretical backgrounds and who work within different methodologies. The many areas that are covered include clinical research, epidemiology, neuro-imagining, evolutionary psychology, psychoanalysis, sociology, medical anthropology, philosophy, and translational research.

The volume contains 12 papers. The first five chapters (including this introductory the chapter, "Introduction: Depression, One and Many") deal with overarching conceptualizations of depression.

In the chapter, "The Current Status of the Diagnosis of Depression", British professor of psychiatry Sir David Goldberg presents an overview of recent clinical, epidemiological and genetic studies. He argues that depression is vaguely defined and covers a heterogeneous mix of conditions, and overlaps with a wide range of mental as well as somatic disorders that merge clinically with normality. Goldberg concludes that recognizing this extreme heterogeneity – which contrasts with the apparent homogeneity represented in classificatory systems and textbooks – is critical for working clinicians.

In the chapter, "The Continuum of Depressive States in the Population and the Differential Diagnosis Between "Normal" Sadness and Clinical Depression", Italian professor of psychiatry Mario Maj addresses the problem of distinguishing normal sadness from clinical depression. Observing that recent clinical and epidemiological studies fail to establish clear diagnostic boundaries for depression, Maj contrasts two rival approaches, the "pragmatic" versus the "contextual," to establishing such a boundary. The pragmatic approach, favored by both the DSM-5 and ICD-10 (World Health Organization 1992) diagnostic systems, claims that clinical utility (e.g., usefulness in prognosis and treatment) is the major criterion for establishing the boundary between normal sadness and depression. The contextual approach, by contrast, aims at better taking into account all the contextual factors that indicate whether sadness is a proportionate response to environmental circumstances, and insists on the importance of the *conceptual validity* of the distinction. Maj examines the strengths and weaknesses of both approaches, and concludes that neither approach is completely satisfactory, thus that further qualitative research is needed for resolving the issue.

In the chapter, "Beyond Depression: Personal Equation from the Guilty to the Capable Individual", French sociologist Alain Ehrenberg examines the "global idiom" of depression that cuts across contemporary societies. He argues that the replacement of psychoanalytic theories by the cognitive neurosciences has led to a reconceptualization of depression, with a new emphasis on individual autonomy and the capacity for emotional self-control. Whereas at the end of the nineteenth century the depressed individual was conceived of as a guilty individual, he or she is now seen as an individual whose emotional and action capacities are dysfunctional and need to be restored. This transformation has influenced our view of people's responsibility for their physical and psychological health. Ehrenberg concludes that depression should be seen not only as *an individual disorder* but as one profoundly connected with our ways of being affected by others and our ways of acting as autonomous individuals in our contemporary societies.

In the chapter, "Depression as a Problem of Labor: Japanese Debates About Work, Stress, and a New Therapeutic Ethos", Japanese professor of anthropology Junko Kitanaka traces the evolution of the Japanese national debate about depression during the 1990s, which she argues was connected to feelings of increasing stress in the workplace. She describes and evaluates the recent transformation in Japanese culture in which depression became the target of public surveillance. This shift in the conceptualization of depression, from a "private matter" to a "public illness" sheds light on the social nature of depression, and especially its relationship with recent development of the neoliberal economy.

The chapters "Darwinian Blues: Evolutionary Psychiatry and Depression", "Is an Anatomy of Melancholia Possible? Brain Processes, Depression, and Mood Regulation" and "Loss, Bereavement, Mourning, and Melancholia: A Conceptual

Sketch, in Defence of Some Psychoanalytic Views" examine depression from three very different theoretical perspectives: evolutionary, neurophysiological, and psychoanalytic.

In the chapter, "Darwinian Blues: Evolutionary Psychiatry and Depression", Canadian philosopher Luc Faucher critically examines two recent evolutionary models of depression: Nesse's low mood model, and Andrews and Thomson's "analytical rumination" model. The author describes the strength and weaknesses of these two models, and their links with previous models (like the "social competition" model developed by Price or the "bargaining model" proposed by Hagen). He concludes that, despite the fact that the speculative nature of these models prevents us from applying them as established doctrine in the clinic, evolutionary scenarios still can play a "heuristic function" in psychiatry. Faucher argues, however, that it is doubtful that evolutionary psychology can one day constitute the "basic science" that some psychiatrists, such as Nesse, envision.

Could future neuroscience shed more light than evolutionary psychology on the understanding of depressive mechanisms? In the chapter, "Is an Anatomy of Melancholia Possible? Brain Processes, Depression, and Mood Regulation", French philosopher Denis Forest identifies many weaknesses in the current neurobiological approach to depression, but argues that these problems can be addressed. The author calls for further conceptual analysis of mood and affective states, and advocates for a more elaborate epistemological reflection on the interdependence between physiological and emotion regulation mechanisms. Finally, he argues for a multidisciplinary approach including neuroscience, moral philosophy and social science that would encompass the several kinds of explanations provided in different disciplines.

In the chapter, "Loss, Bereavement, Mourning, and Melancholia: A Conceptual Sketch, in Defence of Some Psychoanalytic Views", French philosopher and psychoanalyst Pierre-Henri Castel, through an examination of Henry James' story, "Altar of the Dead", appraises the psychoanalytic conceptions of melancholia and mourning put forward by Karl Abraham, Sigmund Freud, Melanie Klein and Jacques Lacan. Castel insists that the central dimension of any depressive state – commonly neglected in behavioral approaches – is the intentionality of the patient's loss. *What* is lost *to whom*? What determines the choice to mourn and live with the loss versus in effect to die with the lost person? These simple questions are crucial for clinical practice and offer a complex view that illuminates the parallel that often exists between mourning and melancholia concerning the lost object. This chapter also offers an implicit argument that clinicians can benefit greatly from studying not only science articles and medical textbooks, but also literature and humanities.

The chapters "Suffering, Meaning and Hope: Shifting the Focus from Depression in Primary Care", "An Insider View on the Making of the First French National Information Campaign About Depression" and "Extrapolation from Animal Model of Depressive Disorders: What's Lost in Translation?" examine depression in specific contexts: primary care, public health, and animal research.

In the chapter, "Suffering, Meaning and Hope: Shifting the Focus from Depression in Primary Care", British physician and medical philosopher Christopher

Dowrick argues that, despite its being one of the most frequently diagnosed mental disorders in primary care settings, "the diagnosis of depression is not fit for the purposes of primary care." The author lists and analyses the defects of the "depression" label: it lacks validity, it lacks utility, it has iatrogenic effects, and it lends itself to a reductionist perspective. Dowrick encourages the development of a new conceptual framework, nourished with medical knowledge as well as philosophical and political insights. Dowrick concludes by highlighting the centrality of two concepts for clinical settings: coherence (as opposed to the *fragmented individual* that medical textbooks deal with) and engagement (as a remedy for the neglect of the intersubjective structure of our emotional states in medical literature). This new perspective, the author claims, would help develop "a theory of the person based not on passivity but on agency and creative capacity".

In the chapter, "An Insider View on the Making of the First French National Information Campaign About Depression", French sociologist Xavier Briffault investigates the implications of depression diagnosis for public health strategies. Briffault draws on his personal experiences working on the implementation of the first French national information campaign on depression in 2007, to identify methodological difficulties related to such national campaigns. To positively impact the population, a national information campaign must rely on a broad consensus amongst experts as well as rigorous scientific evaluation. Unfortunately, neither of these goals were attained at the end of the French national campaign process. Given the harsh ideological controversies that exist concerning depression (especially in France, where psychoanalytic theories are still influential), the national campaign turned into a battle ground amongst professionals. Briffault provides many illustrations of the negotiations between the different parties that occur in such a campaign, and describes the largely hidden yet important role played by DSM in the French debate.

In the chapter, "Extrapolation from Animal Model of Depressive Disorders: What's Lost in Translation?", French philosopher Maël Lemoine explores the theoretical underpinnings of animal models of depression, identifying the main epistemological and methodological difficulties confronting such models. Lemoine asks when, and on what grounds, we can say that an animal model is successful, arguing that the main difficulties lie not in the *mental* nature of depression but in its fuzzy clinical characterization (its *exophenotype*). He takes the example of the monoamine hypothesis of depression, which is supported by a variety of animal models related to each other in complex ways. Lemoine distinguishes between *mosaicism* of animal models (the modelling of a disease by the way different animal models operate at different levels of explanation) versus *chimerism* of animal models (different animal models are used in order to instantiate one specific aspect or part of a disease explanation). His analysis illuminates the complex ways animal models and translational psychiatry may help to lead to a progressive reconceptualization of our prescientific notion of depression.

Finally, the volume ends with the chapter, "Psychiatry's Continuing Expansion of Depressive Disorder", an **epilogue** in which American philosopher of psychiatry and clinician Jerome C. Wakefield and sociologist Allan Horwitz review recent developments and provide a retrospective account of the controversial influence of their book, *The Loss of Sadness*, initially published in 2007, on the North-American debate concerning depression. Although their critical analysis of the decontextualized symptom-based definition of major depression in DSM-IV was widely praised, the revision of the DSM-5 moved in the opposite direction to the one they suggested: DSM-5 removed the one contextual criterion in the definition of major depression, i.e. the bereavement exclusion criteria. Wakefield and Horwitz, in this final chapter, give a comprehensive overview of the recent scientific debate concerning depression, and document the ever-increasing tendency of modern societies to pathologize normal sadness.

**Acknowledgment**  This volume grew out of a conference held in Paris in June 2010 on the occasion of the publication of the French translation of Horwitz and Wakefield's book, *Loss of Sadness,* titled "Tristesse ou depression?" [*Sadness or Depression*?]. This international conference, organized by Françoise Parot and Steeves Demazeux, was financed by the project PHS2M ('Philosophie, Histoire et Sociologie de la Médecine mentale') and supported by the Agence Nationale pour la Recherche (ANR-08-BLAN-0055-01). We want to express our deep gratitude to the director of the PHS2M, Pierre-Henri Castel, to Françoise Parot – who translated the *Loss of Sadness* into French, and who led this collective project – and to all the participants in this initial event: Derek Bolton, Xavier Briffault, Pierre-Henri Castel, Françoise Champion, Christopher Dowrick, Alain Ehrenberg, Luc Faucher, Denis Forest, Bernard Granger, David Healy and Fernando Vidal. We are grateful to David Goldberg, Allan Horwitz, Junko Kitanaka, Maël Lemoine and Mario Maj who later accepted invitations to join the project. Finally, we would like to thank co-editor Philippe Huneman and Springer's Ties Nijssen for their complete support and confidence in this project throughout this long publication process.

# References

American Psychiatric Association. (2013). *Diagnostic and statistical manual of mental disorders* (5th ed.). Arlington: American Psychiatric Association.
Aristotle. (1927). Problemata (E. S. Forster, Trans.). In J. A. Smith & W. D. Ross (Eds.). *The works of Aristotle translated into English: Vol. 7*. Oxford: Clarendon Press.
Aristotle. (2000). Brilliance and melancholy. In J. Radden (Ed.), *The nature of melancholy: From Aristotle to Kristeva* (pp. 55–60). New York: Oxford University Press.
Barthes, R. (2005). *The neutral: Lecture course at the Collège de France (1977–1978)*. New York: Columbia University Press.
Barthes, R. (2010). *Mourning diary*. New York: Hill and Wang.
Burton, R. (1621/2001). *The anatomy of melancholy*. New York: New York Review Books.
Fink, M., & Taylor, M. A. (2007). Resurrecting melancholia. *Acta Psychiatrica Scandinavica, 115*(Suppl. 433), 14–20.
Fink, M., Bolwig, T. G., Parker, G., & Shorter, E. (2007). Melancholia: Restoration in psychiatric classification recommended. *Acta Psychiatrica Scandinavica, 115*(2), 89–92.
Galen. (1929). On prognosis (A. J. Brock, Trans.). In A. J. Brock (Ed.), *Greek medicine, being extracts illustrative of medical writing from Hippocrates to Galen* (pp. 200–220). London: J. M. Dent and Sons.
Hacking, I. (1999). *The social construction of what?* Cambridge, MA: Harvard University Press.
Hippocrates. (1923). *Epidemics III* (W. H. S. Jones, Trans.). In *Hippocrates, Vol. I* (pp. 213–287). Cambridge, MA: Harvard University Press.

Hippocrates. (1931). *Aphorisms* (W. H. S. Jones, Trans.). In *Hippocrates, Vol. IV* (pp. 97–222). Cambridge, MA: Harvard University Press.

Horwitz, A. V., & Wakefield, J. C. (2007). *The loss of sadness: How psychiatry transformed normal sorrow into depressive disorder*. New York: Oxford University Press.

Hume, D. (1767). *Letter to the Comtesse de Boufflers*, 19 of June.

Jackson, S. W. (1986). *Melancholia and depression: From Hippocratic times to modern times*. New Haven: Yale University Press.

Johnson, S. (1755). *Dictionary of the English language*. London: J. F. & C. Rivington.

Kendell, R. E. (1976). The classification of depressions: A review of contemporary confusion. *British Journal of Psychiatry, 129*, 15–28.

Klein, D. F., & Thase, M. (1997). Medication versus psychotherapy for depression: Progress notes. *American Society of Clinical Psychopharmacology, 8*, 41–47.

Kraepelin, E. (1915). Clinical psychiatry: A text-book for students and physicians. In A. Ross Diefendorf (Ed. & Trans.), *The seventh German edition of Kraepelin's Lehrbuch der Psychiatrie* (2nd ed.). New York: Macmillan. (Original work published 1907)

Lantéri-Laura, G. (2003). Introduction historique et critique à la notion de dépression en psychiatrie. *PSN, 1*(3), 39–47.

Lewis, A. J. (1934). Melancholia: A clinical survey of depressive states. *The British Journal of Psychiatry, 80*(329), 277–378.

Medin, D., & Ortony, A. (1989). Psychological essentialism. In S. Vosniadou & A. Ortony (Eds.), *Similarity and analogical reasoning* (pp. 179–195). New York: Cambridge University Press.

Moffitt, T. E., Caspi, A., Taylor, A., Kokaua, J., Milne, B., Polanczyk, G., & Poulton, R. (2010). How common are common mental disorders? Evidence that lifetime prevalence rates are doubled by prospective versus retrospective ascertainment. *Psychological Medicine, 40*(6), 899–909.

Parker, G., Fink, M., Shorter, E., et al. (2010). Issues for DSM-5: Whither melancholia? The case for its classification as a distinct mood disorder. *The American Journal of Psychiatry, 167*, 745–747.

Rohde, P., Lewinsohn, P. M., Klein, D. N., Seeley, J. R., & Gau, J. M. (2013). Key characteristics of major depressive disorder occurring in childhood, adolescence, emerging adulthood, and adulthood. *Clinical Psychological Science, 1*(1), 41–53.

Shorter, E. (2007). The doctrine of the two depressions in historical perspective. *Acta Psychiatrica Scandinavica, 115*(s433), 5–13.

Starobinski, J. (2012). *L'encre de la mélancolie*. Paris: Seuil.

Wakefield, J. C. (1992). The concept of mental disorder: On the boundary between biological facts and social values. *American Psychologist, 47*, 373–388.

Wakefield, J. C. (2009). Mental disorder and moral responsibility: Disorders of personhood as harmful dysfunctions, with special reference to alcoholism. *Philosophy, Psychiatry and Psychology, 16*, 91–99.

Wakefield, J. C. (2010). False positives in psychiatric diagnosis: Implications for human freedom. *Theoretical Medicine and Bioethics, 31*(1), 5–17.

World Health Organization. (1992). *The ICD-10 classification of mental and behavioural disorders: Clinical descriptions and diagnostic guidelines*. Geneva: World Health Organization.

# The Current Status of the Diagnosis of Depression

David Goldberg

**Abstract** The term "depression" is an umbrella that covers a large number of heterogeneous depressive disorders, with symptoms overlapping with other common mental disorders on the one hand, and chronic systemic disease on the other. It covers both disorders that definitely benefit from recognition and treatment by the clinician, and those that can be thought of as homeostatic reactions to adverse life events, which will remit spontaneously whether or not they are detected. The former group includes depressions following severe loss events in vulnerable individuals.

Typical bereavement reactions can readily be distinguished from depressive disorders, and requires only supportive care from clinicians. However, bereavement can also precipitate a depressive disorder in vulnerable people which most definitely benefits from treatment, and has additional features not usually seen in the more usual bereavement reactions. Vulnerability factors include genes, early maternal attachment, adverse childhood experiences and personality factors.

In their relationships with other physicians, what has come to be known as "major" depression is the flagship of psychiatry – the condition that general physicians commonly neglect to detect, but which co-occurs with many chronic physical disorders that produce disability. It is often referred to as though it is a homogenous concept, and many countries have mounted national campaigns aimed at improving detection rates (Regier et al. 1988a; Paykel et al. 1997; Jorm et al. 2006).

In several other areas of the classification of mental disorders, we have come to acknowledge that there are spectrums of disorder, for example, schizophrenias, autistic disorders and eating disorders. It will be argued in this chapter that there are a wide range of depressive disorders, and that the manifestations of depressive disorders are influenced by genetic factors, early childhood adversity and pre-morbid personality. These factors help to determine which of the overlapping syndromes of depression a particular individual is likely to develop. Depression also merges into normality and frequently occurs as a transient reaction to a wide range of adverse

D. Goldberg (✉)
Psychiatry Research Trust, Institute of Psychiatry, London, UK
e-mail: davidpgoldberg@yahoo.com

© Springer Science+Business Media Dordrecht 2016                                    17
J.C. Wakefield, S. Demazeux (eds.), *Sadness or Depression?*
History, Philosophy and Theory of the Life Sciences 15,
DOI 10.1007/978-94-017-7423-9_2

circumstances. The current concept is a blunderbuss approach which gathers together a heterogeneous collection of common disorders under a single umbrella.

## The Case for Heterogeneity

When once recalls that the DSM diagnosis should be made when a patient – in addition to one of the required symptoms – has any four out of eight other symptoms, and then recalls that several of these are opposites of one another, it is easy to see how this heterogeneity might arise. For example, a patient who has psychomotor retardation, hypersomnia and gaining weight is scored as having identical symptoms as another who is agitated, sleeping badly and has weight loss. Lux and Kendler (2010) studied depression in a sample of twins and distinguished between "cognitive" and "neuro-vegetative" symptoms, and show that these had different relationships to a larger set of potential validators. They conclude that their results "challenge our understanding of major depression as a homogeneous categorical entity". Others have been able to separate the various depressive symptoms, and to compare the relative efficiency of each symptom to making the diagnosis (McGlinchey et al. 2006). Jang et al. (2004) factor analysed a larger set of depressive symptom scales, and found that they could identify 14 different subscales, which had rather low inter-correlations, and very different heritabilities. Given these findings, to declare that all those satisfying the DSM-5 criteria for the diagnosis of "Major Depressive Disorder" are suffering from the same disorder seems like magical thinking.

## Can Homeostatic Responses to Adverse Circumstances Be Included as Cases of Depression?

Epidemiological studies (Regier et al. 1988b; Melzer et al. 1995; Andrews et al. 2001) reveal such high prevalence of depression in the developed world that some have supposed that such syndromes in the community often represent transient homeostatic responses to internal or external stimuli that do not represent true psychopathologic disorders (Regier et al. 1998). It is certainly true that many people develop an episode of depression after a loss event, or in response to some other transient, adverse circumstance. In a paper prepared in the preparations for DSM-5, it is clearly stated that a mental disorder must not merely be an expectable response to common stressors and losses (Stein et al. 2010). It has also been shown that the public does perceive depressive symptoms as an indication of mental disorder when occurring in the context of adverse life events (Holzinger et al. 2011). Maj (2011) has considered the differentiation between a depressive illness and normal sadness, and argues that the latter is always triggered by a life event and appears to be proportionate to that event. By contrast if depression is triggered by a life event it is disproportionate to that event in its intensity and duration, and in the degree of the functional impairment it produces.

We know, from the large placebo response to antidepressants that many milder cases remit without specific treatment, suggesting that they are indeed homeostatic responses to life stress, as others have suggested (Wakefield 1997). Even cases of moderate severity may respond to non-specific psychological interventions like problem solving (Gath and Catalan 1986). All these arguments appear to support the idea that what passes for depression in community surveys are often merely gloomy people with transient disorders, whose distress should not be medicalised.

The concept of "disproportionate" depression is a slippery concept, as the clinician may suppose that if he or she had experienced that particular event they would not have developed the particular set of symptoms of the patient before them: but the clinician may well be much less vulnerable to developing symptoms, and may not justifiably know how stressful the situation was to that individual. The link between severe loss events and depression was first conclusively demonstrated by Brown and Harris (1967), who showed that severe loss events occurred in 68 % of community onset cases of depression among a population of working class women, in contrast to 23 % of normal controls. While this undoubtedly establishes severe loss events as precipitants of depressive episodes, we may make two further observations: 32 % of onsets of depression do not follow severe loss events, and the fairly high rate of loss events in the control population is not followed by an onset of depression for a substantial proportion of those so exposed. In other words, many people are relatively *resilient* in the face of loss, or at any rate to not develop depression.

It is also important that while sadness is a single, very common experience, that the *diagnosis* of depression refers to the development of a set of at least five symptoms, present for most of the time in the previous two weeks, and is associated with disability and distress. This goes well beyond the simple experience of sadness, and frequently persists for much longer than two weeks. Furthermore, a range of psychological and pharmacological interventions produce much better results than a simple placebo (NICE 2004).

Only a small minority of depressed people are seen by psychiatrists, the great majority are seen in primary care and general hospital settings, usually presenting to doctors with somatic symptoms. Having excluded a physical cause for these symptoms, the doctor needs to recognise the depressed state, and offer an intervention for depression. The presenting somatic symptoms often remit provided the depression responds to the intervention offered.

## How Can Bereavement Be Distinguished from Depression?

The psychological sequelae of the death of a loved one are themselves quite heterogeneous. In most cases, there is very little difficulty, since a normal bereavement consists of quite distinctive phenomena which are quite unlike depression. Sigmund Freud (1917) pointed this out in a famous paper called "Mourning and Melancholia" (see Castel, this volume), and made the point that whereas in mourning, time is needed for reality-testing to "free the ego of its libido of the lost object, the complex of melancholia behaves like an open wound, drawing to itself energies…from all directions, and emptying the ego until it is totally impoverished". In more prosaic language, during bereavement the person grieves for the lost person, and the grief comes in waves, rather than being a constant phenomenon. Nor does the survivor usually experience self hatred and wish to die. The following excerpt is from an authoress (Jamison 2009) who has experienced both depression and bereavement:

> Time alone in grief proved restorative. Time alone when depressed was dangerous. The thoughts I had of death after (my husband's) death were necessary and proportionate. They were of his death, not my own. With depression, however, it was my own death I sought out. In grief, death occasions the pain. In depression, death is the solution to the pain….My mood, fixedly bleak during depression, was not so during grief. It was mutable and commonly rose in response to the presence of my family and friends. I was generally able to meet the demands of the world. ….Even during the worst of my grief I had some sense that this would happen, that the weather would clear. I did not have this faith during the merciless months of depression.

However, medical classifiers love these polarities, and like to describe these two phenomena as though they are quite different. Unfortunately real life is more complex, since a bereavement can also precipitate a depressive illness, so the clinician must listen carefully to the patient's experience before deciding that this is a typical case of bereavement, deserving of sympathy and perhaps symptomatic and supportive help, rather than treating a depressive episode. The people with typical bereavement are much less vulnerable to loss events than those who become depressed when bereaved, and it is important to understand what is known about the determinants of vulnerability. Some people develop depression after adverse events that cause only transient reactions in more resilient people, while others do not become depressed until they have experienced prolonged and severe adverse experiences.

## Some Determinants of Vulnerability to Depression

Caspi et al. (2002) used the Dunedin birth cohort to show that the extent to which stressful life events were followed by depression is partly determined by the 5HT transporter gene on chromosome 17. With two long version of the gene, there was only a slight relationship, so that the probability of later depression rose from about 9 % with no stressful events, to about 12 % with four or more events. With the gene heterozygous (one long, and one short version) the probability rose to about 24 %, and with a double short version of the gene the probability rose to nearly 39 %. There have been several replications of this finding since the original paper (Eley et al. 2004; Kendler et al. 2005; Wilhelm et al. 2006). It would therefore appear that part of the explanation for the greater vulnerability of some individuals to life stress is the presence of a particular version of a gene – about a third of the Dunedin population have the double short version of the gene, with a further 51 % being heterozygous, and therefore less highly susceptible to stressful events.

This genetic variant – having either a double short (ss), or one long and one short gene (ls) – has also been shown to interact with the quality of maternal responsiveness to the child. Barry, Kochanska, and Philibert (2008) also showed by prolonged naturalistic observation of 88 mother infant pairs, that there was no such relationship for those homozygous for the long gene (ll). However, with ss and ls infants, low maternal responsiveness was associated with very poor attachment, while high responsiveness was associated with high infant attachment (similar to those with the ll gene); medium maternal responsiveness was intermediate between the two. Negative early experience amplified the risk conferred by the short 5-HTT allele, whereas positive early experience, while it served to buffer that risk, did not appear to lead to better outcomes than outcomes for children without the genetic risk.

If the mother is responsive to her infant, normal attachment occurs whatever the maternal genes, but the combination of an unresponsive mother and either ss or ls in the 5HT transporter genes produces insecure attachment. Disorders of maternal attachment may occur as a result of maternal depression, or a failure of the mother to bond with the infant for other reasons.

There is also evidence that adversity in the form of either neglect and physical abuse in early and middle childhood may further increase vulnerability to stressful events. As genetic contributions have been introduced into research designs it has become increasingly clear that some individuals contribute to the onset of their own adverse environments and that genetic effects may contribute to psychopathology indirectly through their influence on the child's behaviour (Rudolph et al. 2000).

## The Importance of Anxiety in Depressive States

Epidemiological studies of mental disorders in the community all show substantial co-morbidity between depression and generalized anxiety disorder (GAD). This occurs despite the fact that GAD has to last 6 months before it is counted, whereas depression only needs to have lasted 2 weeks. In a large study of patients attending primary care in 11 countries, if the duration of symptoms required for GAD is shortened from 6 months to 1 month, the prevalence of "co-morbid" depression and GAD goes up from 3.4 to 5.7 %, while the prevalence of depression without anxiety drops from 4.7 to 2.3 % (Goldberg et al. 2011). Provided that anxious depression refers to the simultaneous experience of symptoms of both anxiety and depression, it is therefore more than twice as common as depression without anxiety. Anxious forms of depression are indeed the commonest forms of depression in general medical settings, although the anxious symptoms are frequently missed. Longitudinal studies have shown that co-morbid cases of depression and anxiety have experienced more severe adversity in early childhood (Moffitt et al. 2007; Richards and Goldberg 2008).

These co-morbid cases (major depression plus generalized anxiety disorder) have a worse outlook and a longer course than depression occurring on its own, and the suicide rate is also higher in these cases. These differences are consistent for both major depression and bipolar disorder when anxious symptoms are present

(Goldberg and Fawcett 2012). There is consistent evidence that there are personality differences when anxious symptoms are also present, with higher score on negative affect (neuroticism) (Goldberg et al. 2009). When anxious symptoms are absent, the depressive disorders is likely to have less severe depressive symptoms, and to have parents with an excess only of depressive symptoms on their own; in contrast, anxious depressives have parents with a wide range of common mental disorders, also including mania (Goldberg et al. 2014). Using Cloninger's personality constructs, this study also showed that while non-anxious depressives were no more likely to be harm avoidant than controls, the anxious depressives were likely to be high on harm avoidance and reward dependence.

There is some suggestive evidence that there are also biological differences between anxious and non-anxious depression. In an early study (Meller et al. 1995). adrenocorticotrophic hormone (ACTH) and cortisol levels were measured in 14 patients with anxious depression following exogenous cortisol releasing hormone (CRH) challenge. Compared to 11 patients with non-anxious depression and 27 healthy controls, subjects with anxious depression exhibited a significantly attenuated response. However, patients were not required to be medication free at the time of testing, and depressed patients could meet criteria for either major depression or bipolar disorder. In a structural neuro-imaging study, 49 patients with anxious depression were compared with 96 patients with depression without anxiety and 183 healthy controls. Those with anxious depression had increased grey matter volume in the superior temporal gyrus, extending into the posterior middle temporal gyrus and inferior temporal gyrus in the right hemisphere when compared to the depressed group without anxiety (Inkster et al. 2011).

Cases of depression with apathy, psychomotor slowness low energy therefore appear to have quite different characteristics than the more common anxious depressives, yet both are given the same name: major depressive disorder. This is perhaps the most important sub-form of depression, with fundamental differences from the anxious forms of depression. This important group of depressions has been much less well studied than the anxious depressions, partly because they have been defined by exclusion, and partly because they are buried in the overall concept of "major depression".

## Multiple Co-morbidity, or Depressive Syndromes Influenced by Personality?

The term "co-morbidity" was applied by Alvan Feinstein (1970) to refer to those cases in which a '*distinct additional* clinical entity' occurred during the clinical course of a patient having a particular illness (*italics added*). In its original meaning, it referred to "a medical condition existing *simultaneously but independently* of another condition". If the two disorders are completely unrelated, for example ischaemic heat disease and carcinoma of the prostate, this makes good sense, but it is also used to refer to conditions which are highly related to each other, such as anxiety and depression. It is also extended to the overlapping syndromes of common mental disorders, so that a person who develops a depressive illness with obsessional symptoms and panic attacks will be said to suffer from 'co-morbid' major depression, obsessional compulsive disorder and panic disorder.

There is nothing wrong with this, provided it is used merely to catalogue the symptoms that are present in a particular patient, and to direct the clinician to particular interventions. Unfortunately it tends to create the idea in the clinician's mind that the patient is suffering from three independent disorders, which happen to be present at the same time.

Karl Jaspers (1923) argued that below the severe group of disorders (*psychoses and organic disorders of the brain*) were the '*psychopathien*', which comprise abnormal personalities and the neuroses. These are "phenomena which continually keep merging into one another...there is no sharp dividing line between types (of neuroses and personality disorders) nor is there a decisive borderline between what is healthy and what is not. A diagnosis remains typological and multi-dimensional, including a delineation of the type of personality".

There are two different ideas here: rather than different diseases, we should think of overlapping syndromes; and in making sense of these we should consider the pre-morbid personality of the patient. These provide a key to some of the various depressive syndromes.

People who are normally punctual, orderly and conscientious and who are vulnerable to affective disorders will, when faced with a severe life event, develop severe and distressing obsessional and compulsive symptoms. When the accompanying depressive symptoms have been treated, these will disappear. The person has been suffering from one disorder, not two.

In similar manner, a habitually anxious person may develop panic attacks when depressed, and an introspective person with mild health concerns may develop quite severe hypochondriacal symptoms when depressed. The combinations of symptoms experienced by depressed individuals are by no means as neat as medical textbooks suggest – these are *overlapping syndromes*, rather than independent disorders (Goldberg 2011).

However, there are four other, important forms of depressive illnesses.

## *Depression Presenting with Somatic Symptoms*

In general medical settings, this is by far the most common presentation of depressive illness. These patients are experiencing the symptoms that occur in depression, but their main reason for consulting is to find the cause, and obtain alleviation for, distressing somatic symptoms. When no cause can be found for these symptoms, the clinician may consider the depressive symptoms as a cause for these pains and discomforts. There is now impressive evidence for inflammatory changes in depression, and one possible explanation for these pains are pro-inflammatory cytokines (Capuron and Miller 2004; Zunszain et al. 2011).

Whatever the cause, the most rational management of these patients is to help them with their depressive symptoms, and to explain that their pains are real, and not imaginary. The best management strategies for these forms of depression are described elsewhere (Rosendal et al. 2009; Olde Hartman et al. 2013).

## Depression Accompanying Chronic Physical Illnesses

These depressions are often poorly recognised by generalists, whose attention is largely for the real physical disorder, and typically confine themselves to the treatments for it. Rates of depression are at least double that among the healthy in a wide range of chronic physical disorders, and in some may be five times the usual rate (Goldberg 2010).

Diagnosis of these depressions is complicated by the fact that four of the "diagnostic features" of depression may well be caused by the physical illness, including *fatigue, poor sleep, poor appetite and weight loss.* This may cause confusion since no clear threshold for the numbers of symptoms needed for a diagnosis seems to exist if such symptoms are to be discounted. However, if there is a positive reply to either of the usual two screening questions, it is only necessary to ask three additional questions dealing with poor concentration, ideas of worthless and thoughts of death. A total of three symptoms or more from this list of five symptoms allows depression to be diagnosed with high sensitivity and specificity, when assessed against the full list of criteria (Zimmerman et al. 2006; Andrews et al. 2008). Successful treatment of the depression is associated with a lower mortality and better collaboration with the necessary physical treatments.

Such patients report a poor quality of life, and experience more pain from their physical illness than they would if there depression was treated. The special task of the physician is to reach agreement with the patient that he or she is indeed depressed, and to explain the effects that this is having on the quality of the patient's life, the severity of any pains that are experienced, and the disability associated with the physical illness. The range of treatments that are effective in depression among the healthy are all effective in these patients, and the only special measure required of the clinician should an antidepressant drug be used is to guard against harmful interactions between the antidepressant and drugs used for the physical illness.

## Pseudo-demented Depression

In older people, depression may present as an apparent dementia, but the presenting symptoms turn out to be due to inattention and impaired concentration, while symptoms of depression are undoubtedly present and may be elicited by direct enquiry. It is important to grasp that there is no clear dividing line between early dementia and the apparent dementias referred to here: there may well be mild, early signs of organic damage, but when a depressive process is added the clinical picture may resemble a definite dementing illness.

The special task here is to reassure both patient and carer that the memory problems are not due to advanced cerebral disease, and are likely to improve a great deal with treatment of the depression.

## *Depression Due to Drugs, Both Licit and Illicit*

The list of drugs that can themselves cause depression is a long one, and includes drugs prescribed by doctors, excessive use of alcohol, as well as a wide variety of 'recreational' drugs and other toxic agents. Many drugs have been said to cause depression on slender evidence, but among those for which the evidence is good are included β-blockers, steroids, some anti-viral agents and digoxin (Patten and Love 1993; Zdilar et al. 2000). Among legal drugs, alcohol is easily to most important agent producing depression.

## Conclusion

While these various forms of depressive illness need to be known and recognised by all working clinicians who are not trained psychiatrists, there are in fact strong arguments for continuing to see them all as different varieties of depressive illnesses, despite their aetiological and clinical heterogeneity. While many cases of depression can be regarded as homeostatic reactions to adverse circumstances, it is important to recognise that such reactions can be prolonged, and are accompanied by both distress and disability.

It must also be recognised that an individual's vulnerability to adverse circumstances is determined by factors both inherited and acquired by interactions between genes and environment, and by various forms of child abuse. This helps to explain the wide variety of reactions to a bereavement, ranging from any culturally sanctioned bereavement reaction to typical depressive illnesses.

## References

Andrews, G., Henderson, S., & Hall, W. (2001). Prevalence, co-morbidity and disability in the Australian National Mental Health Survey. *British Journal of Psychiatry, 178*, 145–153.

Andrews, G., Anderson, T. M., Slade, T., & Sunderland, M. (2008). Classification of anxiety and depressive disorders: Problems and solutions. *Depression and Anxiety, 25*(4), 274–281.

Barry, R. A., Kochanska, G., & Philibert, R. A. (2008). G·E interaction in the organization of attachment: Mothers' responsiveness as a moderator of children's genotypes. *Journal of Child Psychology and Psychiatry, 49*, 1313–1320.

Brown, G. W., & Harris, T. (1967). *The social origins of depression*. London: Tavistock (1978, 1986).

Capuron, L., & Miller, A. H. (2004). Cytokines and psychopathology: Lessons from interferon-alpha. *Biological Psychiatry, 65*, 819–824.

Caspi, A., Sugden, K., Moffitt, T., et al. (2002). Influence of life stress on depression. Polymorphism on the 5HTT gene. *Science, 301*, 386–389.

Eley, T. C., Sugden, K., Corsico, A., Gregory, A. M., Sham, P., McGuffin, P., Plomin, R., & Craig, I. W. (2004). Gene-environment interaction analysis of serotonin system markers with adolescent depression. *Molecular Psychiatry, 9*(10), 908–915.

Feinstein, A. R. (1970). Pre-therapeutic classification of co-morbidity in chronic disease. *Journal of Chronic Diseases, 23*(7), 455–468.

Freud, S. (1917). *Mourning and Melancholia. Collected papers* (Vol. 4, p. 589). London: Hogarth Press.

Gath, D. H., & Catalan, J. (1986). The treatment of emotional disorders in general practice - psychological metohds versus medication. *Journal of Psychosomatic Research, 30*, 381–386.

Goldberg, D. (2010). The detection and treatment of depression in the physically ill. *World Psychiatry, 9*(1), 16–20.

Goldberg, D. P. (2011). The heterogeneity of "Major depression". *World Psychiatry, 10*(3), 226–228.

Goldberg, D. P., & Fawcett, J. (2012). The importance of anxiety in both major depression and bipolar disorder. *Anxiety and Depression, 29*(6), 471–478.

Goldberg, D. P., Krueger, R. F., Andrews, G., & Hobbs, M. J. (2009). Emotional disorders: Cluster 4 of the proposed meta-structure for DSM-V and ICD-11. *Psychological Medicine, 39*, 2043–2059.

Goldberg, D. P., Simms, L. J., Gater, R., & Krueger, R. F. (2011). Integration of dimensional spectra for depression and anxiety into categorical diagnoses for general medical practice. In D. Regier, W. E. Narrow, E. A. Kuhl, & D. J. Kupfer (Eds.), *The conceptual evolution of DSM-5*. Washington, DC: American Psychiatric Publishing Inc.

Goldberg, D. P., Wittchen, H.-U., Zimmermann, P., Pfister, H., & Beesdo-Baum, K. (2014). Anxious and non-anxious forms of major depression: Familial, personality and symptom characteristics. *Psychological Medicine, 44*(6), 1223–1234.

Holzinger, A., Matschinger, H., Schomerus, G., et al. (2011). The loss of sadness: The public's view. *Acta Psychiatrica Scandinavica, 123*, 307–313.

Inkster, B., et al. (2011). Structural brain changes in patients with recurrent major depressive disorder presenting with anxiety symptoms. *Journal of Neuroimaging, 21*(4), 375–382.

Jamison, K. R. (2009). *Nothing was the same: A Memoir*. New York: Knopf. ISBN 0-307-26537-4, 2009.

Jang, K., Livesley, W., Taylor, S., Stein, M., & Moon, E. (2004). Heritability of individual depressive symptoms. *Journal of Affective Disorders, 80*, 125–133.

Jaspers, K. (1923). *Allgemeine Psychopathologie*, 5 Aufl., Springer, S. 507; Translated into English as General psychopathology. Manchester: Manchester University Press, 1963.

Jorm, A. F., Christensen, H., & Griffiths, K. M. (2006). Changes in depression awareness and attitudes in Australia: The impact of beyondblue: The national depression initiative. *Australian and New Zealand Journal of Psychiatry, 40*(1), 42–46.

Kendler, K. S., Kuhn, J. W., Vittum, J., Prescott, C. A., & Riley, B. (2005). The interaction of stressful life events and a serotonin transporter polymorphism in the prediction of episodes of major depression: A replication. *Archives of General Psychiatry, 62*(5), 529–535.

Lux, V., & Kendler, K. S. (2010). Deconstructing major depression: A validation study of the DSM-IV diagnostic criteria. *Psychological Medicine, 40*, 1679–1690.

Maj, M. (2011). When does depression become a mental disorder? *The British Journal of Psychiatry, 199*, 85–86.

McGlinchey, J. B., Zimmerman, M., Young, D., & Chelminski, I. (2006). Diagnosing major depressive disorder VIII are some symptoms better than others? *The Journal of Nervous and Mental Disease, 194*, 785–790.

Meller, W. H., et al. (1995). CRH challenge test in anxious depression. *Biological Psychiatry, 37*(6), 376–382.

Melzer, H., Gill, B., Pettigrew, M., et al. (1995). *OPCS surveys of psychiatric morbidity in Great Britain. The prevalence of psychiatric morbidity among adults in private households*. London: Her Majesties Stationary Office, Office of Population Censuses and Surveys.

Moffitt, T. E., Caspi, A., Harrington, H. L., et al. (2007). Generalized anxiety disorder and depression: Childhood risk factors in a birth cohort followed to age 32. *Psychological Medicine, 37*, 1–12.

NICE (National Collaborating Centre for Mental Health). (2004). Depression: The treatment and management of depression in primary and secondary care, Gaskell, also available from www.nccmh.org.uk

Olde Hartman, T. C., Blankenstein, A. H., Molenaar, A. O., Bentz van den Berg, D., Van der Horst, H. E., Arnold, I. A., Burgers, J. S., Wiersma, T., & Woutersen-Koch, H. (2013). NHG guideline on Medically Unexplained Symptoms (MUS). *Huisarts Wet, 56*(5), 222–230.

Patten, S. B., & Love, E. J. (1993). Can drugs cause depression? A review of the evidence. *Journal of Psychiatry and Neuroscience, 18*(3), 92–99.

Paykel, E. S., Tylee, A., Wright, A., et al. (1997). The defeat depression campaign: Psychiatry in the public arena. *American Journal of Psychiatry, 154*(Festschrift supplement), 59–65.

Regier, D. A., Hirschfeld, R. M., Goodwin, F. K., et al. (1988a). The NIMH depression awareness, recognition, and treatment program: Structure, aims, and scientific basis. *The American Journal of Psychiatry, 145*, 1351–1357.

Regier, D., Boyd, J., Burke, J., et al. (1988b). One month prevalence of mental disorders in the United States. *Archives of General Psychiatry, 45*, 977–985b.

Regier, D. A., Kaelber, C. T., Rae, D. S., et al. (1998). Limitations of diagnostic criteria and assessment instruments for mental disorders: Implications for research and policy. *Archives of General Psychiatry, 55*, 109–115.

Richards, M., & Goldberg, D. P. (2008). Are there early adverse exposures that differentiate depression and anxiety risk? In D. Goldberg, K. S. Kendler, P. Sirovatka, & D. A. Regier (Eds.), *Diagnostic issues in depression and generalized anxiety disorder: Refining the research agenda for DSM-V*. Arlington: American Psychiatric Association.

Rosendal, M., Burton, C., Blankenstein, A. H., Fink, P., Kroenke, K., Sharpe, M., Frydenberg, M., & Morriss, R. (2009). Enhanced care by generalists for functional somatic symptoms and disorders in primary care. *Cochrane Database of Systematic Reviews, 4*, CD008142. Wiley, Chichester.

Rudolph, K. D., Hammen, C., Burge, D., et al. (2000). Toward an interpersonal life-stress model of depression: The developmental context of stress generation. *Development and Psychopathology, 12*(2), 215–234.

Stein, D. J., Phillips, K. A., Bolton, D., et al. (2010). What is a mental/psychiatric disorder? From DSM-IV to DSM-V. *Psychological Medicine, 40*, 1–7.

Wakefield, J. C. (1997). Diagnosing DSM-IV. 1. DSM-IV and the concept of disorder. *Behaviour Research and Therapy, 35*, 633–649.

Wilhelm, K., Mitchell, P. B., Niven, H., et al. (2006). Life events, first depression onset and the serotonin transporter gene. *British Journal of Psychiatry, 188*, 210–215.

Zdilar, D., Franco-Bronson, K., Buchlar, N., et al. (2000). Hepatitis C, interferon α, and depression. *Hepatology, 31*(6), 1207–1211.

Zimmerman, M., Chelminski, I., McGlinchey, J. B., & Young, D. (2006). Diagnosing major depressive disorder. Can the utility of the DSM-IV symptom criteria be improved? *The Journal of Nervous and Mental Disease, 194*, 893–897.

Zunszain, P. A., Anacker, C., Cattaneo, A., Carvalho, L. A., & Pariante, C. M. (2011). Glucocorticoids, cytokines and brain abnormalities in depression. *Progress in Neuro-Psychopharmacology and Biological Psychiatry, 35*(3), 722–729.

# The Continuum of Depressive States in the Population and the Differential Diagnosis Between "Normal" Sadness and Clinical Depression

Mario Maj

**Abstract** One of the principles of the "neo-kraepelinian credo", articulated in the 1970s, was that "there is a boundary between the normal and the sick". In other terms, it was maintained that there is a clear, qualitative distinction between persons who have a mental disorder and persons who do not. A corollary to this principle was the statement that "depression, when carefully defined as a clinical entity, is qualitatively different from the mild episodes of sadness that everyone experiences at some point in his or her life". Apparently in line with this statement was the observation that tricyclic antidepressants were active only in people who were clinically depressed; when administered to other people, they did not act as stimulants nor did they alter the subjects' mood. Today the picture has changed dramatically. Taxonomic studies have failed to support the idea that a latent qualitative difference exists between major depression and ordinary sadness, arguing instead in favor of a continuum of depressive states in the general population. We are left, therefore, with two competing approaches: a "contextual" approach, which assumes that the differential diagnosis between "true" depression and "normal" sadness should be based on the presence or not of a triggering life event and on whether the response is proportionate to that event in its intensity and duration; and a "pragmatic" approach, positing that the boundary between depression and "normal" sadness should be based on issues of clinical utility (i.e., thresholds should be fixed – in terms of number, intensity and duration of symptoms, and degree of functional impairment – which are predictive of clinical outcomes and treatment response). This chapter summarizes the strengths and weaknesses of these two approaches.

M. Maj (✉)
Department of Psychiatry, University of Naples SUN, Naples, Italy
e-mail: majmario@tin.it

© Springer Science+Business Media Dordrecht 2016                    29
J.C. Wakefield, S. Demazeux (eds.), *Sadness or Depression?*
History, Philosophy and Theory of the Life Sciences 15,
DOI 10.1007/978-94-017-7423-9_3

# The Evolving Target of Psychiatry

There was a time when the target of the psychiatric profession was very clear and widely accepted. It was "madness", that is, a few patterns of behaviour and experience which were clearly beyond the range of normality (Maj 2012a). The crucial characteristic of those patterns, easily recognizable also by non-professionals, was the apparent lack of meaning: ideas or perceptions without any foundation in reality; emotions or behaviours that were clearly irrational. This "breakdown of rationality" (Bolton 2008) was more or less explicitly ascribed to some alteration in the functioning of the brain ("mental illnesses are diseases of the brain").

In the perception of part of the general public, of some colleagues of other medical disciplines, and, paradoxically, of some fervent critics of old asylums, this traditional target of psychiatry has remained unchanged: psychiatry only deals with people who are "mad".

However, the actual target of the psychiatric profession has changed dramatically in the past decades. It has become a wide range of mental disorders, several of which do have a "meaning" that can be reconstructed. The presence of a "dysfunction" in these conditions is still hypothesized but, according to the DSM-5, it is "a dysfunction in the psychological, biological, or developmental processes underlying mental functioning" (American Psychiatric Association 2013). So, the presence of an alteration in the functioning of the brain is no longer a prerequisite.

Since several of these disorders are obviously on a continuum with normality, fixing a boundary between what is normal and what is pathological has become problematic. This boundary is often determined on pragmatic grounds, or on the basis of "clinical utility" (i.e., prediction of clinical outcomes and response to treatment), although this pragmatism may involve some tautology (in fact, requiring that a diagnostic threshold be predictive of response to treatment seems to imply that a condition becomes a mental disorder when there is an effective treatment available for it) (Maj 2012b). Furthermore, there are mental disorders (depression is a good example) for which several different treatments are available, the response to which may be predicted by different diagnostic thresholds (e.g., the threshold predicting response to interpersonal psychotherapy is likely to be different from that predicting response to selective serotonin reuptake inhibitors (SSRIs), which in its turn is different from those predicting response to tricyclic antidepressants and to electroconvulsive therapy).

In this new scenario, psychiatry has become the focus of opposite pressures.

On the one hand, the profession is being accused of unduly pathologizing ordinary life difficulties in order to expand its influence (e.g., Horwitz and Wakefield 2007; Stein 2010). This criticism becomes harsher when the above-mentioned evolution of the target of psychiatry from "madness" to a range of mental disorders is, in good or bad faith, ignored: pathologizing ordinary life difficulties becomes "making us crazy" (Kutchins and Kirk 1997). Of course, the argument is presented with greater fervor when the perceived undue "pathologization" occurs in children or adolescents, or when it is considered to be a consequence of an alliance between psychiatry and the pharmaceutical industry.

On the other hand, the psychiatric profession is being pressured to go beyond the diagnosis and management of mental disorders, acting towards the promotion of mental health in the general population (e.g., World Health Organization 2001; World Health Organization Regional Office for Europe 2005). Within this framework, especially in those countries in which community mental health services are most developed and psychiatrists are leading such services, there is a call for dealing with "mental health problems" that are not proper mental disorders, such as the serious psychological distress occurring as a consequence of a natural disaster or the ongoing economic crisis. Furthermore, psychiatrists are being pressured to diagnose and manage proper mental disorders as early as possible, which means dealing with a variety of conditions that may be "precursors" or "prodromes" of those disorders, but more frequently are not, with the unavoidable risk of, again, pathologizing situations that are within the range of normality.

Indeed, the ongoing economic crisis is having a significant impact on the mental health of the population in many countries, especially where scarce social resources are available to protect people who become unemployed, indebted or poor due to the crisis (Wahlbeck and McDaid 2012). Mental health services are often called to intervene, in a situation of uncertainty and confusion about roles and competences. A couple of recent episodes from my own country, Italy, are emblematic in this respect. In 2012, a group of widows of entrepreneurs who had committed suicide, allegedly as a consequence of economic ruin, marched in an Italian town under the slogan "Our husbands were not crazy". "It was despair, not mental illness, which brought my husband to do that", one of them said (Alberti 2012). In the same period, in another Italian town, the widow of an entrepreneur who had committed suicide blamed the professionals of a mental health service because they had not hospitalized him compulsorily. They had found him worried about his economic problems, but they had thought he did not have a mental pathology. "He was depressed. They should have hospitalized him", the widow said (Di Costanzo 2012). So, psychiatry is being blamed on the one hand for unduly pathologizing and stigmatizing understandable psychological distress, and on the other for not pathologizing that same distress and not managing it as if it were a proper mental disorder.

Equally emblematic is the recent discussion on "attenuated psychosis syndrome" and "juvenile bipolar disorder" (the former proposed for inclusion in the DSM-5 and finally included only in the Section III for conditions requiring further study; the latter never included in the DSM, despite considerable lobbying). On the one hand, the need is emphasized to diagnose and manage schizophrenia and bipolar disorder as early as possible, even before the typical clinical picture becomes manifest, in order to improve the outcome of those disorders; on the other, concern is expressed about the risks involved in false-positive diagnoses, especially in terms of social stigma and self-stigmatization, and of misuse of medications (e.g., Corcoran et al. 2010; Parens et al. 2010).

# The Differentiation between "Normal" Sadness and Clinical Depression

The issue of the boundary between "normal" sadness and "true" depression should be considered in the light of the above scenario.

One of the principles of the "neo-kraepelinian credo", articulated by Gerard Klerman in the 1970s (Klerman 1978), was that "there is a boundary between the normal and the sick" (i.e., there is a clear, qualitative distinction between persons who have a mental disorder and persons who do not). A corollary to this assumption was the statement that "depression, when carefully defined as a clinical entity, is qualitatively different from the mild episodes of sadness that everyone experiences at some point in his or her life" (Blashfield 1984). Apparently in line with this statement was the observation that tricyclic antidepressants were active only in people who were clinically depressed; when administered to other people, they did not act as stimulants nor did they alter the subjects' mood.

Today the picture has changed dramatically. Taxonomic studies, carried out in clinical and non-clinical samples, have failed to support the idea that a latent qualitative difference exists between major depression and ordinary sadness, arguing instead in favor of a continuum of depressive states in the general population (e.g., Ruscio and Ruscio 2000). The only possible exception is a nuclear depressive syndrome, roughly corresponding to what is currently called melancholia, which does seem to differ qualitatively from normal sadness in some respects (Grove et al. 1987). Whether this condition represents a distinct disease entity, as advocated by some experts, or corresponds to the most profound states of depression, in which there is probably the recruitment of further neuronal circuits, so that the clinical picture is more complex and with a more prominent biological component, remains open to research. The fact that in many people with recurrent depression some episodes are melancholic and some are not (Melartin et al. 2004) seems to support the latter notion, i.e., that melancholia is a marker of the severity of depression. Anyway, the notion that there is always a qualitative difference between "true" depression and "normal" sadness appears today very hard to maintain.

So, given the current state of knowledge, we are left with two competing approaches, which I have called, respectively, "contextual" and "pragmatic" (Maj 2011). The "contextual" approach assumes that there is a basic difference between depression and "normal" sadness: the latter is always triggered by a life event and appears to be proportionate to that event; the former is either not triggered by a life event or, if triggered by an event, is disproportionate to that event in its intensity and duration. The "pragmatic" approach posits that the boundary between depression and "normal" sadness should be based on pragmatic grounds (i.e., thresholds should be fixed – in terms of number, intensity and duration of symptoms, and degree of functional impairment – which are predictive of clinical outcomes and treatment response).

The "contextual" approach is certainly more appealing to the general public. In fact, a recent population study carried out in Germany (Holzinger et al. 2011) concluded that ordinary people do not tend to perceive depressive symptoms as an indication of the presence of a mental disorder when they occur in the context of adverse life events. In contrast, nearly two-thirds of the almost 5,000 psychiatrists participating in a recent survey of the World Psychiatric Association and the World Health Organization (Reed et al. 2011) stated that the diagnosis of depression should be made if the syndrome is present, even if it appears to be a proportionate response to an adverse life event.

Indeed, the "contextual" approach has several weaknesses.

First, the presence itself of a depressive state can lead to a significant increase in reports of recent stressful events (Cohen and Winokur 1988), since many depressed people tend to attribute a meaning to events that are likely to be neutral. Second, the presence of a depressive state may expose a person to adverse life events: in fact, the relationship between depression and so-called "dependent" events (i.e., events which can be interpreted as a consequence of the depressive state, such as being fired from a job or being left by a fiancé) is much stronger than the relationship between depression and other events (Williamson et al. 1995).

Third, whether an adverse life event has been really decisive in triggering a depressive state may be difficult to establish in many cases, and in any case requires a subjective judgment by the clinician, likely resulting in poor reliability. This has been well known since the 1930s, when Sir Aubrey Lewis, testing a set of criteria aimed to distinguish between "contextual" and "endogenous" depression, concluded that most depressive cases were "examples of the interaction of organism and environment", so that "it was impossible to say which of the factors was decidedly preponderant" (Lewis 1934).

Fourth, the few studies comparing definitely situational with definitely non-situational major depressive disorder, defined according to Research Diagnostic Criteria (RDC, Spitzer et al. 1975), reported that the two conditions were not different with respect to demographic, clinical, and psychosocial variables (e.g., Hirschfeld et al. 1985). Similarly, in a study comparing five groups of depressed patients differing by the level of psychosocial adversity experienced prior to the depressive episode, Kendler et al. (2010) found that the groups did not differ significantly on several clinical, historical, and demographic variables.

Finally, the clinical utility of the proposed contextual exclusion criterion in terms of prediction of treatment response appears very uncertain. Currently available research evidence suggests that the response to antidepressant medication in major depressive disorder is not related to whether or not the depressive state was preceded by a major life event (Anderson et al. 2000). Furthermore, interpersonal psychotherapy is based on the assumption that depression is often understandably related to a disturbing life event, and that "if the patient can solve the life problem, depressive symptoms should resolve as well" (Markowitz and Weissman 2004). This begs the question of whether we should conclude that all cases in which interpersonal psychotherapy is effective are not "true" cases of depression (Maj 2012b).

The "pragmatic" approach, however, is not free from problems. The duration criterion fixed by the DSM-5 (at least two weeks of depressive symptoms) has not been supported by research (e.g., Kendler and Gardner 1998), while the functional criterion (a clinically significant degree of distress or psychosocial impairment) has been found to be redundant by most clinical and epidemiological studies (e.g., Mojtabai 2001; Zimmerman et al. 2004; Wakefield et al. 2010).

The symptomatological threshold (presence of at least five depressive symptoms) has been extensively tested by empirical research, but has not received a convincing validation. Actually, an increasing number of depressive symptoms has been found to correlate in a monotonic fashion with a greater risk for future depressive episodes, a greater functional impairment, a higher physical comorbidity, and a more frequent family history of mental disorders (Kessler et al. 1997). When a point of rarity has been reported, it usually corresponded to a threshold higher than that fixed by the DSM-5. For instance, Kendler and Gardner (1998) found that the risk for future depressive episodes was substantially greater in subjects with seven or more symptoms than in those with six symptoms, while Klein (1990) reported that the risk for mood disorder was significantly higher in relatives of patients with six or more depressive symptoms than in both those with four or five symptoms and those with non-affective disorder.

The notion that the threshold fixed by the DSM-5 may be too low is also supported by some research concerning the prediction of response to pharmacological treatment. Paykel et al. (1988) found that the superiority of amitriptyline over placebo was more substantial when the initial score on the 17-item Hamilton Rating Scale for Depression (HRSD-17) was between 16 and 24, less substantial when it was between 13 and 15, and non-significant when it was between 6 and 12. The authors reported that 13 % of patients with RDC major depression were among those with HRSD-17 scores between 6 and 12, while 34 % had a score between 13 and 15. So, almost one half of the patients with a diagnosis of major depression according to RDC (which are almost identical to DSM-5 criteria) were in the groups showing a non-significant or "less substantial" response to pharmacotherapy. Similarly, Elkin et al. (1989) found that, among patients with an RDC diagnosis of major depressive disorder, those with an initial score of less than 20 on the HRSD-17 (more than 60 % of the sample) did not recover more frequently with imipramine than with placebo plus clinical management, whereas patients with an initial score of 20 or more did significantly better.

However, other studies, using psychosocial impairment as a validator, reported that this impairment was not different in people with two to four depressive symptoms compared to those with five or more symptoms (e.g., Broadhead et al. 1990), which seems to suggest that the threshold proposed by the DSM-5 may be too high. Notably, the RDC and the DSM-III and its successors assume that all depressive symptoms (with the only exception of depressed mood and loss of interest or pleasure) have the same "weight" for diagnostic purposes, which may not actually be the case (e.g., Wakefield and Schmitz 2013).

It is worthwhile to observe that the ICD-10 definition of a depressive episode (World Health Organization 1999) is not consistent with the DSM-5 criteria. In fact, the ICD-10 fixes a threshold for mild depressive episode requiring the presence of at least four depressive symptoms (including at least two of the core symptoms of depressed mood, loss of interest and enjoyment, and increased fatiguability), none of which should be present to an intense degree, and a threshold for severe depressive episode requiring the presence of at least seven depressive symptoms, including all the above mentioned core symptoms, some of which should be of severe intensity. It is further specified that "an individual with a mild depressive episode is usually distressed by the symptoms and has some difficulty in continuing with ordinary work and social activities, but will probably not cease to function completely", whereas "during a severe depressive episode it is very unlikely that the sufferer will be able to continue with social, work, or domestic activities, except to a very limited extent". So, although the "pragmatic" approach is adopted by both our main diagnostic systems, the thresholds they provide are not consistent, and a person may have a depressive episode according to the ICD-10 but not to the DSM-5.

It is clear that neither the "contextual" nor the "pragmatic" approach, in their current formulations, are really able to guide the clinician in the differential diagnosis between "true" depression and "normal" sadness.

Excluding the diagnosis of depression simply because the depressive state looks understandable and proportionate to a recent life event involves the risk of automatically depriving people with a severe and disabling condition of a treatment they may require. Every experienced clinician is able to recall several cases in which he himself or a colleague made that mistake, with serious, sometimes tragic, consequences. On the contrary, making the diagnosis of depression if clinical criteria are fulfilled does not necessarily imply that the person will receive a treatment, and certainly not that he will receive a pharmacological treatment. It will be in the phase of the clinical characterization of the individual case, which follows the phase of the diagnosis, that the circumstances in which the depressive state emerged will be considered, along with many other variables, and this may lead to the decision not to treat (watchful waiting), or to prescribe a psychotherapy which may be just supportive, or to prescribe a pharmacological treatment chosen among the many available, or to prescribe a combination of a psychotherapy and a pharmacotherapy.

On the other hand, the thresholds currently fixed for the diagnosis of major depression following the "pragmatic" approach are not consistent and not convincingly validated, and the notion itself of a single symptomatological threshold being predictive of response to whatever treatment seems now unreasonable. It is clear that the introduction of several evidence-based psychotherapies and of SSRIs has contributed to lower the threshold for the diagnosis of depression in ordinary clinical practice, because those interventions seem to work in milder depressive states which did not respond to tricyclic antidepressants (or in which the risk-benefit ratio of those medications was clearly unfavorable). So, response to different interventions may be predicted by different diagnostic thresholds. That the availability of new effective treatments may influence the perceived boundary between what is normal and what is pathological is certainly not unique to psychiatry. For instance, infertility has been regarded as a fact of life for many centuries, being acknowledged as a disease only when effective reproductive techniques became available (Elliott 1999).

Overall, an analogy seems to emerge between depression and some common physical diseases such as hypertension and diabetes, which also are on a continuum with normality in the general population, with at least two thresholds identifiable along that continuum: one for a condition deserving any kind of clinical attention (which may just be watchful waiting) and another for a state requiring pharmacological intervention. In the case of depression, the former threshold is likely to be lower than that fixed by the DSM-5, while the latter is certainly higher. Both thresholds may need to be based on the overall severity of depressive symptoms in addition to their number.

Contrary to our colleagues diagnosing and treating hypertension and diabetes, we do not have laboratory tests on which to base the above thresholds. This makes the role of the experience and wisdom of the clinician, and the need for diagnostic manuals to guide clinical practice, much more significant in psychiatry than in other medical disciplines.

The detailed description of proper mental disorders provided by current diagnostic systems, however, may not be sufficient, especially for psychiatrists working in a community setting. We may also need a description of ordinary responses to major stressors (such as bereavement, economic ruin, exposure to disaster or war, disruption of family by divorce or separation) as well as to life-cycle transitions (e.g., adolescent emotional turmoil). The DSM-5 attempt to describe "normal" grief as opposed to bereavement-associated depression, in order to guide differential diagnosis, is a first step in this direction.

Furthermore, we may need a characterization of the more serious responses to the above stressors that can be brought to the attention of mental health services although not fulfilling the criteria for any mental disorder. The serious and potentially life-threatening psychological distress related to economic ruin, in which shame and despair are the most prominent features and the diagnostic criteria for depression are often not fulfilled, is a good example. The current delineation of "adjustment disorders" in both the DSM-5 and ICD-10 is too generic and ambiguous to be useful for differential diagnostic purposes and as a guide for management.

Of course, other mental health professionals (and perhaps other professionals outside the health field) will have to collaborate with psychiatrists or even take the lead in those characterizations. This may hopefully contribute to the construction of a transdisciplinary, clinically relevant, body of knowledge in the mental health field, whose existence is at present arguable (Maj 2012a).

Further research is clearly needed to refine the thresholds for the diagnosis of depression and for the assessment of the severity of a depressive episode. Further qualitative studies are also needed to explore the subjective experience of depressed persons, and the possible differences between this experience and that of ordinary sadness. A more precise characterization of individual depressive symptoms is required, as well as an exploration of the predictive value of individual symptoms and specific symptom clusters, with respect to different outcome measures and response to different treatments. Further research on the validity and clinical utility of the construct of melancholia is also warranted.

Meanwhile, however, it should be clarified that the fact that a diagnosis of depression is made does not imply that the person is "mad", nor that his brain is not functioning well, nor that he necessarily needs an intervention, and certainly not that he must be treated with a psychotropic drug. This clarification is likely to reduce significantly the philosophical, social, and ethical implications that the debate on this issue obviously has at the moment.

# References

Alberti, F. (2012, May 5). Le vedove della crisi in corteo: i nostri mariti non erano pazzi. *Corriere della Sera*

American Psychiatric Association. (2013). *Diagnostic and statistical manual of mental disorders* (5th ed.). Arlington: American Psychiatric Association.

Anderson, I. M., Nutt, D. J., Deakin, J. F. W., et al. on behalf of the Consensus Meeting and endorsed by the British Association for Psychopharmacology. (2000). Evidence-based guidelines for treating depressive disorders with antidepressants: A revision of the 1993 British Association for Psychopharmacology guidelines. *Journal of Psychopharmacology, 14*, 3–20.

Blashfield, R. K. (1984). *The classification of psychopathology*. New York: Plenum.

Bolton, D. (2008). *What is mental disorder? An essay in philosophy, science and values*. Oxford: Oxford University Press.

Broadhead, W. E., Blazer, D. G., George, L. K., et al. (1990). Depression, disability days, and days lost from work in a prospective epidemiologic survey. *JAMA, the Journal of the American Medical Association, 264*, 2524–2528.

Cohen, M. R., & Winokur, G. (1988). The clinical classification of depressive disorders. In J. J. Mann (Ed.), *Phenomenology of depressive illness* (pp. 75–96). New York: Human Sciences Press.

Corcoran, C. M., First, M. B., & Cornblatt, B. (2010). The psychosis risk syndrome and its proposed inclusion in the DSM-V: A risk-benefit analysis. *Schizophrenia Research, 120*, 16–22.

Di Costanzo, A. (2012, April 26). Imprenditore suicida, la moglie accusa. *La Repubblica*.

Elkin, I., Shea, T., Watkins, J. T., et al. (1989). National Institute of Mental Health Treatment of Depression Collaborative Research Program. General effectiveness of treatments. *Archives of General Psychiatry, 46*, 971–982.

Elliott, C. (1999). *A philosophical disease: Bioethics, culture and identity*. London: Routledge.

Grove, W. M., Andreasen, N. C., Young, M., et al. (1987). Isolation and characterization of a nuclear depressive syndrome. *Psychological Medicine, 17*, 471–484.

Hirschfeld, R. M. A., Klerman, G. L., Andreasen, N. C., et al. (1985). Situational major depressive disorder. *Archives of General Psychiatry, 42*, 1109–1114.

Holzinger, A., Matschinger, H., Schomerus, G., et al. (2011). The loss of sadness: The public's view. *Acta Psychiatrica Scandinavica, 123*, 307–313.

Horwitz, A. V., & Wakefield, J. C. (2007). *The loss of sadness. How psychiatry transformed normal sorrow into depressive disorder*. Oxford: Oxford University Press.

Kendler, K. S., & Gardner, C. O., Jr. (1998). Boundaries of major depression: An evaluation of DSM-IV criteria. *The American Journal of Psychiatry, 155*, 172–177.

Kendler, K. S., Myers, J., & Halberstadt, L. J. (2010). Should the diagnosis of major depression be made independent of or dependent upon the psychosocial context? *Psychological Medicine, 40*, 771–780.

Kessler, R. C., Zhao, S., Blazer, D. G., et al. (1997). Prevalence, correlates, and course of minor depression and major depression in the National Comorbidity Survey. *Journal of Affective Disorders, 45*, 19–30.

Klein, D. N. (1990). Symptom criteria and family history in major depression. *The American Journal of Psychiatry, 147*, 850–854.

Klerman, G. L. (1978). The evolution of scientific nosology. In J. C. Shershow (Ed.), *Schizophrenia: Science and practice* (pp. 99–121). Cambridge: Harvard University Press.

Kutchins, H., & Kirk, S. A. (1997). *Making us crazy. DSM: The psychiatric bible and the creation of mental disorders*. New York: Free Press.

Lewis, A. (1934). Melancholia: A clinical survey of depressive states. *The Journal of Mental Science, 80*, 277–378.

Maj, M. (2011). When does depression become a mental disorder? *The British Journal of Psychiatry, 199*, 85–86.

Maj, M. (2012a). From "madness" to "mental health problems": Reflections on the evolving target of psychiatry. *World Psychiatry, 11*, 137–138.

Maj, M. (2012b). Differentiating depression from ordinary sadness: Contextual, qualitative and pragmatic approaches. *World Psychiatry, 11*(Suppl. 1), 43–47.

Markowitz, J. C., & Weissman, M. M. (2004). Interpersonal psychotherapy: Principles and applications. *World Psychiatry, 3*, 136–139.

Melartin, T., Leskelä, U., Rytsälä, H., et al. (2004). Co-morbidity and stability of melancholic features in DSM-IV major depressive disorder. *Psychological Medicine, 34*, 1443–1452.

Mojtabai, R. (2001). Impairment in major depression: Implications for diagnosis. *Comprehensive Psychiatry, 42*, 206–212.

Parens, E., Johnston, J., & Carlson, G. A. (2010). Pediatric mental health care dysfunction disorder? *The New England Journal of Medicine, 362*, 1853–1855.

Paykel, E. S., Hollyman, J. A., Freeling, P., et al. (1988). Predictors of therapeutic benefit from amitriptyline in mild depression: A general practice placebo-controlled trial. *Journal of Affective Disorders, 14*, 83–95.

Reed, G. M., Mendonça Correia, J., Esparza, P., et al. (2011). The WPA-WHO global survey of psychiatrists' attitudes towards mental disorders classifications. *World Psychiatry, 10*, 118–131.

Ruscio, J., & Ruscio, A. M. (2000). Informing the continuity controversy: A taxometric analysis of depression. *Journal of Abnormal Psychology, 109*, 473–487.

Spitzer, R. L., Endicott, J., & Robins, E. (1975). *Research Diagnostic Criteria (RDC). Biometrics research*. New York: New York State Psychiatric Institute.

Stein, R. (2010, February 10). Revision to the bible of psychiatry, DSM, could introduce new mental disorders. *Washington Post*.

Wahlbeck, K., & McDaid, D. (2012). Actions to alleviate the mental health impact of the economic crisis. *World Psychiatry, 11*, 139–145.

Wakefield, J. C., & Schmitz, M. F. (2013). When does depression become a disorder? Using recurrence rates to evaluate the validity of proposed changes in major depression diagnostic thresholds. *World Psychiatry, 12*, 44–52.

Wakefield, J. C., Schmitz, M. F., & Baer, J. C. (2010). Does the DSM-IV clinical significance criterion for major depression reduce false positives?: Evidence from the NCS-R. *The American Journal of Psychiatry, 167*, 298–304.

Williamson, D. E., Birmaher, B., Anderson, B. P., et al. (1995). Stressful life events in depressed adolescents: The role of dependent events during the depressive episode. *Journal of the American Academy of Child and Adolescent Psychiatry, 34*, 591–598.

World Health Organization. (1999). *International classification of diseases and related health problems* (10th revision). Geneva: World Health Organization.

World Health Organization. (2001). *The world health report 2001. Mental health: New understanding, new hope*. Geneva: World Health Organization.

World Health Organization Regional Office for Europe. (2005). *Mental health: Facing the challenges, building solutions*. Report from the WHO European Ministerial Conference, 2005. World Health Organization Regional Office for Europe, Copenhagen.

Zimmerman, M., Chelminski, I., & Young, D. (2004). On the threshold of disorder: A study of the impact of the DSM-IV clinical significance criterion on diagnosing depressive and anxiety disorders in clinical practice. *The Journal of Clinical Psychiatry, 65*, 1400–1405.

# Beyond Depression: Personal Equation from the Guilty to the Capable Individual

**Alain Ehrenberg**

**Abstract** The aim of this chapter is to propose a sociological definition of mental health problems and practices. Due to the wide range of practices (from psychosis to self-help), this task is approached as a global idiom, enabling the formulation of multiple tensions and conflicts of contemporary modern life, and providing answers for acting on them—in the family, work and workplace, between couples, in education, etc. The centrality of emotional issues in our society can be described as a form of "mandatory expression" (Marcel Mauss), which characterizes an attitude toward contingency or adversity in a global context where autonomy is the supreme value. From this perspective, mental health can be seen as an individualistic way of dealing with what the ancients called the 'passions'; it is the name individualistic society has given to what was referred to as the 'passions'. Mental health is concerned with our ways of being affected by our ways of acting, and our ways of acting on these afflictions. A transversal viewpoint is presented, of which depression is only one aspect, at three intertwined levels of changes regarding: (1) the configuration of values and norms; (2) the concept of mental health; (3) the type of knowledge that dominates psychiatry and mental health fields, that is, the progressive replacement of psychoanalysis by cognitive neuroscience as the main type of knowledge of the human mind since the 1980s.

Reports on mental health published by health and political organizations, generally indicate that between 20 and 25 % of the population of any developed society is affected by a "mental illness", but primarily by anxiety and mood disorders, and most notably, depression. The area of mental health refers to a large spectrum of problems, ranging from psychosis to personal development, self-help, and enhancement, or what psychiatrists have called "positive mental health" (Vaillant 2008). So, it comes as no surprise that the number of persons affected and, consequently, the cost to society are huge – from 3 to 4 % of the GDP of EU countries (European Commission 2005). Today, mental health certainly is a central public health issue, but contrary to cancer for instance, it is not only such an issue.

A. Ehrenberg (✉)
CNRS (Centre National de la Recherche Scientifique), Université Paris-Descartes, Cermes3
(Centre de recherche, médecine, sciences, santé, santé mentale, société), France
e-mail: alain.chrcnbcrg@parisdescartes.fr

© Springer Science+Business Media Dordrecht 2016                                        39
J.C. Wakefield, S. Demazeux (eds.), *Sadness or Depression?*
History, Philosophy and Theory of the Life Sciences 15,
DOI 10.1007/978-94-017-7423-9_4

The main difference between traditional psychiatry and modern mental health can be expressed very simply: psychiatry is a *local idiom*, specialized in the identification of particular problems. Mental health, because of large domain it encompasses, is a *global idiom*, enabling the identification of multiple tensions and conflicts of contemporary modern life, and, moreover, providing solutions. That is, the practice of mental health is concerned with identifying problems generally linked to social relationships, seeking reasons to explain them, and finding solutions. Today, mental health is not only about the struggle against mental illness, it is also a way of addressing multiple problems in ordinary society—in the family, work and workplace, between couples, in education, etc. Mental health concerns not only health, but also the socialization of the modern individual. It addresses the essential elements of individualistic society, such as self-value, the opposition between responsibility and illness, and the ability to succeed in life. It raises moral questions concerning good and evil, justice and injustice, dignity and shame.

One has to elaborate further about the central place mental health has come to occupy in our way of life.

In "Understanding a Primitive Society", a discussion on the concept of objective reality with anthropologist Edward Evans-Pritchard and philosopher Alasdair McIntyre, published in 1964, Peter Winch explains that the magical rites of the Azandes observed by Evans-Pritchard "express an attitude to contingencies; one, that is, which involves recognition that one's life is subject to contingencies, rather than an attempt to control these". These rites:

> emphasize the importance of certain fundamental features of their life [...] We have a drama of resentment, evil-doing, revenge, and expiation, in which there are ways of dealing (symbolically) with misfortunes and their disruptive effects on man's relations with his fellows, with ways in which life can go on despite such disruption (Winch 1964, 321).

The idea I'll develop here is that the centrality of emotional issues in our society can be described as a form of "mandatory expression" (Mauss 1921/1969), which characterizes an attitude toward contingency or adversity in a global context where autonomy is our supreme value. From this perspective, mental health can be seen as an individualistic way of dealing with what the ancients called the 'passions'; it is the name individualistic society has given to what was referred to as the 'passions'. Mental health, as we shall see, is about our *ways of being affected* by our *ways of acting*, and about our *ways of acting on these afflictions*.

Here I present a transversal viewpoint, of which depression is only one aspect, at three intertwined levels of changes regarding: (1) the configuration of values and norms; (2) the concept of mental health; and (3) the type of knowledge that dominates psychiatry and mental health fields, that is, the progressive replacement of psychoanalysis by cognitive neuroscience as the main type of knowledge of the human mind since the 1980s.

## The Configuration of Values and Norms: Guilt and Discipline, Capability and Autonomy

In attempting to understand the anthropological place of mental health issues today, one should primarily consider the encompassing values and norms of society. Following a Durkheimian perspective, human and social affairs have to be approached in terms of collective representations. Collective representations are not constraints that come from outside; they are *expectations* that determine, or rather constitute, *us* by affecting us in a *total manner*. For instance, and to put it briefly, in traditional African lineage society, it is of crucial importance to respect one's ancestors (and the social ideal is to become an ancestor); in traditional Indian caste society, it is to abide by one's degree of purity; in modern individualistic society, it is to become someone by oneself. Recently, this question of becoming oneself has changed. I would summarize the change as follows: we have witnessed a shift from the guilty and disciplined individual to the capable and autonomous individual. This shift occurred during the second part of the twentieth century.

The concept of autonomy today designates many aspects of social life and has to be historically described in two steps. Autonomy first emerged as a collective aspiration in developed societies between the end of Second World War and the 1970s, an aspiration towards greater choice or independence and more equality—in which equality between men and women, and therefore the rise of woman as individual, is the epicenter. Between the 1970s and the 1980s it has become the common condition and has pervaded social relationships beyond the dynamic of emancipation: it has widened to action itself where individual initiative is highly valued, notably through the transformations of the workplace and capitalism where flexible work implies the autonomy of workers. Values and norms of choice, self-ownership, and individual initiative value the three dimensions of independence, cooperation, and competition. This change modifies the relationships between the agent and his or her action; it increases the responsibility of the agent regarding his or her own action. The consequence is that everything that concerns individual behavior, the mobilization of personal dispositions, and notably the ability of the individual to change by himself, to be the agent of his own change (in short, "personality") is a major social and political preoccupation.

I summarize this change as a shift from autonomy-aspiration to autonomy-condition. It must be added that these aspects can be understood and valued differently according to a given society: for instance, autonomy unifies the US, where the self-motivated individual is a major collective representation, but divides France, where it tends to represent an abandonment of the individual and society to market forces (Ehrenberg 2010, Italian version 2010, German 2011).

Today autonomy has become our common condition; it is a normative expectation for everyone, and not a choice you have the liberty to make.

The history of depression incarnates this change. It accompanied the shift from guilt and discipline to capability and autonomy during the second half of the twentieth century. It has progressively occupied the place of Freudian neurosis, that is, the pathology of guilt, and has become the shadow of the individual normed by autonomy. I will summarize the shift as follows. In a form of life organized by traditional discipline, the question was: *am I allowed to do it?* When reference to autonomy dominates the concept of society, when the idea that everyone can become someone by oneself becomes an ideal embedded in our mores, the question is: *am I able to do it?* Neurotic guilt has not disappeared; it has taken the form of depressive insufficiency. My hypothesis is that, if melancholy was the illness of the exceptional man during the sixteenth century Renaissance, and if during the Romantic Era, it was at the crossroads of creation or genius and unreason (Klibanski et al. 1964), it is now the situation of everyone, because contemporary individualism consists in having democratized the idea that any one could be exceptional. In fact, the history of contemporary depression must be approached in two steps: from the 1940s to the beginning of the 1970s, depression was considered to be a subfield of neurosis, and hence remained attached to the categories of conflict, guilt, and desire; since then, it has been reconceptualized by psychoanalysts as a narcissistic pathology where topics centered on desire lost ground in favor of a problematic centered on object loss, subjective identity, and shame, which subordinated feelings of guilt. It seems it is less desire that was at stake than a feeling of permanent insecurity. Depression has become a pathology of greatness, developing feelings of insufficiency regarding social ideals. It has been a major expression of the democratization of the exceptional. This shift of our configuration of norms and values has set the individual on an axis that goes from capability to incapability (Ehrenberg 1998 English translation 2010). In this shift, personal assertion, or the capability to assert oneself, appropriately becomes a core element of socialization at every level of the social hierarchy.

We have been faced with new life trajectories and new ways of living affecting the family, employment, education, relationships between generations, and so on. Along with this we have witnessed the end of the welfare state of the twentieth century. This change indicates that we are living in a type of society where we all have to invest ourselves personally in numerous and heterogeneous social situations. Individual capability to act as an autonomous self has become a major point of reference. It embodies our ideals of personal accomplishment.

This is a change in what can be called "personal equation". In the previous discipline-based system, the aim of behavior regulation was the docile individual, and values of autonomy, like choice or individual initiative, were subordinated: in this light, personal equation was weak. In the new autonomy-based system, the aim of regulation is one's personal initiative, and each person has to adopt a line of conduct: personal equation is strong. For instance, think of the shift from *qualifications* in the Taylorian/Fordian workplace to *skills* in the flexible workplace, and notably social skills with which an emotional dimension has emerged related to increased self-control. These skills condition the possibility to adopt a line of conduct in a type of management of the workforce where the problem is no longer how to coordinate the action from a centralized direction, but how to make people cooperate with each other. In the discipline-based system, the regulation of action consisted of a discipline of the body; in the flexible organization it consists of a mobilization of their personal commitment. In both cases, the individual has to "self control", to "self regulate", but the style of social constraint is different. Today, work is constituted by interdependent relationships between human beings. The source of efficiency in the workplace is both the relationship *and* the individual. These capacities are required at every hierarchical level of companies because we are faced with a type of temporality characterized by uncertainty. In this context, emotional control is a major *skill*.

The meaning of discipline itself has changed: it is subordinated to the design of getting individual initiative, therefore abilities to self-motivate and self-activate. It tends to self-discipline. Where the problem previously was to render the individual docile and useful, as philosopher Michel Foucault put it (Foucault 1975), now it is to develop abilities to self-activate *and* to self-control. The aim of discipline is not obedience mainly; it is a means to develop abilities of empathy and self-reliance (Ehrenberg 2010).

Capacities for good socialization have a triple aspect: cognitive, social, and emotional. There is a new dimension of personal responsibility in social life. Consequently, relations between responsibility, capability, and emotional self-control are crucial for public policies.

The point I want to make here is that the contemporary concern about the treatment of personality is not primarily about an upsurge in psychological disorders. It is about the normative changes of our ways of acting in society, therefore about our new forms of socialization and its consequences for inequalities and poverty. In this society, individual subjectivity has become a major issue because it emphasizes problems of *self-structuring*. Without this self-structuring, it is difficult to act by oneself in an appropriate manner. It was never a central concern in a society of mechanical discipline. The consequence of the shift from discipline to autonomy is a demand for an increased capacity of emotional self-control. At the same time, our social relationships are more frequently formulated in a language of affect and emotions, distributed between the good of mental health and the bad of psychic suffering. This leads me to the second level of change.

## From Psychiatry to Mental Health: The New Morbidity

Self-motivation, self-activation, self-control, self-discipline, self-regulation: there is, of course, a strong relationship between these notions and the predominant place occupied nowadays by mental health issues in social life. Generalized attention to mental health and psychic suffering is a major reference point for individualization.

Depression certainly is the clinical entity through which changes appear in guilt and in reasons to feel guilty in society. But since its reconceptualization 40 years ago, numerous entities have appeared that have made up the field of mental health. Changes in personal equation have been accompanied by a *new morbidity* of a behavioral nature, which is the pathology of the capable individual, of which the depression reconceptualized, either by psychoanalysis or biological psychiatry. Capable individual is an expression of a system of social relationships where choice, individual initiative, self-ownership, and ability to act as an agent of one's own change are supreme values.

This new morbidity, which is not only a matter for the *particular* area of mental illness, but above all for the *general* field of social life, has been instituted as a major issue in the workplace, education, and family—stress and burnout, ADHD, school phobia, and intra family violence. It highlights two major changes. The first change is the status of symptom: the mental disorder is an expression of difficulties related to socialization in one way or another, and criteria related to social functioning have become essential—this is the rise of axis five in the DSM-III, dedicated to the assessment of adaptive functioning in the past year (Millon 1983). Though axis 5 was removed from the fifth version, functioning remains at the center of professionals' concern. The second change is related to the style of unhappiness: the feeling of not being able to be good enough or not being able to mobilize oneself into action is at the core of the evil; the inability to act and to project oneself in the future is at the core of the difficulties of the subject.

The evolution of American pediatrics is typical of the change regarding functioning. In 1975, the American Academy of Pediatrics introduced the concept of « new morbidity » to designate non-infectious problems affecting children and families whose prevalence were on the rise. In 1991, it released a report on the role of the pediatrics in the future. Its first sentence asserts that "societal changes have engendered significant changes in the delivery of health care" (American Academy of Pediatrics Task Force 1991, 401) in which social dimensions have a central place. The new morbidity is behaviorial, and the concept of *behavioral health* earns a new value, from toddlers to young adults. Now, social, developmental, and behavioral problems are the core of the profession of pediatrics. Two other reports followed, in 2001 and 2012, which went in the same direction. This morbidity represents a "shift in the understanding of what has an impact on children and families health" (American Academy of Pediatrics, Committee on Psychosocial Aspects of Child and Family Health 2001, 1228). Disparities, claims the 2012 report, "threaten the democratic ideals of our country in weakening the national creed of equality of opportunity". This is a "significant change of paradigm" (Shonkoff et al. 2012): through developmental approaches, which aim to reducing pathologies of adulthood with early intervention in childhood, a shift occurred from a *sick-care* model to a *health-care* one.

In a nutshell, the new morbidity and the new health is behavior, and behavior is individual autonomy. It is less disobedience that counts than lack of empathy for others and lack of self-reliance, which are disclosed by the behavior, and have long-term disadvantageous consequences for socialization.

The accent put on early intervention and the developmental approach highlights a fundamental element of autonomy: the relationship with time. Because mental health deals with pathologies of relational life that disable individual freedom, it appears to be an ensemble of practices where personal transformation is a key value, which amounts to practices conceived in terms of a relation to time centered on uncertain and unstable futures. Changes in our relationship to time and the rise of our worry for emotional and drive control are closely connected.

Regarding the most common disorders (mainly depression and anxiety disorders), let's take some examples in the UK to illustrate the idea of a global idiom in which emotional self-control and autonomy are intertwined. For instance, the famous report on depression published by economist Richard Layard (professor at the LSE&PS) in 2006, in the context of "Initiative for Improving Access to Psychological Therapy" (IAPT) prepared by National Health Service and launched in 2008, claims that anxiety and depression disorders are the main social issue today and that the primary cause of misery is not poverty, but "mental illness". Why? Because "mental illness" is related to behavior, and behavioral problems are considered to be the most challenging aspects of our society by Layard and other "happiness economists". The report proposed recruiting 10,000 therapists specialized in CBT to alleviate this new social scourge (Center for Economic Performance's Mental Health Policy Group 2006). The same year, the Institute for Public Policy Research (IPPR), a progressive British think tank, published *Freedom's Orphans*. In this report, the authors "used two large surveys that followed young people born in 1958 and 1970, and shows that in just over a decade, personal and social skills became 33 times more important in determining relative life chances" (Margo et al. 2006, viii). Several reports were published in the UK on the topic of "character capabilities" as targets for early intervention public policy against child poverty. For instance, Demos, and its "Character Inquiry" of 2011:

> The aim of The Character Inquiry is to investigate the potential of focusing on character, and character development, to help achieve greater levels of wellbeing in society and among individuals [...] The capabilities that enable individuals to live ethically responsible and personally fulfilling lives [...] consist of the ability to apply oneself to tasks, to empathize with others and to regulate one's emotions (Lexmond and Grist 2011, 10).

Focus, empathy, and self-control are three key words of autonomy. Another report published by IPPR in 2009 about personal advisers, who have a pivotal role in welfare-to-work, is entitled *Now it's Personal. Personal Adviser and the New Work Public Service*. It notably underlines:

> [...] evidence that new training techniques such as the Cognitive Behavioral Interviewing technique can encourage a more open and productive dialogue between adviser and client, enabling discussions to move onto employment related goals more quickly (McNeil 2009, 6).

The same year a report was published by Carol Black, director of NHS (National Health Service), which proposed changing the conception of fitness and disability at work from a "sick" to "fit for work" model. Following these various reports and recommendations, a plan for developing psychotherapy training and access has been launched in 2010. As the Minister for care service put it in his foreword, "talking therapies are a major element of our cross-government mental health strategy" (Department of Health 2011, 2).

This example highlights an extension of psychotherapy to problem-solving, that is, a form of coaching: social functioning is added to and intertwined with psychopathology. Such interventions are conceived as forms of empowerment to develop individual's capacities to rely on themselves by helping them to support themselves through accompaniments whose purpose is to make them the agents of their own change. It is crucial to understand that mental health issues are at the core of today's public policy, which have larger targets than strictly psychiatric problems. The shift from a sick-model to a health model means mental health is about how to achieve good socialization in a world where ability to decide and act by oneself pervades social relationships, and is the common condition. Mental health acts on our mores and habits. Similarly to civil religion for Rousseau, it fosters a "feeling of sociability" (Rousseau 1762/2001).

Regarding psychiatric patients affected by severe and enduring mental illnesses, like schizophrenia, new approaches have also emerged since the 1970s that are centered on the idea of autonomy. They result from a major change in psychiatric institutions, one that makes the autonomy of the patient the goal and the means of the treatment. This change is the end of the "total institution" described by sociologist Erving Goffman half a century ago (Goffman 1961). The paradox is that Goffman published his book at a point when the dynamic of deinstitutionalization was just beginning. Today, the psychiatric patient has to live in a community and not in a hospital. The issue of being able to live an autonomous life is at the heart of treatments; that is, *social relationships* have become a major aim. Psychosocial interventions (self-management, psychoeducation, cognitive remediation, etc.) aim to improve a patient's skills to live in ordinary social life. The emergence of his or her voice has accompanied a double change in the style of action: from "acting *on*" the patient to "acting *with*" him or her, on one hand; and from the emphasis put on the pathology (on the deficit, on the handicap) to the potential to enhance his or her strengths, on the other. To enhance the patient's potential is a means to better fight against the pathology, the handicap or the deficit. Beyond the clinical stability of the patient, a new goal appeared about 30 years ago, supported by the so-called Recovery movement: the possibility to have a more accomplished and rewarding life as a person, despite the illness (see notably Hopper 2007). Here, also, social functioning is a major concern.

This new understanding of mental illness—as involving the general domain of social life—has been instituted as an organizing vision in workplaces, education, and family life. This vision obviously implies that mental health practices deal with the relations between *individual afflictions* and *social relationships*. A mental disorder is typically seen as the expression of difficulties linked to socialization, that is, with social functioning viewed as essential for individual well-being. This is not so much a "medicalization" of behaviors (as sociologists have too often implied [see Conrad 2007, for instance]). What it represents, rather, is a complementary change both in medical practices and in social relationships, an understanding of which requires a descriptive approach.

## From Psychoanalysis to Cognitive Neuroscience

During the last three or four decades, psychoanalysis has declined in favor of the rise of cognitive neuroscience. The word "cognitive" means that neuroscience aims to combine two areas: neurophysiology and psychology. The concept of emotion is conceived of as information processing, hence its cognitive dimension.

The general issue I explore is the following: through neuroscience there is a change of the relationships between neuropathology and psychopathology, pathologies of lesion and pathologies of function. Notably, there is a strong trend today to merge these two kinds of pathology into a single neuropsychiatric kind, one in which reference to the brain as the biological system on which one can explain as much psychopathology as neuropathology, is the supreme value (See Ehrenberg 2004, 2008/2010). In this context, my aim is to understand how references to the brain and cognition have entered into social life and the collective imagination, how people use them and if it makes a difference in their life.

Following the model of total knowledge that psychoanalysis has pretended to be, cognitive neuroscience has become a psychology, sociology, and a philosophy. Total knowledge has an anthropological nature, in the sense that it addresses the question: what is man made up of? Today, it seems that a genuine science of human behavior tends to replace a psychoanalytic science, regarding which the status of science has remained doubtful. A genuine science is a science able to prove its propositions in the laboratory with the use of standardized methods without which there is no such thing as science. The therapeutic hopes invested in cognitive neuro-science seem analogous to those of psychoanalysis a few decades ago.

This transformation occurred for many reasons, but I want to underscore the anthropological one, from the guilty to the capable individual.

For Freud, civilization is based on the repression of drives, and, as he wrote in "the Id and the Ego" (Freud 1981), the superego is like a garrison in a town. I would qualify his claim: it is the form of life on which psychoanalysis was born which was based on this repression, and not civilization in general. The core moral feeling of Freud's thought is guilt; as he wrote in the same article, the patient doesn't feel guilty, he feels sick. Freud's thought was about guilt and desire. Guilt feelings are disguised in symptoms, which are the expression of forbidden desires. Desire is a conflicting entity for Freud. Psychoanalysis was founded on an anthropology of the guilty individual at a time when the social normative and value systems were based on mechanical discipline. What is at stake in psychoanalysis and in the practice of the talking cure is a set up for "passionate utterance", to use an expression by Stanley Cavell, "an invitation to improvisation in the disorders of desire" (Cavell 2005). Where one's own conflicting desire can appear, desire and conflict being necessarily intertwined—desire being something closer to passion and passivity than to action and activity. When this form of life began to be shaken, psychoanalysts started to think that Narcissus had replaced Oedipus, the ideal ego, and the surperego. They deemed that their patients were subjected more to anxieties of loss rather than of conflict. If the Oedipal patient suffers from anxieties of castration, the narcissistic patient is affected by anxieties of loss. The shift from Oedipus to Narcissus corresponds to the confrontation of psychoanalysis with autonomy.

Cognitive neuroscience developed in a context where the shift from Oedipus to Narcissus had *already* occurred, a context where mores had been emancipated from the old taboos, where flexible work had started to spread, and where workfare was in the process of replacing welfare. For this reason, cognitive neuroscience is founded on a slightly different anthropology, an *anthropology of the capable individual*. For cognitive neuroscientists, civilization is derived not from the repression of drives, but from the expansion of empathy, and related concepts like decision-making or trust, all concepts which are framed by "theory of mind" and are a stand-in for social relations.

I'll end this chapter by presenting cognitive neuroscience as an *echo maker* of values and norms of autonomy. Decision making, trust, empathy, cognitive bias, etc., on which cognitive neuroscience develops its demonstrations in the laboratory are among the core social concepts of today. Empathy is a necessary attitude in the flexible workplace where people have to cooperate one with another; this was not the case in the Fordian workplace. Now, empathy is a *skill*, not just a moral attitude. Right decision-making and avoidance of cognitive bias are a huge market for a multitude of personal advisers and coaches who are supposed to help people choose. Cognitive neuroscience is not in search of mechanisms of obedience, but of decision-making; anti-social behaviors are defined as wrong decision-making. The brain and cognitive neuroscience are not pervaded by collective representations of the mechanical discipline (who is in search of an obedient brain?), but by that of autonomy.

Of course, this doesn't mean that cognitive neuroscience can be reduced to a reproduction of values and norms. I mean something analogous to what Marcel Mauss said in his famous speech, "A Category of the Human Mind: the Notion of Person, the Notion of Self" (1938). At the end of the speech, talking about Kant, Mauss underlined that the

> importance of sectarian movements during the seventeenth and eighteenth centuries on the formation of philosophical and political thought. It is there that the issues of individual liberty, of individual consciousness, of the right to communicate directly with God, of being one's own priest, of having an inner God were raised. The notions promoted by the Morave Brothers, Puritans, Wesleyans, Pietists were those which formed the basis on which the notion [of person] was established: person = self; self = consciousness, and consciousness is the key category. [...] It is only with Kant that it has taken an accurate form. Kant was a Pietist [...]. *The indivisible ego, he found it around him* [my emphasis].[1] (Mauss 1950/1968, 360–361)

Mauss underlines the social origins of Kant's thought, but of course this doesn't mean that Kant's thought is only a reproduction of ordinary categories. It means that there is an internal relationship, an interdependent relationship between concepts, categories, and symbols and the lives of those who use them. In the same manner, I suggest that cognitive neuroscience is loaded with values and social ideas, with

---

[1] My translation.

collective representations of autonomy that it found around it; it expresses, through the language of biology, ways of being in society that have spread during the last third of the twentieth century in terms of autonomy. Social and scientific ideas are intertwined. According to me, it is of a fundamental importance to acknowledge that this claim aims to provide a sociological alternative—and more precisely both a Durkheimian and Wittgensteinian alternative—to naturalistic and post-Foucaldian approaches to these problems.

In most naturalistic approaches, it is science that provides criteria to define objective reality (for a discussion about science and objective reality, see Winch 1964); more precisely, I should say, the material basis of reality, and in the case of emotional issues, is the brain. So, real = material = brain.

In the legacy of Foucault, and as a sociological alternative to naturalistic approaches, many speak of the "objective person", of "biosociality", of the "neuro-chemical self", etc. They think that there is a paradigm of "brainhood" that is pervasive in media. Without going deeper, I will only say that post-Foucaldian approaches only offer a counter mythology to the new scientific mythology of cognitive neuroscience. Following Wittgenstein, I want "to *understand* something which is in plain view. For *this* is what we seem in some sense not to understand" (Wittgenstein 1953, §89). What is in plain view that we don't see?

The echo maker hypothesis means that cognitive neuroscience is loaded with values and social ideas, that is, it is pervaded by our current collective representations, to use a Durkheimian formula. Consequently, we should approach it by thinking of its concepts less as criteria defining an objective reality than as *the new language game* that has subordinated psychoanalysis to treat the afflictions of autonomy. With this language game, human beings try to understand their predicament, deal with them, and create a meaningful life in the age of autonomy-condition.

How do people recognize themselves through their brain and cognitive patterns? How do they refer to cognition, the brain, etc. in the description of what is going on for them? How do these references take their place in the tapestry of their lives?

For instance, the trend to merge neuropathology and psychopathology in the same kind of illness has led people to ask themselves: is it intentional or mechanical? Is it both? How are these two aspects related to one another? Here I'm thinking of new kinds of narratives that can be called "neuropsychoanalytic". I'll mention one by the composer and pianist Allen Shawn, *Wish I Could Be There. Notes from a Phobic Life* (2007), and another by the American novelist Siri Hustvedt, *The Shaking Woman or a History of my Nerves* (2009) (for a more detailed analysis see Ehrenberg 2014). The two narratives are "neuropsychoanalytic" because they unfold through a tension between neurobiology and psychoanalysis, a tension that can sometimes transform itself into something more complementary. Research in neuroscience is necessarily from a mechanical perspective: scholars are in search of causes. But in real life, people are looking for a global understanding of their situation and of themselves. Consequently, they need causes *and* reasons, they need to understand if there is something intentional in their symptoms (an unconscious intention, for instance), but also if they are produced by a dysfunctional mechanism;

they need to know if it is either/or (either intentional/or mechanical), if it is of bit of each, and so on. In real life, causes and reasons are not separate entities; they are mainly practical distinctions between which there are tensions, intricacy, and uncertainty.

Being neuropsychoanalytic, these narratives try to make allowances for both the hidden intentionality of the symptom and the involuntary movement of the neurological disorder. The shaking of Siri Hustvedt seems to be a manifestation of a mysterious relationship with her father. In Allen Shawn's life there is the "missing part" of his autistic twin sister whose absence, since she was put into an institution when they turned eight, was progressively replaced by his main symptom, that is, agoraphobia; he wrote a sequel devoted to this relationship, *Twins: a memoir* (2011).

Hustvedt and Shawn appear as *individuals* having subordinated their patient statuses. The story of her nerves and the story of his agoraphobia are those of the subordination of their tremors and phobia to their own individuality—their own self— thanks to an elaboration enabling them to create something *singular* in lieu of being subjected to a *disability*. Of course, Hutsvedt is a writer and Shawn a composer, but today this new individualism is part and parcel of the life of masses of people subjected to various chronic conditions (with autism, with schizophrenia, etc.). Before defining it, one has to say something about the context, which is the following: these people (again, those with autism, schizophrenia, etc.), who half a century ago were into closed and total institutions, now live in the community; therefore, they need the various skills necessary to live a "normal" life, be it with drugs, psychosocial rehabilitation, cognitive behavior therapy, self-help and coach support, etc., which compensate for their handicaps. In this new context, the new individualism goes a step further: the condition is subordinated to a creation of a personal attitude which is not conceived of in terms of adaptation, but of a different style of life. Here autonomy is shaped in relation to the idea that there is a *creative aspect* in a long term or chronic illness—this subject is the connecting thread of the popular narratives by Oliver Sacks (1995). I earlier mentioned the topic of strengths about the psychiatric patient. This notion has recently gained a new meaning: the meaning of a *different cognitive style* related to or implying a different form of life. This is a new collective or common meaning.

This implies a context in which illness is not only approached as a handicap or a disability, but *as a constraint from which you can create something*—which was also a stance claimed by writer Georges Perec and the OULIPO movement in the French literature half a century ago. It makes a creative aspect of the illness stand out. Think of neurodiversity for people affected by autism or Voice Hearers for schizophrenia. Instead of deficient lives, which were lived in closed institutions, new forms of life are developing in the new context of a community. Today, there is an extension to other conditions, like ADHD or dyslexia, as having strengths or advantages.[2] The multiplication of different forms of life is a

---

[2] A recent example among many: "In recent years, however, dyslexia research has taken a surprising turn: identifying the ways in which people with dyslexia have skills that are superior to those

strong trend: it is an expression of values of choice, self-ownership, and initiative, *in* the constraint of the disease. It is a style of being affected, a style of living the illness in a certain way.

These narratives can be linked up to the tradition of German individualism, which is, as Georg Simmel wrote, an individualism of uniqueness, a singularity for which Gœthe is the figurehead and *Bildung* (a rich German word, coming from German Enlightment and Romanticism, which means literally "education" in the sense of an education of the inner self that links together the processes of education, edification, and culture) (Dumont 1994) the form this singularity has adopted. This is what is in "plain view" (ordinary practices with new objects).

The aim of Peter Winch's work was "to suggest that the concept of *learning from* which is involved in the study of other cultures is closely linked with the concept of *wisdom*. We are confronted not just with different techniques, but with new possibilities of good and evil, in relations to which men come to terms with life". This wisdom is about what Winch calls "limiting notions"—birth, death, sexuality—"which give shape to what we understand by 'human life'" (Winch 1964, 322). We can add long term and chronic illnesses to these three limited notions. These illnesses, because they're chronic, are accompanied by a certain suffering and confusion. Considering one's own life as a whole from the perspective of its limitations and, eventually, living a different form of life which can be fulfilling, this is what these narratives are about. In this sense, they express an individualistic attitude toward adversity—an attitude unimaginable at the time of the "total institution" (Goffman 1961). This is what we are in search of when we read these narratives, as when we study other cultures, and to follow Winch, "we may learn different possibilities of making sense in human life" (Winch 1964, 321). These autobiographies of psychiatric, neurologic, or neuropsychiatric patients do a similar work in showing how to live, sometimes a rewarding life, despite the evil to which these people are subjected. The patient appears mainly as an individual having subordinated his patient status, because he extricates himself from the disease with his or her strength of singular creativity. He has subordinated the disease to his own individuality by shaping it with a personal style enabling him to create something. We might increase the possibility to live singular lives.

---

of typical readers. The latest findings on dyslexia are leading to a new way of looking at the condition: not just as an impediment, but as an advantage, especially in certain artistic and scientific fields." A. M. Paul, The Upside of Dyslexia, *The New York Times*, February 4th, 2012. One week later, John Tierney published a "What's New? Exuberance for Novelty Has Benefits", *The New York Times*, February 13th, 2012: "Those are the kinds of questions used to measure novelty-seeking, a personality trait long associated with trouble. As researchers analyzed its genetic roots and relations to the brain's dopamine system, they linked this trait with problems like attention deficit disorder, compulsive spending and gambling, alcoholism, drug abuse and criminal behavior. Now, though, after extensively tracking novelty-seekers, researchers are seeing the upside. In the right combination with other traits, it's a crucial predictor of well-being." "It can lead to antisocial behavior," declares a psychiatrist, "but if you combine this adventurousness and curiosity with persistence and a sense that it's not all about you, then you get the kind of creativity that benefits society as a whole ."

# Conclusion

There is an apparent paradox of autonomy: the diminishing social value of guilt has been replaced by a situation where issues of emotional and drive control seem much more decisive than when autonomy was a secondary value. This paradox is resolved when we situate it in our current relationship to time. Here, we have to follow Norbert Elias: "To assert oneself as an adult in society structured like ours [...] demands a high level of anticipation and of self-control of intermittent impulses in order to reach long run goals and to accomplish one own desires. The level of constraint demanded corresponds to the length of interdependent chains one forms, as individuals, with other persons. In other words, to assert oneself as an adult in our society requires a high degree of self-control of one's own drives and affects". (Elias 1980/2010, 99). The more social complexity increases, notably the uncertainty of the future and the length of interdependent chains (of a now global society), the more our concern for self-control rises. But this concern rises, as I already underscored it, as a skill. Actually, this is a utilitarian idea of morality, that of Bentham and Mill: as skills needed to accomplish a good life, their lack is a consequence of lack of character that is to the disadvantage of the subject who lacks of them. The form of life of the capable individual is much more consequentialist than the one of the guilty individual for which Kantian moral philosophy fits best.

Mental health and psychic suffering are connected to the autonomy-based system as follows: changes in our *ways of acting* in society, symbolized by the notion of autonomy, correspond to changes in our *ways of being affected* symbolized by the notion of psychic suffering—a notion which is everywhere today through the rich vocabulary of mental health. Autonomy consists of an emphasis on the activity of the individual, but, at the same time, it is something to which one is subjected, which one has to put up with: affect, affection, passion, passivity, all of these words are about being subjected to or affected by something.

The value granted today to mental health, psychic suffering, affect and emotions is the fruit of a context through which injustice, failure, deviance, dissatisfaction, etc., tend to be appraised according to their impact on individual subjectivity, and the capacity to lead an autonomous life. In the mental health field, we find a genuine individualistic drama where mistakes, failures, misfortune, and illness, all intertwined, are represented. Autonomy logically highlights an affective and emotional dimension, one that used to have a secondary value and occupied a subordinated place in a disciplined-based system. In this sense, mental health is a social form adopted to deal with passions when norms and value are entirely oriented toward individual action.

Mental health, then, is more than the antonym of mental illness. It is an equivalent of good socialization because being in good mental health is to be able to act by oneself in an appropriate manner in most situations in life. In other words, it is to be able to self-activate in displaying enough emotional self-control. In a style of social life which confronts the individual less with the drama of desire than with the tragedy of self-esteem, mental health appears as an ensemble of practices aiming to render the individual able to control his emotional functioning and whose behavior is regulated by technique resorting to autonomy.

It is thus possible now that a good life might be defined by the best score on the Global Assessment of Functioning (GAF) of axis 5 of the DSM-IV: "91–100. No symptoms. Superior functioning in a wide range of activities, life's problems never seem to get out of hand, is sought out by others because of his or her many positive qualities."

# References

American Academy of Pediatrics Task Force. (1991). Report on the future role of the pediatrician in the delivery of health care. *Pediatrics, 87*(3), 401–409.

American Academy of Pediatrics, & Committee on Psychosocial Aspects of Child and Family Health. (2001). The new morbidity revisited: A renewed commitment to the psychosocial aspect of pediatric care. *Pediatrics, 108*(5), 1227–1230.

Cavell, S. (2005). *Philosophy the day after tomorrow.* Cambridge, MA/London: Harvard University Press.

Center for Economic Performance's Mental Health Policy Group. (2006). *The depression report. A new deal for depression and anxiety disorders.* LSE&PS/ESRC.

Conrad, P. (2007). *The medicalization of society. On the transformation of human conditions into treatable disorders.* Baltimore: The John Hopkins University Press.

Department of Health. (2011). *Talking therapies: A four years plan of action.* www.dh.gov.uk/publications

Dumont, L. (1994). *German ideology. From France to Germany and back.* Chicago: The University of Chicago Press.

Ehrenberg, A. (1998). *La Fatigue d'être soi. Dépression et société.* Paris: Odile Jacob. English translation: *The weariness of the self. diagnosis the history of depression in the contemporary age.* Montreal: McGill University Press, 2010.

Ehrenberg, A. (2004, November). Le sujet cérébral, *Esprit*, pp. 130–155.

Ehrenberg, A. (2008/2010). Le "cerveau social". Chimère épistémologique et vérité sociologique, *Esprit*, January 2008, pp. 79–103. Translated in English in a slightly extended version, The 'social' brain. An epistemological chimera and a sociological fact. In F. Ortega & F. Vidal (Eds), *Neurocultures. Glimpses into an expanding universe* (pp. 117–140). New York/Frankfurt/Berlin: Springer.

Ehrenberg, A. (2010). *La Société du malaise.* Paris: Odile Jacob, *La Societa del Disaggio*, Trino, Einaudi, 2010, *Das Unbehagen in der Gesellschaft*, Berlin, Suhrkamp, 2011.

Ehrenberg, A. (2014). Suis-je malade de mes idées ou de mon cerveau? In B. Chamak & B. Moutaud (Eds.), *Neurosciences et société. Enjeux des savoirs et des pratiques sur le cerveau* (pp. 255–286). Paris: Armand Colin.

Elias, N. (2010). La civilisation des parents (1980). In N. Elias (Ed.), *Au-delà de Freud. Sociologie, psychologie, psychanalyse.* Paris: La Découverte.

European Commission, Health and Consumer Protection DG. (2005). *Green paper. Improving the mental health of the population: Toward a strategy on mental health for the European Union.*

Foucault, M. (1975). *Surveiller et punir.* Paris: Gallimard. American translation, 1977.

Freud, S. (1981). « Le moi et le ça ». In: *Essais de psychanalyse* (pp. 219–275). Paris: Petite Bibliothèque Payot.

Goffman, E. (1961). *Asylums: Essays on the social situation of mental patients and other inmates.* New York: Doubleday.

Hopper, K. (2007). Rethinking social recovery in schizophrenia: What a capability approach might offer. *Social Science and Medicine, 65*, 868–879.

Hustvedt, S. (2009). *The shaking woman or a history of my nerves*. New York: Picador.

Klibanski, R., Panovski, E., & Saxl, F. (1964). *Saturn and melancholy: Studies in the natural history of philosophy, religion and art*. London: Thomas Nelson and Sons.

Lexmond, J., & Grist, M. (Eds.). (2011). *"Character should be at the heart of our responses to social problems..." The character inquiry*. London: Demos.

Margo, J., Dixon, M., Pearce, N., & Reed, H. (2006). *Freedom's Orphans. Raising youth in a changing world*. London: Institute for Public Policy Research (IPPR).

Mauss, M. (1938, July–December) Une Catégorie de L'Esprit Humain: La Notion de Personne Celle de "Moi". *The Journal of the Royal Anthropological Institute of Great Britain and Ireland, 68*, 263–281.

Mauss, M. (1950). Une catégorie de l'esprit humain: la notion de personne, celle de "moi", M. Mauss, *Sociologie et anthropologie*, Paris, PUF, 1968.

Mauss, M. (1969). L'expression obligatoire des sentiments, (*Journal de Psychologie*, 1921), in : *Œuvres* 3, Paris, Ed. de Minuit, pp. 269–279.

McNeil, C. (2009). *Now it's personal. Personal adviser and the New Work public service*. London: Institute for Public Policy Research (IPPR).

Millon, T. (1983). DSM-III: An insider's perspective. *American Psychologist, 38*, 804–814.

Rousseau, J.-J. (1762/2001). *Du Contrat Social*, Paris: Garnier-Flammarion.

Sack, O. (1995). *An anthropologist on Mars. Seven paradoxical tales*. New York: Knopf.

Shawn, A. (2007). *Wish I could be there. Notes from a phobic life*. New York: Viking.

Shawn, A. (2011). *Twin: a memoir*. New York: Viking.

Shonkoff, J. P., Garner, A. S., et al. (2012). The lifelong effect of early childhood adversity and toxic stress, Technical report, *Pediatrics*, http://intheloop.aap.org, pp. 233.

Vaillant, G. E. (2008, August). Mental health. *The American Journal of Psychiatry, 160*(8), 1373–1384.

Winch, P. (1964, October). Understanding a primitive society. *American Philosophical Quarterly, 1*(4), 307–324.

Wittgenstein, L. (1953). *Philosophical investigation*. Oxford: Blackwell.

# Depression as a Problem of Labor: Japanese Debates About Work, Stress, and a New Therapeutic Ethos

**Junko Kitanaka**

**Abstract** The global rise of depression is often linked to the spread of neoliberalism, which urges workers to constantly design and (re)make themselves in order to advance their careers through their ever-widening social networks. Depression can be read as both the pathological breakdown of this self-production and an adaptive response against the increasing demand for affective communication. The fundamentally social nature of depression has been heatedly debated in Japan, where, since the 1990s, it has surfaced as a "national disease" that disrupts the workplace. Many workers are said to have become depressed as a result of their traditional work ethic, notable for its loyalty and diligence, which is less valued in a neoliberal economy. Using this argument, a workers' movement has successfully established depression as an illness of work stress, thereby winning economic compensation and long-term sick leave for afflicted workers. Yet, this radical reconceptualization of depression as socially produced has also created an impetus to collectively manage workers' mental health, with the government's much-disputed plan to impose "stress checks" on all workers in order to screen out the vulnerable. The emerging psychiatric science of work also questions the traditional clinical approach to depression that emphasizes "natural" recovery through rest; instead, it is cultivating modes of restoring health in ways that render workers more efficient and productive for business. This paper examines Japanese debates about the nature of workers' psychopathology, their vulnerabilities, and their recovery – or even their potential for further transformation – against the backdrop of the new therapeutic ethos.

## Depression as a Problem of Labor

In a teachers' strike in Chicago in 2012, American workers debated whether they should join a "wellness plan" that would enable employers to observe and intervene in the realm of workers' physical health (Finamore 2012). In Japan, where workers

J. Kitanaka, Ph.D. (✉)
Department of Human Sciences, Faculty of Letters, Keio University, Tokyo, Japan
e-mail: kitanaka@flet.kcio.ac.jp

© Springer Science+Business Media Dordrecht 2016
J.C. Wakefield, S. Demazeux (eds.), *Sadness or Depression?*
History, Philosophy and Theory of the Life Sciences 15,
DOI 10.1007/978-94-017-7423-9_5

have long accepted annual physical health checks as a routine matter, they are now debating who has the right to intervene into workers' *mental* health. This question has become imminent over the last decade, as Japan has witnessed an "epidemic" of depression (with its patient number exceeding a million) and a surge in national suicide rate (hitting historical highs of more than 30,000 per year for fourteen consecutive years), both of which are seen as related to the long-lasting recession (Cabinet Office 2014). Depression, which has been labeled by the World Health Organization as an important part of the "global burden of disease" impeding productivity (WHO 2002), seems to be afflicting Japanese workers on a massive scale. As many in Japan are said to have become depressed and even suicidal from excessive work stress, the government recently announced a plan to introduce stress checks on all workers across the nation (Asahi 2010). This has stirred up heated opposition from workers, psychiatrists, and occupational doctors (Asahi 2014), many of whom argue that such a move is an insidious form of psychiatric surveillance and a sign of the neoliberal order that puts a new demand of responsibility on individuals for their own health.

What is ironic about this national call for stress checks, however, is that it is partly a product of a hugely successful workers' movement. Since the 1990s, left-wing lawyers, doctors, workers, and their families have been engaged in legal battles concerning what they call "overwork suicide" and "overwork depression", whereby workers have allegedly been driven to depression and/or suicide from excessive work stress (Kawahito 1998). With the 2000 Supreme Court verdict that held a company liable for a worker's suicide and ordered the highest amount of compensation ever paid for a worker's death in Japan, the government has begun to discuss mental health as a matter of social responsibility (Kuroki 2002). This is a significant change, as depression had long been regarded in Japan as a constitutionally determined, biological disease, and, moreover, a private matter. Recognizing how excessive fatigue, stress, and sleep deprivation can destroy a healthy mind, the government has created Stress Evaluation Tables, which lists 31 typically stressful work events, including demotion, relocation, and harassment, along with standardized scores, to aid Labor Standards Offices to objectively measure workers' stress levels and provide worker's compensation for stress-induced psychopathology (Okamura 2002). Reconceptualizing the workplace as a potential psychological minefield, the government has also begun to implement other policy changes, including the revision of the Labor Safety Law and the creation of the Suicide Prevention Law, thereby acknowledging the responsibility of the state and corporations for keeping workers mentally healthy (Asahi 2005; Kōsei Rōdōshō 2001). In this context, the government's latest call for stress checks might even seem like an inevitable evolution of its Durkheimian stance, which regards psychiatric breakdown and the increased number of suicides as a product of society.

Yet, the government's stance is also conflicted, insofar as it encompasses two perspectives on depression as a problem of labor – that is, as an impediment to work and a product of work itself. This also points to the inherent tension in today's global discourse about depression, that is, as an illness of productivity in the way it involves competing politics of causality (cf. Young 1995; Martin 2007). The first perspective sees depression mainly as a biological anomaly, to be detected and located within the individual, who then becomes primarily responsible for ensuring his or her own mental health. The second regards depression as a kind of normal response to a pathogenic work environment, for which the employer and the government become accountable. While the lawyers and doctors in Japan involved in the workers' movement concerning suicides related to workplace-induced stress and depression are strongly committed to the latter perspective, they have also grappled with the fact that suicide, at its core, is an agentive act, and they realize they cannot completely disregard the role that workers – including their subjectivity – play in the development of depression (Okamura 2002). Particularly in cases where workers appear as if they have driven themselves to pathogenic overwork, those involved in the movement have had to ask about workers' agency and their self-subjugation – that is, how they become complicit in structuring a pathogenic situation (Kawahito 1998). As such concerns are increasingly voiced in Japan by those outside the worker's movement, I want to examine what political consequences are brought about by the understanding of depression as a problem of labor. More specifically, I want to explore how the shift in the conceptualization of depression from a "private matter" to a "public illness" has come to make individual workers responsible for both their physical and psychological health, thereby recreating the realm of the psychological as a new object of self-governance and public surveillance.[1]

## A Brief History of Depression as an Illness of Fatigue

While the legal conceptualization of depression as an illness of labor is a product of the recent workers' movement, Japanese psychiatrists have long explored the link between work, fatigue, and depression. Fatigue had initially emerged as an important object of investigation for nineteenth century European scholars of the "science of work", who saw it as an indication of the utmost limits of production (Rabinbach 1990). While some of these scholars searched for ways to cultivate "bodies without fatigue," other, more socially oriented scholars began to examine fatigue as an innate defense mechanism that would protect people "against the danger of a work pursued to the extreme" (Rabinbach 1990, 141). Joining this line of inquiry at the turn of the twentieth century, Japanese psychiatrists also scrutinized illnesses of

---

[1] My analysis of the rise of depression in Japan is based upon anthropological research that stretches from 1998 to 2012, a period that covers before and after the onset of the medicalization. This included two years of intensive ethnographic fieldwork conducted at three psychiatric institutions, observing the proceedings of several overwork death/overwork suicide court cases at the Tokyo District Court, and attending conferences and a series of study groups held by the lawyers and psychiatrists involved in such cases. For archival research, I examined the *Japanese Journal of Psychiatry and Neurology* from its first issue in 1902 to the present as well as a number of popular journals and a few of national newspapers from the 1870s to the 2000s. I also used Japanese legal journals such as *Jurist* and *Hanrei Times* in order to investigate the legal discourses regarding overwork depression and overwork suicide.

fatigue such as neurasthenia, which was said to be affecting elites at the forefront of modernity. As neurasthenia became discredited as a legitimate disease category and came to be seen as a sign of psychological weakness, some Japanese psychiatrists turned their attention to investigating depression, which they regarded as a *real* biological disease, affecting, in particular, hardworking men in their prime years (Kitanaka 2008). Prominent psychiatrist Mitsuzō Shimoda elaborated on how these people – who exhibited a strong sense of responsibility, diligence, and thorough- ness – seemed constitutionally unable to sense their fatigue and pushed themselves beyond their limits, only to collapse at the height of exhaustion. In his view, depres- sion functions like an internal thermostat built into a machine that, when overheated, shuts down the system so as to protect itself. Thus depression, for Shimoda, is a "biological response for self-preservation", a protective mechanism of adaptation (Shimoda 1950, 2; 1941). The depressed were thus conceptualized in terms of the body-as-machine and as a product of their inherent constitution, with little agency or power to enact personal change.

While this early twentieth century theory of depression as an illness of fatigue had a strong flavor of biological determinism, later Japanese theorists – many of whom were influenced by the vehement antipsychiatry movement from the 1960s – began to offer an alternative interpretation. As they witnessed the discovery of anti- depressants and a surge in the number of depressed persons in the community, they began to ask why so many seemingly normal, even "ideal" workers were suddenly driven to this affliction. Recalling how Shimoda observed the depressed to be responsible, diligent, and thorough workers, these theorists argued that such a "pre- morbid melancholic personality" is not only an inborn constitution but also a latent product of Japanese socialization. This would explain why there seemed to be an increase in the number of people with depression at a time of social change, when these people's core values were no longer as appreciated as before, as the changing structure of the workplace might have turned their inflexible diligence and blind loyalty into something maladaptive, or even self-destructive (Hirasawa 1966; Iida 1974). Thus, relocating its cause from biology to psychology and from individual to society, these psychiatrists portrayed depression as an illness of labor and pathologi- cal of Japanese work ethic (Nakai 1976). Their argument was later adopted by law- yers and doctors involved in litigation regarding overwork suicide, through which they have done much to reconceptualize psychiatric vulnerability from something inherent, static, and biological to something historical, malleable, and social.

This reconceptualization of depression also raised questions about what psychia- trists can do to cure socially pervasive, *collective* vulnerability. Given that the aim of clinical practice is not to voice social critiques but to provide a remedy for the dis- ruptions in individuals' lives, psychiatrists began to ask how they should direct patients' awareness about the nature of their affliction. Seeing how antidepressants alone did not seem to entirely cure depression, some psychiatrists in the 1970s turned to psychotherapy in order to encourage patients to reflect on the social roots of their depression and the nature of their self-subjugation (see Hirose 1979). This was an exceptionally experimental time in Japanese psychiatry, given that Freudian psychoanalysis – though introduced in 1912 – had never taken root in this country, and most forms of psychological intervention had generally been "viewed with deep suspicion" (Lock 1980, 258). Perhaps it is not surprising, then, that these psychiatrists soon began to observe, in their clinical practice, that not only was such introspection often too threatening for patients but that it left them "worse off" than before (Iida 1978). Criticizing this as a form of "iatrogenesis" – an illness of doctors' own making (Iida 1978; Yoshimatsu 1987) – and suggesting how this form of confessional technology might be too alien, destabilizing, and even intrusive for many Japanese patients (cf. Doi 1972; Kandabashi 1974/1988), prominent experts began to caution against intervening into the intimate realm of psychology. They emphasized how depressed persons tend to eventually recover, with medication and ample rest. Their recommended approach was instead to let patients disconnect from the pathogenic relations in the workplace, and to retreat into a space of their own inner freedom (Kasahara 1978, 1989; Yokoyama and Iida 1998). As they intentionally left the question of patients' agency unexplored, insight-inducing psychotherapy became a matter of interdiction for most Japanese psychiatrists for decades to come.

## Problematizing Workers' Psychology

In the current medicalization of depression, there has been a renewed interest in workers' psychology, a concern that has emerged from legal, governmental, industrial, and popular discourses. This was first articulated through legal disputes, particularly in the 2003 Toyota case involving the suicide of an employee who was, by all accounts, an ideal "Toyota Man". Emphasizing how this man's objective stress level (as indicated by the recorded hours of overtime) was not necessarily more than that of his peers, the defense argued that the worker's alleged depression was caused by his own vulnerability (i.e., melancholic premorbid personality), which they argued must have driven him to take on more tasks than he was able to accomplish. The plaintiff, while emphasizing how this man was respected for his good leadership and a strong sense of responsibility and was driven to suicide by impossible work demands, asserted that what should matter is not the "objective" level of stress but rather how the worker himself experienced the stress. The judges accepted the latter argument that it is not the *quantity* but rather the *quality* of work that should be considered. The judges even went so far as to declare that the standards for work conditions should not be set to accommodate the "average" worker – as the government's guidelines state – but rather to those who are "most vulnerable to stress" (that is, as long as their personalities remain within an acceptable range found among the workers doing the same kind of job and having a similar age and experience (Asahi 2003; Daily Yomiuri 2004). While this radical "subjectivist" stance, which challenged the government's approach, was reported as another "victory for the weak" (Asahi 2001), it may have also provoked the government's interest in the realm of workers' psychology.

The growing interest in workers' psychology has also come from industry, which is bound by the system of lifetime employment and thus faced with the high costs of depressed workers on extended sick leave. This concern has been shared by some psychiatrists and occupational doctors involved in the field of "psychiatric science of work," who, since the mid-2000s, have questioned the idea that initially made depression a common illness category in Japan – namely, that depression is an illness of fatigue and stress. Pointing out that there is in fact no definitive scientific evidence that demonstrates the causal link between stress and depression (see a systematic review by Fujino et al. 2006), they have emphasized instead how depression is a product of the interaction between the environment and individuals, and the fact that how individuals experience and interpret the stress plays an equally important role (e.g., Onishi and Kondō 2008). To further question the medico-legal discourse that had shifted responsibility from depressed persons by promoting a "blame-free self of the therapeutic model" (Douglas 1992, 230), these doctors have instead problematized workers' agency by redefining depression as not only a product of stress but also a form of risk that every worker is subjected to (see the report by Nihon Sangyō Seishin Hoken Gakkai or the Japan Society for Occupational Mental Health 2006). Depression, defined in this way, becomes something preventable by rational management both at collective and individual levels – an idea that is becoming more emblematic of the stance of the government and corporations as they search for effective means of dealing with the rapid increase in the number of depressed workers. Industry has also begun to find ways to assess and manage workers' recovery, not in terms of infinitely malleable and unpredictable *clinical time*, but rather in terms of standardized and more strictly controlled *industrial time* with the hope of more speedily restoring workers' health as well as productivity. As both personnel staff and workers are coming under increasing pressure to return the afflicted to a healthy state, they have to negotiate the ideals of clinical time that prioritizes a "natural' recovery and the demands of industrial time that constantly seeks, even for a therapeutic process, the principle of efficacy. The new demand for workers' individual "self care" has also served to blur the distinction between "private illness" – which is dealt with as a personal and family problem – and "public illness" (Nomura et al. 2003), calling for social responsibility as well as surveillance in Japan.

These legal, governmental, and industrial concerns have also resonated with the changing tone of the popular discourse about depression through the 2000s, when the initial hype around new antidepressants quickly waned and was replaced by a growing sense of disillusionment with psychiatric care (Yomiuri 2010). Particularly after the mid-2000s, the media began to problematize the rapidly growing number of depressed patients – many of whom seemed to be developing the problem chronically, and remaining on sick leave, sometimes for years – as a social problem (e.g., NHK 2009). Critics of psychiatry (many of whom are themselves psychiatrists) pointed out how ambiguous a psychiatric diagnosis can be, and how lay people seemed all too willing to embrace a diagnosis of depression without fully realizing what physiological, psychological, social, and economic consequences it might bring (e.g., Kayama 2008). Indeed, social scientists have long debated the ill effects of being labeled as mentally ill, as well as the ways in which a socially stigmatized identity becomes internalized, even to the point of eroding a person's core sense of self (Becker 1960; Goffman 1963).

What the current medicalization of depression has brought seems even more complex: what Ian Hacking calls a "looping effect"; in this case, where the nature of "depression" is altered by the way people start to live as (and conform to the idea of) "depressed patients". As they do so, these people's lives also evolve in ways that alter the classifications, descriptions, and experiences of "depression" itself (Hacking 1999). For instance, some of the depressed persons I met in Tokyo in 2008 and 2009 had been diagnosed as "depressed" and given antidepressants by doctors who likely would have been more cautious with such a diagnosis 10 years prior. Despite the fact that some of these patients initially felt uncertain about the diagnosis, they continued to take antidepressants, even when they felt the pills were not helping, but rather aggravating, their condition. Remaining uncured and homebound, some of them eventually became part of the growing number of "intractable" patients, for whom a traditional treatment of antidepressants and ample rest was apparently ineffective. As psychiatrists were confronted with these "new types" of patients (or what Hacking would call "moving targets": Hacking 1999), they began to discuss the limits of conceptualizing depressed patients as mere victims of biological and social forces, and to increasingly problematize patients' psychology.

## A New Therapeutic Ethos

While most psychiatrists have remained hesitant to get involved beyond prescribing antidepressants, in part because they know that past psychotherapeutic attempts with the depressed have a bad track record, others, who work more closely with industry, have begun to criticize the traditional psychiatric approaches. Arguing how the traditional rest cure, which often results in long-term sick leave, may have adverse effects on patients and emphasizing that the "workplace is no place for rehabilitation" (Onishi and Kondō 2008), they have devised a more aggressive treatment program called Rework, which rapidly is becoming, in many companies, a prerequisite for depressed persons to return to work (Utsubyō Riwaku Kenkyukai 2009). In contrast to the legal conceptualization of depressed persons as passive victims, driven to depression by stressful social relations, Rework borrows from cognitive therapy and re-defines patients as active agents who drove themselves to depression through distorted interpretations of stressful social relations. For instance, at a leading center of Rework in Tokyo, patients are first urged to manage their depression by closely keeping track of their bio-rhythms and affective changes. Second, they are placed with other patients in a mock-office environment and given communal tasks in order to analyze and correct the patterns of their miscommunication and distorted cognition. Third, patients are re-trained in affective labor through group therapy, where they are encouraged to try alternative communication skills and learn how to control their emotions. Through these daily activities, therapists carefully control the level of stress that patients are exposed to, and they gradually increase its level to see how much stronger and healthier patients have become. They also closely monitor the patients' biological, cognitive, and affective changes in order to decide when patients are ready to return to their own workplace (Utsubyō Riwaku Kenkyukai 2009, 2011).

As Rework urges patients to heal themselves by being re-immersed in the thick of social relations, it clearly departs from the traditional psychiatric approach that emphasizes therapeutic isolation. Particularly in the way it tries to get inside the patients' minds and reshape them as more productive workers, Rework might also be accused of operating as a "factory of correction" (cf. Scull 1979) that seeks to instill a new form of self-governance. Such accusations are rarely heard, however, even among leftwing doctors involved in the workers' movement. This is partly because psychiatrists have been pressed to respond to growing criticism of therapeutic ineffectiveness, and to adopt a seemingly scientific, managerial program to restore workers' health. But more importantly, it may also be a result of Rework beginning to serve as a place for patients to voice their dissent. As a medical anthropologist, I conducted interviews with patients and doctors in 2000–2003 and 2008–2009, and found that, despite Rework's explicit emphasis on distorted cognition, the numerous testimonies of illness-inducing workplaces across industries that both therapists and patients encounter serve to undermine the assumption that the problem mainly lies with individual workers. With its own introspective technology turned on its head, Rework's therapeutic aim is constantly destabilized by those who ask what may lie beneath what appears to be socially induced vulnerability.

In the process, Rework seems to provide patients with an opportunity to critically examine the nature of their self-subjugation and ask if their relentless pursuit of personal advancement through the current system is really the way to pursue happiness. In fact, some of their reflections seem to parallel the narratives of depressed workers I met in a self-help depression group during 2000–2003, many of who told me how they had reached, through bitter struggles with depression, a sense of liberation in embracing their vulnerabilities, reexamining their worldly obsessions, and relinquishing their desire to be in control. Yet, a key difference is also apparent, as patients today no longer seem able to afford the kind of quiet resignation and detachment that their older counterparts had chosen as a cure for depression; they know all too well that lifetime employment is crumbling, and that social security, as indicated by the quickly eroding pension and the national health insurance systems, is disappearing from under their feet. In order to escape unemployment, they need to learn to mask their vulnerabilities and appear resilient to stress. Thus, while Rework does not impose on workers a set of ethics one might follow and limits itself in offering workers a set of standardized skills with which to protect themselves, it does seem to cultivate in them a belief in *resilience* as a new kind of morality – even if it is not at all clear what sense of personal fulfillment, if any, that could ultimately bring.

## Changing Forms of Self-Governance

The call for collective and individual management of mental health in Japan suggests changing demands for self-governance. The rising interest in the psychological realm has been cited as a hallmark of modernity (Rieff 1966; Giddens 1991) and a sign of the changing nature of political surveillance and possible forms that agency can take in contemporary society (Marcuse 1970; Foucault 1975; Rose 1996). This has been particularly pertinent to societies like the United States, where psychoanalysis had a strong influence over the course of the twentieth century, and where organizations like the National Institute of Mental Health (NIMH) have done much to promote public awareness of psychological health. The rise of Prozac from the 1990s – portrayed as a "happy pill" that would not only cure depression but also transform people's personality – was widely seen to be putting an end to the dominance of the psychological. Liberating the meaning of the "biological" in psychiatry from its old connotation of genetic determinism and instead presenting it as something infinitely flexible and malleable, Prozac seemed to displace the psychological from its previous role (see Elliott and Chambers 2004). While some critics have pointed out how the Prozac narrative insidiously promotes an idealized image of the neoliberal worker as self-directed, flexible, and productive, its attraction certainly lay in its celebration of individual autonomy, self-enhancement, infinite growth, and possibilities of transcending nature by means of neurobiological technology (Elliott 2003). Thus helping redefine the biological as the new location of agency, the Prozac discourse of the 1990s offered a new vision of biological self-governance.

Yet, despite the concern that the Prozac narrative is sweeping the globe, instilling a single vision of the "neurochemical self" fit for the new economic order, global medicalization has instead emerged as a fertile ground for local critiques against the imposition of a homogenizing view of personhood (Rose 2007; Metzl 2003; Ecks 2005; Kitanaka 2012). In this regard, it is notable how the Japanese discourse about depression as a work hazard is quickly becoming a part of the global reality as other nations have begun to suffer the same kind of stagnating recession that Japan has been affected by for the last few decades. For instance, in France, where Japanese cases of overwork death were once discussed with a sense of curiosity (Brice 1999), there have been growing reports of suicides among employees of France Telecom, attributed to the stress they were under due to the company's radical restructuring (BBC News, September 12, 2009). Rising rates of suicide and psychopathology in the workplace have raised public concern elsewhere in Europe – particularly in Germany, Italy, and Finland – where these are often discussed as products of the increasing pressure people face in the new economic order (e.g., Mole 2010). Like their Japanese counterparts, European commentators tend to emphasize how typical victims are not "deviants" but people who have led well-adjusted lives, and that their pathologies should not be explained away by their individual biological/psychological weakness but rather interpreted, a la Durkheim, as social problems, even forms of social protest (Moerland 2009). By linking depression to the "socials ills" brought on by neoliberalization –including the perils of privatization, the collapse of lifetime employment, and the crisis in national health care – people seem to be addressing their sense of alienation as real and concrete, as something that requires resolution through political intervention beyond Prozac. Yet, this conceptualization of depression as an illness of labor has already produced inconsistent effects in Japan, where workers' calls for social restructuring seem to have invited a national call for restructuring – even reprogramming[2] – of workers themselves. They are now expected to not only overcome depression but also to transcend their former selves, to become resilient.

Resilience has become a dominant concept in the recent global mental health movement partly because of its seemingly "benign" connotation (Howell and Voronka 2012). Its appeal lies in the fact that it glamorizes the transcendental ability of the individual even as it serves to mask an underlying economic rationality or the fact that it has risen in the context of the "retrenchment of state services through neo-liberal restructuring and cost-cutting measures" (Howell and Voronka 2012, 1). These politics are clearly embodied in the emerging discourse about stress and resilience in post-9/11 America, where, as Allan Young has shown, the notion of resilience "as something to be achieved with the help of experts" has come to threaten "to displace effortless 'normality' as the default condition of human life" (Young 2012). At this historical moment, Japan's national call for stress checks might begin to seem not so much a preventative measure for depression and suicide *per se* as it is an ominous sign of a coming era of "positive mental health", with its infinitely expansive meanings and growing demands for bio-psychological self-governance.

**Note**  This study is supported by JSPS Grant-in-Aid for Scientific Research (No. 24300293). This chapter is based on additional empirical material and new theorizing of what was presented in my 2012 book *Depression in Japan: Psychiatric Cures for a Society in Distress* (Princeton University Press).

# References

*Asahi Shimbun*. (2001). *Shokuba no "jakusha" ni hikari, karō jisatsu ni rōsai nintei hanketsu* (Light on the "weak" in workplaces: workers' compensation granted in overwork suicide lawsuit). June 18.

*Asahi Shimbun*. (2003). *Rōsai nintei no handan shishin "gutaiteki ni", Toyota karō jisatsu Soshō* (The standard for determining workers' compensation "should be more concrete"): Toyota overwork lawsuit). July 9.

*Asahi Shimbun*. (2005). *Jisatsu Yobō e Sōgō Taisaku* (Comprehensive measures For preventing suicide). July 16.

*Asahi Shimbun*. (2010). *Seishin shikkan chōsa gimuka miokuri* (Mandatory mental health examination deferred). July 15.

*Asahi Shimbun*. (2014). *Utsubyō yoō kensa kibōshanomini kōrōshō hōkaiseian o shūsei* (Depression screening only for those who wish to have it, the Ministry of Health, Welfare and Labor revises its legislative proposal). March 6.

*BBC News*. (2009). *French unease at Telecome suicides*. September 12.

Becker, H. (1960). *Outsiders: Studies in the sociology of deviance*. New York: Free Press.

Brice, P. (1999). Au Japonpersonne ne respecte les limites legales. *Le Monde*. May 22.

Cabinet Office, the Government of Japan. (2014). *Jisatsu taisaku hakusho* (Suicide prevention white paper). http://www8.cao.go.jp/jisatsutaisaku/whitepaper/index-w.html, Accessed 8 July 2014.

---

[2] I owe this phrase to Ann Laura Stoler (2012).

*Daily Yomiuri.* (2004). *Worker's comp claim filed over Osaka judge's suicide.* March 30.

Doi, T. (1972). Bunretsubyō to himitsu (Schizophrenia and secrets). In T. Doi (Ed.), *Bunretsubyō no seishinbyōri* (The psychopathology of schizophrenia). Tokyo: Tokyo University Press.

Douglas, M. (1992). *Risk and blame: Essays in cultural theory.* London: Routledge.

Ecks, S. (2005). Pharmaceutical citizenship: Antidepressant marketing and the promise of demarginalization in India. *Anthropology and Medicine, 12*(3), 239–54.

Elliott, C. (2003). *Better than well: American medicine meets the American dream.* New York: W. W. Norton.

Elliott, C., & Chambers, T. (2004). *Prozac as a way of life.* Chapel Hill: University of North Carolina Press.

Finamore, C. (2012). *Getting healthy at work: Who do you trust?* http://labornotes.org/2012/09/getting-healthy-work-who-do-you-trust. Accessed 11 Sept 2013.

Foucault, M. (1975). *The birth of the clinic: An archeology of medical perception.* New York: Vintage Books.

Fujino, Y., Horie, S., Hoshuyama, T., Tsutsui, T., & Tanaka, Y. (2006). Rōdōjikan to seishintekifutan tono kanren ni tsuite no taikeiteki bunken review (A systematic review of working hours and mental health burden. *Sangyo Eiseishigaku Zasshi* (Journal of Japan Society for Occupational Health), *48*, 87–97.

Giddens, A. (1991). *Modernity and self-identity: Self and society in the late modern age.* Cambridge: Polity Press.

Goffman, E. (1963). *Stigma: Notes on the management of spoiled identity.* Englewood Cliffs: Prentice-Hall.

Hacking, I. (1999). *The social construction of what?* Cambridge, MA: Harvard University Press.

Hirasawa, H. (1966). *Keishō utsubyō no rinshō to yogo* (Clinical practice and prognosis of mild depression). Tokyo: Igaku shoin.

Hirose, T. (1979). Utsubyō no seishin ryōhō (Psychotherapy for depression). *Rinshō Seishinigaku* (Clinical Psychiatry), *8*(11).

Howell, A., & Voronka, J. (2012). Introduction: The politics of resilience and recovery in mental health care. *Studies in Social Justice, 6*(1), 1–7.

Iida, S. (1974). Sōutsubyō (Manic depression). *Gendai no Esupuri* (L'esprit d'aujourd'hui), *88*, 5–15.

Iida, S. (1978). Utsubyō no seishinryōhō (Psychotherapy for depression). *Kikan Seishinryōhō* (Japanese Journal of Psychotherapy), *4* (2), 114–117.

Kandabashi, J. (1988/1974). "Himitsu" no yakuwari (The role of the "secret"). *Hassō no Kōseki* (Trajectory of thoughts). Iwasaki Gakujutsu Shuppansha.

Kasahara, Y. (1978). Utsubyō no shōseishinryōhō (Brief psychotherapy for depression). *Kikan Seishinryōhō* (Japanese Journal of Psychotherapy), *4*(2), 6–11.

Kasahara, Y. (1989). Utsubyō no seishinryōhō. In Y. Narita (Ed.), *Seishinryōhō no jissai* (Practice of psychotherapy). Tokyo: Shinkōigaku Shuppansha.

Kawahito, H. (1998). *Karō jisatsu* (Overwork suicide). Tokyo: Iwanami Shoten.

Kayama, R. (2008). *Watashi wa utsu" to iitagaru hitotachi* (People who like to say 'I'm depressed'). PHP Kenkyujo.

Kitanaka, J. (2008). Questioning the suicide of resolve: Disputes regarding 'overwork suicide' in 20th century Japan. In: J. Weaver & D. Wright (Eds.), *Histories of suicide: Perspectives on self-destruction in the modern world.* Toronto: University of Toronto Press.

Kitanaka, J. (2012). *Depression in Japan: Psychiatric cures for a society in distress.* Princeton: Princeton University Press.

Kōsei Rōdōshō (The Ministry of Health, Welfare, and Labor) (Ed.). (2001). *Kōsei Rōdō hakusho* (The white paper of the Ministry of Health, Welfare, and Labor). Tokyo: Gyōsei.

Kuroki, N. (2002). Jisatsu to seishin shikkan ni kansuru rōsai hoshō no dōkō (Recent trends in work-related compensation involving job-related suicide and mental disease). *Seishin Shinkeigaku Zasshi* (Psychiatria et Neurologia Japonica) *104*(12), 1215–1227.

Lock, M. (1980). *East Asian medicine in urban Japan.* Berkeley: University of California Press.

Marcuse, H. (1970). *Five lectures: Psychoanalysis, politics, and utopia.* Boston: Beacon Press.

Martin, E. (2007). *Bipolar expeditions: Mania and depression in American culture.* Princeton: Princeton University Press.

Metzl, J. (2003). *Prozac on the couch: Prescribing gender in the era of wonder drugs.* Durham: Duke University Press.

Moerland, R. (2009). In France, suicide can be a form of protest. *NRC Handelsblad.* October 9, 2009.

Mole, N. (2010). *Labor disorders in neoliberal Italy: Mobbing, well-being, and the workplace.* Bloomington: Indiana University Press.

NHK. (2009). *NHK Supesharu: Utsubyō chiryō jōshiki ga kawaru* (NHK Special: Changing the beliefs about depression treatment). Tokyo: Takarajimasha.

Nakai, H. (1976). Saiken no rinri to shite no kinben to kufū (Deligence and innovation as an ethic of reconstruction). In Y. Kasahara (Ed.), *Sōutsubyō no seishinbyōri I (Psychopathology of manic depression I).* Tokyo: Kōbundō.

Nihon Sangyō Seishin Hoken Gakkai (Japan Society for Occupational Mental Health). (2006). "Karō jisatsu" o meguru Seishinigakujō no mondai ni kakawaru kenkai (Views on psychiatric problems concerning "overwork suicide"). http://mhl.or.jp/kenkai.pdf. Accessed 8 July 2014.

Nomura, Y., Kinomoto, N., Hiranuma, T., Sugita, M., Kuroki, N., Katō, M., Itō, F., Kodama, Y., & Ōno, Y. (2003). Karōshi to kigyō no songai baishō sekinin: Dentsū karōshi jisatsu jiken (Overwork death and corporate liability: Dentsu overwork suicide case). *Baishō Kagaku* (Journal of Compensation Science), *30*, 115–36.

Okamura, C. (2002). *Karōshi karōjisatsu kyūsai no riron to jitsumu* (Theory and practice of providing relief to overwork death and overwork suicide). Tokyo: Junpōsha.

Onishi, M., & Kondō, N. (2008). Shokuba de no mentaru herusu katsudō o "shikaru" (Scolding the mental health activities in the workplace). *Kokoro no Kagaku* (Science of the Mind), *142*, 123–126.

Rabinbach, A. (1990). *The human motor: Energy, fatigue, and the origins of modernity.* New York: Basic Books, Harper Collins.

Rieff, P. (1966). *The triumph of the therapeutic.* Chicago: University of Chicago Press.

Rose, N. (1996). *Inventing our selves: Psychology, power, and personhood.* Cambridge: Cambridge University Press.

Rose, N. (2007). *The politics of life itself: Biomedicine, power, and subjectivity in the twenty-first century.* Princeton: Princeton University Press.

Scull, A. T. (1979). *Museums of madness: The social organization of insanity in nineteenth-century England.* London: Allen Lane.

Shimoda, M. (1941). Sōutsubyō no byōzen seikaku ni tsuite (On premorbid personality of the manic depressive). *Seishin Shinkeigaku Zasshi (Psychiatria et Neurologia Japonica), 45*, 101.

Shimoda, M. (1950). Sōutsubyō ni tsuite (On manic depression). *Yonago igaku zasshi* (Yonago Medical Journal), *2*(1), 3–4.

Stoler, A. L. (2012). Commentary on Kitanaka's paper titled Isolating the vulnerable: National debates about workers' depression in recession-plagued Japan on the panel on Refusal of Relation, Organized by Lucas Bessire and David Bond. In American Anthropological Association Annual Meeting, San Francisco, November 16.

Utsubyō Riwaku kenkyukai. (2009). *Utsubyō Riwaku puroguramu no hajimekata* (How to start Rework program for depression). Tokyo: Kōbundō

Utsubyō Riwaku kenkyukai. (2011). *Utsubyō Riwaku puroguramu no tsuzukekata* (How to continue Rework program for depression). Tokyo:Nanzandō.

World Health Organization. (2002). *World Health Report 2002. Reducing risks, promoting healthy life.* Geneva: WHO.

Yokoyama, T., & Iida, S. (1998). Utsubyō no seishin ryōhō (Psychotherapy for depression). *Seishinka chiryōgaku* (Journal of Psychiatric Treatment), *13*(Suppl), 87–92.

*Yomiuri Shimbun*. (2010). "Utsu hyakumannin" kage ni shinyaku? Hanbaidaka to kanjasū hirei (New medication behind "One million people in depression"? Ratio of sales to number of patients). January 6.

Yoshimatsu, K. (1987). *Isha to kanja* (Doctors and patients). Tokyo: Iwanami Shoten.

Young, A. (1995). *The harmony of illusions: Inventing post-traumatic stress disorder*. Princeton: Princeton University Press.

Young, A. (2012). *Keynote presentation: Stress, cultural psychiatry, and resilience in the 21st century*. In Annual meetings of the Japanese Society for Transcultural Psychiatry, Fukuoka, Japan. June, 23.

# Darwinian Blues: Evolutionary Psychiatry and Depression

Luc Faucher

**Abstract** Psychiatry is in disarray. Case in point: psychiatry's primary classification manual has been under attack almost since the nosological revolution initiated by the DSM-III. The latest version – the DSM-5 – was not even published when criticism of it began. From many corners of psychiatry, voices were heard that urged a reclassification of mental disorders based on research in neuroscience and genetics as a solution to psychiatry's current situation. A radically different solution has been proposed to 'cure' the DSM of its alleged ailments: to build (or rebuild) it based on an evolutionary understanding of disorders. Indeed, advocates of evolutionary psychiatry believe that psychiatry could benefit from the adoption of an evolutionary perspective by providing a new understanding of specific mental illnesses such as schizophrenia, phobia, autism, etc. In this paper, I will focus my attention on two recent explanations of depression that adopt an evolutionary-style: Nesse's, and Andrews and Thomson's. In this paper, I will present their respective positions in regards to depression. I will then present some reasons as to why one should remain unconvinced by these explanations of depression.

## Introduction

Psychiatry is in disarray, and things seem unlikely to change anytime soon. Case in point: psychiatry's primary classification manual has been under attack almost since the nosological revolution initiated by the DSM-III (see McReynolds 1979; for overviews of some problems affecting various DSM editions, see Cooper 2004; Galatzer-Levy and Galatzer-Levy 2007; Kirk and Kutchins 1992; Mayes and Horwitz 2005; Tsou 2011). The latest version – the DSM-5 – had not even been published when criticism began, accusing the new manual of either not departing radically enough from earlier versions (Frances 2009; Frances and Widiger 2012) or (and possibly as well as) for a lack of empirical support for some of its reforms (Widiger 2011). Worst of all, the National Institute for Mental Health (NIMH) seems

L. Faucher (✉)
Département de philosophie, Université du Québec à Montréal, Montreal, QC, Canada
e-mail: faucher.luc@uqam.ca

© Springer Science+Business Media Dordrecht 2016          69
J.C. Wakefield, S. Demazeux (eds.), *Sadness or Depression?*
History, Philosophy and Theory of the Life Sciences 15,
DOI 10.1007/978-94-017-7423-9_6

to have completely lost faith in the DSM, launching an initiative called the Research Domain Criteria (RDoC), whose goal is to propose a reclassification of mental disorders based on research in neuroscience and genetics (Insel et al. 2010; Morris and Cuthbert 2012). As Steven Hyman puts it: "It now appears that the accreting failures of the current diagnostic system cannot be addressed simply by revising individual criterion sets and certainly not by adding more disorders to DSM-5" (2010, 3).

A radically different solution has been proposed to 'cure' the DSM of its alleged ailments: to build (or rebuild) it based on an evolutionary understanding of disorders (Nesse and Jackson 2011; Nesse and Stein 2012). From the end of the 1970s on, as Nesse and his colleagues observed, a 'medical model' has dominated psychiatry. As one leading advocate of this model put it, psychiatry has placed "the brain and its structure and functions in health and illness at the center of interest and study" (Guze 1992, 54). As a result of this model's adoption (or at least, of an interpretation of it; see Murphy 2009), psychiatry has turned to molecular and cellular neurosciences (Kandel 1998; Akil et al. 2010) or cognitive neurosciences (Andreasen 1997) as the "basic sciences" from which explanations (and category validation) of disorders can be expected (the RDoC initiative is the latest expression of the belief in this model). However, by focusing almost exclusively on the abnormality of brain structures, it is argued that psychiatry has relied on a "crude medical model" of mental disorders (Nesse and Williams 1995, 22), and has neglected to understand the functions of the diverse cognitive components that comprise our minds. As many observers of psychiatry have noted (see Widiger and Sankis 2000; Murphy 2006), psychiatry lacks an explicit (and scientific) image of what constitutes the normal functioning of the mind. Such an image is crucial for the establishment of diagnoses, and psychiatry without it is somewhat blind. According to Nesse and Williams, by providing a framework within which to understand the normal functions of the mechanisms of the mind, the adoption of an evolutionary approach "... would bring the study of mental disorders back to the fold of medicine ..." (idem, p. 22; see also Nesse and Stein 2012, 3). For this reason, evolutionary biology should also be considered as "*an essential basic science* for understanding mental disorders" (Nesse 2005, 903; my emphasis). This is not to say that genetics and cognitive neurosciences should be tossed away, but that they should be incorporated into a larger framework, which includes evolutionary theories. As Nesse put it recently in a paper about depression, "Neuroscience is not enough, evolution is essential" (2009).

What would psychiatry specifically gain by adopting an evolutionary framework? It would gain at least two things, according to the supporters of this approach.

Firstly, considering cognition and affect as being the result of evolutionary processes should prove helpful in both defining and providing an enriched general taxonomy to categorize mental disorders. For instance, Nesse (2002) posits that one of the most useful contributions of an evolutionary approach is the emphasis on the distinction between defects or disorders and "evolved defenses". According to Nesse, cases of evolved defenses are sometimes confused with dysfunctions because they cause pain or discomfort (what he refers to as "the DSM fallacy" [Nesse and Jackson 2011, 182] because the DSM ignores so blatantly this distinction). As will be seen in the next few sections of this paper, some behaviors and mental states that cause pain or discomfort to ourselves or others, and for which help is sought (such as depression), can indeed be normal forms of defensive responses to certain types of situations that reduce our reproductive fitness. In other words, pain and discomfort are not good cues of what is dysfunctional and what is not.

Other cases of fully functional mechanisms that are misconceived as defective by psychiatrists are those where the mechanism has to perform its function in an environment that is completely or radically different from the one in which it has been selected to work. In particular, this is the case in new environments where the cues that previously indicated fitness benefits no longer indicate them. One example of such an "environmental mismatch" is drug addiction in which an artificial substance triggers responses that are usually activated by fitness-related stimuli: like food, sex, etc. (Nesse and Berrige 1997).

The concepts of "evolved defense" and "environmental mismatch" are just two examples of theoretical benefits that could be gained by adopting an evolutionary perspective in relation to mental disorders. Another example of such a benefit is the explanation of the persistence of certain disorders through the invocation of evolutionary phenomena like pleiotropy or polygenic mutation-selection balance (see Keller and Miller 2006).

Secondly, advocates of evolutionary psychiatry believe that psychiatry could benefit from the adoption of an evolutionary perspective by providing a new understanding of specific mental illnesses such as schizophrenia, phobia, autism, etc. (see Burns 2004; Mineka and Öhman 2002; Ploeger and Galis 2011). From among this group of mental illnesses – as Kennair (2003) noted in a review of the field of evolutionary psychiatry – "[t]he disorder that has received most attention recently from an evolutionary perspective is depression: most of the key researchers within EPP [evolutionary psychopathology] are involved in the study of this disorder. Within the review period covered here, papers on depression stand out as most groundbreaking and probably provocative ..." (693). Though more than a decade has elapsed since Kennair's statement, I believe it remains accurate. In the past several years there has been a flurry of papers from some of the main advocates of evolutionary psychiatry as applied to depression (Allen and Badcock 2006; Andrews and Thomson 2009; Gilbert 2006; Hagen 2011; Keller and Nesse 2006; Nesse 2009; Nettle 2004; Price et al. 2007; Sloman 2008; Stein et al. 2006). These papers echoed a growing preoccupation in certain circles concerning the recent and sudden increase in the number of cases of depression in the general population. Indeed, many authors have questioned the ability of current diagnostic criteria as found in the DSM-5 to distinguish the normal from the abnormal, and consider this the source of the depressionepidemic (Horwitz 2011; Horwitz and Wakefield 2007; Mulder 2008; Parker 2005).[1] For instance, Mulder maintains that "[t]he DSM criteria define a heterogeneous group ranging from individuals whose symptoms are dysfunctional,

---

[1] The authors listed here have focused on DSM-IV and DSM–IV TR, but their point carries over to the new version of the DSM. Indeed, according to the APA website of the DSM-5 (www.dsm5.org) there is no notable changes in the core criterion symptoms or in the duration of major depression from DSM-IV to DSM-5. The only major change concerns the omission of the bereavement exclusion from the new version of the DSM. This change will only exacerbate the problem noticed by the authors aforementioned who would rather prefer the exclusion clause to be extended to other kinds of loss than eliminated (see for instance Wakefield et al. 2007; Wakefield and First 2012).

serious and ongoing to those whose symptoms are fleeting and related to social circumstances" (2008, 241). It is precisely the distinction between different groups that evolutionary psychiatry seeks to establish on firmer ground.

In what follows, I will focus my attention on two recent papers about depression that adopt an evolutionary-style explanation: Nesse (2009) "Explaining Depression: Neuroscience is Not Enough, Evolution is Essential" and Andrews and Thomson (2009) "The Bright Side of Being Blue: Depression as an Adaptation for Analysing Complex Problems". My reason for selecting these two papers is the following: despite sharing a common general framework (the evolutionary theory), evolutionary psychiatrists who attempt to explain depression can be divided by the positions they take about the adaptative character of depression, and about the evolved domain of mechanisms involved in depression. Nesse and Andrews and Thomson have differed on both accounts. Nesse considers major depression as the result of dysfunctional adaptive mechanisms, while Andrews and Thomson consider it to be an adaptative response to some varieties of problem.[2]Nesse considers the domain of depression (or of the adaptive mechanisms that break in depression) as general (it is a response to the loss of adaptative resources), while Andrews and Thomson consider the domain of depression as essentially social.

In what follows, I will present their respective positions with regards to depression (section "Evolutionary explanation of depression"). I will then (section "Remarks and problems with evolutionary models of depression") present some reasons as to why I am unconvinced by these explanations of depression.

## Evolutionary Explanation of Depression

As stated in the previous section, evolutionary explanations of depression can be divided along at least two axes: functionality and domain. Evolutionary psychiatrists interested in depression have explored all possible options following this delineation. Though I will briefly recount other positions, in this section I will focus on two particular ways to think about depression along those axes. The first holds that depression is a dysfunction and that it is the result of the malfunctioning of a mechanism that is non-essentially social in nature; the second holds that depression is functional and that its domain is essentially social.

---

[2] In a brief, general-public oriented presentation of their theory, they wrote: "We believe that depression is in fact an adaptation [...]" (Andrews and Thomson 2010, 57). Later in the same paper (as well as in a subsequent paper [2011]), they recognized that depression also exists as a disorder (2010, 61). For instance, they write: "In our article, we argued that while depressive disorder is probably over-diagnosed, it must exist because all body systems are susceptible to malfunctioning" (Andrews and Thomson 2011, 3). This concession would seem to collapse the distinction I am trying to draw with Nesse concerning the dysfunctional aspect of depression. If such was Andrews and Thomson's position after all, it would differ from Nesse's only by the kind of problems depression is designed to deal with. But even if this was the case, the two theories still are different enough in their content to justify to study them both in this paper.

## *Nesse: Low Mood and Depression*

In his "Explaining Depression: Neuroscience is not Enough, Evolution is Essential" (2009), Nesse argues that "… serious depression*is not an adaptation* shaped by natural selection. It has *no evolutionary explanation*. However, we do need an evolutionary explanation for why natural selection left us so vulnerable to a disease as common and devastating as depression. Some abnormal depression is related to normal low mood, so explaining the origins and functions of mood is an essential foundation for understanding depression…" (my emphasis; 21). Thus, an evolutionary perspective does not commit one to assuming that depression is an adaptation; in this case, it instead highlights the necessity of explaining why we are vulnerable to it. It grounds this explanation in the dysfunction of an otherwise functional mechanism, a mechanism in charge of what Nesse calls "low mood". Since low mood is crucial to the explanation of depression, let's say a few words about it.

Nesse's theory of mood is based on a functional theory of moods and emotions (for a statement of his position, see Nesse 1990; more recently Nesse 2006; Nesse and Ellsworth 2009). According to Nesse, emotions and moods are organized adaptative responses to recurrent problems in our ancestral environment.[3] Negative emotions and moods are responses to threatening or loss-type situations, or situations where costs and risks are greater than benefits. More precisely, low mood is elicited by cues indicating loss of resources of adaptative significance: "The losses that cause sadness are losses of reproductive resources […] A loss signals that you may have been doing something maladaptive" (Nesse and Williams 1997, 9). Reproductive resources could be "somatic" (personal health, attractiveness and ability, and material resources), "reproductive" (a mate or an offspring), or "social" (allies and status; Nesse 2009, 27). For example, low mood can be triggered by the sudden loss of a pension fund, parental death, a lost love following departure or rupture, a lost friendship, loss of social status, etc. The patterns of behavior and cognitive characteristics associated with low mood (prostration, lack of motivation, etc.) are consistent with the idea that it is a functional response to problematic features of the evolutionary environment. Following Klinger's (1975) seminal work, Nesse proposes that low mood functions in two stages: "When efforts to reach a goal are failing, low mood motivates pulling back to conserve resources and reconsider options. If conditions do not improve and no other strategy is viable, low mood disengages motivation from the unreachable goal so efforts can be turned to more productive activities. If the individual persists in pursuing an unreachable goal, ordinary negative affect can escalate into pathological depression" (2009, 23). Note that in this theory, low mood is not typically caused by stress or anxiety,[4] but by the inability to disengage from an unreachable goal (for instance, trying to find happiness in an unhealthy relationship). In other words, stress or anxiety is produced by the low-mood mechanism; it is not the cause of low mood.

---

[3] In this context, "[m]ood regulates patterns of resource investment as a function of propitiousness" (Nesse 2009, 24).

[4] Though Nesse sometimes mentions the fact that exposure to repeated episodes of stress might lower the threshold of low mood until it becomes pathological.

A few years ago, Nesse and Keller (Keller and Nesse 2005, 2006; see also Keller et al. 2007) have suggested that selection might have shaped different subtypes of depression to address different types of problems. This prediction was the result of the "situation-symptom congruence hypothesis", according to which symptoms should be adapted to deal with adaptative challenges characteristic of different types of situations. According to the studies that Nesse and Keller conducted, bereavement and romantic rupture would be associated with symptoms differing from those of chronic stress and failures (sadness, anhedonia, appetite loss and guilt in bereavement and fatigue and hypersomnia in romantic rupture).[5]

Now that we understand Nesse's hypothesis about low-mood, we can return to the issue of depression as such. According to Nesse, many cases of what is diagnosed as depression by the DSM are actually cases of low mood – that is, totally normal responses to a loss of resources, which are roughly the equivalent of pain responses to tissue damage. Pain is a defensive response, as is low mood. Pain becomes a pathology when the response is disproportionate to its cause, or when it appears without cause. Similarly, low mood becomes a pathology when it is disproportionate or without cause. In these cases, it indicates that something is wrong with the low mood mechanism.

One consequence of Nesse's position concerning low mood and depression – which I think will be received gladly by some clinicians – is that in order to be able to distinguish between the two, one will have to look past the symptoms (which might well be identical in the two cases) and the brain centers (which also might be identical in the two cases) and look instead at life circumstances and judge if the patient's response is appropriate or proportional as it relates to them. Thus, it means that clinicians should be attentive to context. This is in opposition to the DSM, where a diagnosis is completed only on the basis of the presence or absence of specific signs and symptoms. For instance, a diagnosis of major depression is given to a patient if they have five of nine symptoms for at least two weeks, independently of the context or the precipitating events that took place before the episode. For this reason, Nesse and Jackson argue "DSM-5 should incorporate life events and life situations into main diagnostic categories, where their role as elicitors of emotions will be clearer" (2011, 192). Such a reform (which was not retained by those who worked on DSM-5) would clearly lead to a decrease in diagnostic reliability due to the variability of interpretations of the appropriateness of reactions to circumstances, but according to Nesse et al, it would increase diagnostic validity by eliminating numerous false positives.

Finally, as mentioned earlier, the adoption of evolutionary perspectives is not only motivated by the new testable hypotheses that one can derive from them, but also by the possibility of explaining general vulnerability as well as individual vulnerability. At present, there is no accepted explanation of general vulnerability: Nesse mentions the possibility that we might live in a "depressogenic" world where

---

[5] Other subtypes might include seasonal affective disorder (SAD) which is a recurrent type of depression associated with the winter season, and that is characterized by fatigue, increased appetite, sleeping and carbohydrate craving.

goals are often time unrealistic, or that new physical factors like artificial light, lack of exercise, or changes of diet might influence the brain mechanisms responsible for depression (Nesse 2006, 2009). If this were the case, part of the explanation of the depression epidemic would be a mismatched environmental explanation where the low mood mechanism is activated overtime in the contemporary environment.[6] As for individual vulnerability, evolutionary explanations might refer to the fact that traits such as low mood tend to have a high variance between individuals, so much so that some individuals might be at the pathological extreme of the low-mood spectrum and thus more vulnerable to the development of depressive disorder. Research suggests that there is a genetic polymorphism on the 5-HTT gene that increases the risk of depression (Caspi et al. 2003). Though there is no current hypothesis concerning the possible benefits of having this variant of the 5-HTT gene, an evolutionary perspective suggests that there might be benefits linked to certain circumstances, thus motivating the research in that direction.

To summarize, this position states that the depression epidemic can be explained by the fact that the DSM cannot distinguish between low mood and dysfunctional depression. Low mood might be on the rise because of differences between ancestral environments and present environments, or it might be more frequent in certain individuals because of balanced selection. Real depression is thus less common than thought and is produced by a dysfunction of the low mood mechanism.

## Andrews and Thomson: Rumination and Motivation

In "The Bright Side of Feeling Blue" (2009), Andrews and Thomson proposed what they call a "social navigation hypothesis of depression". Their hypothesis belongs to a family of models that asserts the role of depression in social relationships as well as its functional nature. (I am not arguing here that every social theory of depression also advocates for an adaptative view of depression; see for instance Allen and Badcock 2006). Before turning to their model, we will quickly present some of the other models belonging to this family, which can assist in understanding Andrews and Thomson's highly original proposal.

### Previous Models of Depression as Strategy in Social Competition

The first model is the "social competition" or "social rank" theory of depression. Price et al. (1997) advocated this position, suggesting that depression is an "involuntary subordinate strategy" (sometimes also called "involuntary defeat strategy" [Sloman 2008] or "social defeat hypothesis" [Gilbert 2006]), which evolved from

---

[6] Note that it is unclear if this explains "real cases of depression" as opposed to what Nesse considers false-positives (i.e. low mood).

mechanisms mediating ranking behavior.[7] According to these authors, depression has three functions: (1) preventing a costly attempted 'come-back' of an individual whose defeat in a hierarchical struggle is inevitable; (2) sending a "no threat signal" to dominant individuals; (3) putting the individual in a defeated state which encourages the acceptance of an outcome. As Sloman puts it, depression "[...] is *exquisitely designed* to influence the individual to give up certain aspirations such as winning the affection of a possible mate, or to end a confrontation. It can lead to submission, the development of more realistic goals, and a redirection of energy towards more productive pursuits" (2008, 221; my emphasis). This hypothesis is supported by studies from Raleigh and McGuire who observed that in vervet monkeys, the highest-ranking males (alpha) had serotonin levels twice as high as other males. When an alpha male lost his position, his serotonin levels fell immediately and he huddled and rocked, refusing food – behaviors characteristic of depression in humans. They also found that, if the alpha male was removed from the rest of the group and a randomly chosen male was given anti-depressants, that individual male became the alpha male in every instance (see also, McGuire et al. 1997).

A second model of depression is the "bargaining model" proposed by Hagen (1999, 2002, 2003; Hagen and Barrett 2007). In this model, depression is seen as a sort of strike, i.e. a way for an individual to say that he or she no longer accepts the terms of a relationship, and that he or she demands better treatment. As Hagen puts it: "When simple defection from a costly cooperative venture is socially constrained because, for example, each participant has a monopoly on essential resources or can impose costs on defection, individuals suffering net costs from their participation may benefit by withholding the benefits they are providing until better terms are offered, that is, they may benefit by bargaining or 'going on strike'" (2002, 324).[8] Depression is seen essentially as an unconscious strategy to redress the loss of valuable social assets and elicit help or concern. This strategy works if it results in the modification of the "social environment" (increase in solicitous behavior or parental investment from those whom the strike targets, for instance). Just as some strikes might be disturbing and experienced negatively by those at whom they are targeted, depression might also be experienced negatively by those who are socially close to depressives (and met with indifference or less concern by those who are less close and thus less dependent on the resources they are 'deprived of' by the strike).

---

[7] Note that for advocates of this position, depression is not always adaptative (one wonders if these researchers should not have distinguished low mood from clinical depression, as Nesse has done). As Sloman recently stated: "In general, depression and anxiety are adaptative when they are switched off early before they become too intense. Because a mechanism that is proving ineffective in coping with agonistic conflict tends to become more entrenched which makes it more difficult to switch it off and the continued action of the mechanism may lead to a maladaptative cycle of escalating depression or anxiety" (2008, 222).

[8] In this model, psychic pain "should function to inform individuals that life circumstances ... are imposing a biological fitness cost, motivate individuals to cease activities contributing to the fitness cost, and condition them to avoid similar circumstances in the future" (Hagen and Barrett 2007, 24). Because of the role of psychic pain in depression, Hagen sometimes calls his theory an "evolutionary theory of psychic pain".

Hagen (1999, 2002) has tested his theory using postpartum depression (PPD) as a model for depression in general, which enabled him to make a number of specific predictions and test for them. Among them were: (1) individuals with no other children and few future chances to invest in offspring (those who have everything to lose) should have lower levels of PPD; (2) individuals who, for social reasons (social norms related to abortion, for instance), are forced to have unwanted children should experience higher levels of PPD (new costs are imposed on the individual who may want to renegotiate her current arrangement); (3) PPD in one spouse should be associated with increased parental childcare investment by the other spouse. According to Hagen, all these predictions were confirmed; additionally, there are preliminary indications that they might be valid cross-culturally (Hagen and Barrett 2007).

## Andrews and Thomson's Theory of Depression

Andrews and Thomson's theory has a resemblance to Hagen's; like the latter, they see depression as a type of strategy to extort increased investment from others. Their theory also tries to explain the *cognitive features* of depression, which Hagen's theory leaves unexplained (Watson and Andrews 2002, 3). Using both Andrews and Thomson's recent paper and Watson and Andrews' (2002) earlier statement of their position, I will present their explanation of these cognitive features, after which I will return to the social motivational features of depression.

According to Andrews and Thomson, depression is "an evolved stress response mechanism" (Andrews and Thomson 2009, 621). More precisely, its function is to address two classes of problem: social dilemmas and avoidable stressors.[9] The authors state that these problems are complex and must be dealt with in an analytical fashion, in that they have to be broken down in smaller pieces to be resolved.[10] Thus, if depression is designed to help solve these types of problem, it must "promote an analytical reasoning style in which greater attention is paid to detail and information is processed more slowly, methodically, thoroughly, and in smaller chunks" (idem, 622); this is exactly what most features of depression can be seen as doing.

According to these authors, the central designed feature of depression is rumination, which can be conceptualized as an analytical and methodological way of considering complex problems whose goal is to generate and evaluate possible solutions to these problems. This is consistent with studies that demonstrate that depressive thinking is more analytical in nature and focused on "regretful thoughts", i.e. under-

---

[9] Note that this is a move from Andrews' previous theory, in which he stated that "[t]he functional domain of depression may be social complexity" (Watson and Andrews 2002, 4), in that depression is now not only exclusively devoted to solving social problems. In their more recent paper, they assert: "complex social problems may be *the primary evolutionarily relevant trigger* of depression in human beings" (Andrews and Thomson 2009, 626; my emphasis).

[10] The authors suggest that their position implies the existence of a mechanism that distinguishes simple from complex problems (Andrews and Thomson 2009, 625). The way such a mechanism would work is not explained by them, nor is there any evidence that such a mechanism exists in non-human animals or in humans.

standing why an episode happened and what could had been done to prevent it (Andrews and Thomson call this 'upward counterfactual thinking'). Other features of depression should be understood in the same fashion, such as:

- The depressed tend to attribute more of their failures to their lack of ability and more of their successes to chance, while non-depressive individuals display the inverse pattern. Due to this, some cite a 'depressive attributional style' (Andrews and Thomson 2009, 636). This attributional style would help individuals focus on their possible shortcomings.
- "Depressed people may also seek information that helps them understand why avoidable problems occurred. For instance, relative to non-depressed people, depressed people prefer to interact with people who give them negative evaluations of their personalities. [...] Depressed people's preference for negative evaluations may be an important mechanism for gaining information that helps them understand why they are facing a problem and helps them identify what difficult behavioral changes they may need to make to solve it. Indeed, the depressed are more interested in negative evaluations because they are believed to be more accurate" (ibid.).
- Negative mood also seems to lead to more accurate decisions with regard to complex situations and to conservative implementation strategies for these decisions.
- In certain complex situations, depressed individuals are more competent than non-depressed individuals at estimating the control they exert over a situation (idem, 639).
- "... depressed people are more sensitive to costs of cooperating than non-depressed people and are more likely to defect when it is costly to cooperate" (idem, 634).
- The depressed are less prone to the fundamental attribution error. This error consists of inferring an actor's internal state despite the fact that this inference is not warranted (for instance, to infer that those who are asked in an experiment setting to write a paper defending evolutionary psychiatry really believe that evolutionary psychiatry is true or useful). Watson and Andrews (2002) assert that because the depressed are more socially dependent, they put more effort into making logically correct inferences about other people's beliefs or desires. In supporting this claim, they note that people make fewer errors when their own outcomes depend on being accurate, and that people in more interdependent societies commit this error less frequently.

The other features generally associated with depression (such as anhedonia and psychomotor changes, sleep and eating dysfunctions) are mechanisms that contribute to ensuring undisturbed rumination. For instance, anhedonia would assist rumination by rendering individuals indifferent to pleasures that could distract them from solving their problems. Preference for solitude (a psychomotor change) would allow the individual to avoid social contact that can be cognitively demanding. This account predicts a relationship between rumination and anhedonia such that a need for increased rumination should produce a more intense anhedonia. In the case of psychomotor changes, it predicts that if an environment is conducive to rumination, lethargy will work to keep the individual in that environment; but if the environment is not conducive to rumination, the individual will be motivated to seek out an environment that supports it (which can lead to agitation). This makes sense of the fact that depression can be characterized by psychomotor retardation or by agitation.

What makes their "analytical rumination hypothesis" (ARH; Andrews and Thomson 2009, 623) particularly interesting is the idea that since most cognitive resources are devoted to solving the complex problem(s) that triggered depression, there are none left for other unrelated tasks. This would explain the poor results of depressive individuals on laboratory tasks. Indeed, when distracted from thinking about their problems, depressives' performances on memory tasks or executive control tasks are similar to non-depressives, whether or not they are otherwise impaired. Contrary to what has been traditionally proposed on the basis of laboratory task results, a depressive individual's cognition is not dysfunctional. Rather, it is perfectly tailored to solving a specific kind of problem. For instance, analyzing problems requires the use of working memory (WM). Since depressive individuals consider their problems to be serious, all resources should be devoted to these problems. Thus, irrelevant tasks that would tap WM show poorer results. Yet these poorer results are not explained by a dysfunctional WM, but rather by the fact that this structure has limited resources and is impervious to disruptive conditions — in other words, it is "distraction resistant" (this state may be achieved through attention control structures, as suggested by increased activity in the left VLPFC in people suffering from depression).

So ARH makes four claims:

1. Complex problems (the primary evolutionarily relevant kinds being social) trigger a depressed affect;
2. Depression coordinates changes in body and brain systems that promote sustained analysis of the triggering problem;
3. Depressive rumination often helps people solve the triggering problem;
4. Depression reduces performance on laboratory tasks because depressive rumination takes up limited processing resources.

Let's now turn to the motivational aspect of depression. We have previously seen that authors such as Sloman, Gilbert and McGuire believe that the function of depression is to send a "no threat" message to social dominants. The function of this message is to reduce aggression towards the depressive individual. Andrews and Thomson make a different claim; consistent with Hagen's position, they claim that depression is used as a means to gather social support either by honestly signalling need[11] or by motivating fitness extortion (by demonstrating that one is ready to inflict

---

[11] In this framework, suicidality can be seen as adaptive: a way of signaling the seriousness of intent, or the individuals' level of need. As per Hagen: "Suicide threats are ... threats to impose substantial costs on group members and can be viewed as a means to signal cheaply and efficiently to a large social group that it may suffer such costs if assistance or change is not forthcoming" (2003, 112). Supporting the idea that suicidality is a form of gamble is the fact that most depressives warn others about their intentions, and frequently choose methods known to be unreliable: "Important for this hypothesis, most suicide attempts fail: globally, there are more than 14 attempts for every completion; for young adult US women, there are more than 100 attempts" (Hagen 2011, 722). As the editors of this volume pointed out to me, psychiatrists typically distinguish two situations: suicidality with a warning to others about suicidal intentions; and suicidality without warning to others. The second kind of situations results in successful suicide more often then the first

costs on themselves and others in order to gain additional support or a new social role). A prediction that follows from this model is that depression should end when support is gathered.[12] It also predicts that depression should generate more support from closer social partners than from distant ones, as one does not have the same bargaining leverage with people for whom you are not a resource. Finally, because of the two preceding predictions, it follows that depression should get more intense when one is removed from one's social milieu (for instance, by being hospitalized).

Since depression is conceived as an adaptation to solve a specific kind of problem, "… performance on the triggering problem [should be considered] as a crucial metric for evaluating depressive cognition. … the conclusion that depression impairs social skills depends on accepting the notion that some behaviors, such as friendliness and cooperation, are always better for social problem solving, regardless of the situation or context. A more direct definition of social competence is simply the ability to achieve social goals, especially in situations of social conflict." (Andrews and Thomson 2009, 637). In other words, what appear to be cognitive and social malfunctions because of its disvalued effects might actually be a functional way to achieve adaptative goals.

The previous theory has consequences for the way therapy should be conducted. Firstly, therapies whose effects are longer lasting should be those that encourage rumination and help to solve social dilemmas or stressful, complex problems. Secondly – this being corollary to the first remark – trying to bypass rumination via antidepressant medications (or otherwise) should not lead to long-lasting changes. Thirdly, isolating an individual from their social milieu risks the exacerbation of depressive symptoms.

Finally, in their paper, Andrews and Thomson do not provide an explanation of depression's prevalence, but in Watson and Andrews it is suggested that

> [t]oday's social environments differ from ancestral ones in ways that could affect the prevalence and intensity of depression. Modern social complexity and dynamism probably increases the context for ruminative and motivational depression, because people face an ever-changing array of fitness enhancing opportunities, but are blocked from or do not understand how to access them. Moreover, people tend to have a greater number of positive fitness partners in modern societies and this could increase the incidence of depression. At the same time, these partners become more replaceable and so the average fitness interest amongst them is lower. Reduced fitness interests amongst partners may increase the intensity of depression needed to motivate partners to help (2002, 2).

So depression is not dysfunctional, but the actual prevalence of depression is explained by the fact that we nowadays live in a more "depressogenic" environment (once again, it is a mismatch environment case).[13]

---

kind. Hagen's remarks are directed to the first kind of situations and he has nothing to say about the second one.

[12] "Recovery from depression is hastened by improvements in social relationships and strong social support." (Watson and Andrews 2002, 4).

[13] Hagen explains the biased sex-ratio of depression through the fact that women more often conflict with powerful others (2003, 115).

## Remarks and Problems with Evolutionary Models of Depression

In this section, I will comment on and formulate a few critiques about what has been written thus far. Before going any further, a word about how one should evaluate an evolutionary hypothesis. It seems to me that there are two constraints that such an explanation needs to meet:

1. If one considers a known trait as an adaptation, an evolutionary explanation should assess the central design features of that trait in light of its hypothesized function(s). That is, one should try to explain the multiple features of a given trait (at least its most central and costliest features) as complex and coordinated ways of dealing with a (set of) specific challenge(s) faced by our ancestors in their environment. If one can demonstrate that a trait has these complex and coordinated features and that in virtue of having them it can provide a solution to an adaptive problem this would be evidence (though a rather weak one) that one has identified an adaptation.[14]

2. An evolutionary explanation should be consistent with knowledge in other disciplines (in our case, with knowledge in psychology, neuroscience, ethology, etc.). That is, at minimum, it should not contradict established knowledge in other disciplines (in the event that it does, it should demonstrate that what we believe is firm and established knowledge is indeed false).

Now that we have set our constraints, let us see if the evolutionary models of depression respect them; I will posit seven reasons why it might not.

1. The problem with the various etiological pathways leading to depression: Kendler's work (see Kendler et al. 2006) suggests that there are at least three major pathways that lead to depression: internalizing symptoms, externalizing symptoms, and adversity and interpersonal difficulty. Many of these pathways include events that took place in childhood (sexual abuse, dysfunctional family, a depressed mother, public humiliation, etc.).[15] Moreover, in a recent paper, Kendler and his colleagues (2009) present studies on twin pairs of subjects who suffered from depression, and identified two genetic pathways to major depression: one pathway has been identified among those subjects who had an early age onset of depression

---

[14] It is with this constraint in mind that evolutionary psychiatrists make claims such as: depression is "exquisitely designed" for a certain purpose (Sloman 2008, 221); or that certain results " ... suggest that *symptoms are a functional response* to particular social problems" (my emphasis; Hagen and Barrett 2007, 24); or that depression is an "orderly" syndrome ("there is a *neurological orderliness that appears to specifically and proficiently promote analysis* in depressive rumination and is not likely to have evolved by chance"; Andrews and Thomson 2009, 622). This 'orderliness' of the syndrome is taken as evidence of special design (Andrews 2007, 49; see also Andrews and Thomson 2010, 58; Durrant and Heig 2001, 362).

[15] The mechanism through which depression is thought to develop in these cases is believed to involve the "programming" of the responsiveness of the hypothalamic-pituitary-adrenal (HPA) axis (see Hyman 2009; Krishnan and Nestler 2008; Pariante and Lightman 2008).

(AAO) and one among individuals who had vascular disease (VD). The members of the latter group have a late AAO, thought to be due to ischemic brain lesions.

Neither depression rooted in childhood events nor depression caused by vascular disease (or for that matter, by other physical illness via the inflammatory effects of cytokines on hippocampal cells) strongly supports the idea that depression is the result of a mechanism in charge of disengagement, or that it is in charge of solving complex social problems.

This is not much of a concern for Nesse, who admits that depression is not always adaptative and that it takes many forms. The problem for Nesse is that if many or most cases of depression are explained by either dysfunctional development environments, or by cerebral accidents or infection, he still has to provide us with an "evolutionary explanation of *depression*" (in other words, there would be a great number of cases of depression that are not explained evolutionarily). As for Andrews and Thomson's theory, it does not fit well with that kind of data, since in these cases, depression is apparently not an adaptation nor necessarily (or primarily) caused by complex social problems.

2. The problem with proportionality and understandability: Nesse wants us to consider as "normal" episodes of depression that are "proportional" to their triggering events (the same point is made by numerous people, among them, Horwitz and Wakefield 2007). One obvious problem with proportionality is the fact that the determination of what is proportional is rather subjective (it depends on a general and non-scientific conception of human nature). That situation can be fixed by providing a detailed empirical (and maybe an evolutionary) theory of emotions which would describe their normal range. For the moment, though, such a theory is lacking and we are left without empirical grounds to make our judgments.

Moreover (and this is related the previous point, according to which some episodes of depression might have no external trigger), one should avoid committing what some have called the "fallacy of misplaced empathy", i.e. the "well-intentioned clinicians [who are] missing the diagnosis of MDD because [they] can 'understand' that 'anybody' undergoing a serious life stressor – whether becoming disabled, impoverished, terminally ill, humiliated, or bereaved – might be distraught and upset" (Lamb et al. 2010, 20). Indeed, it does not follow that if one can understand someone's reaction to an event, that the reaction is not pathological (this can be understood as a precautionary principle; it should not be understood as saying that proportionality can or should not be used, but rather that one should be careful not to apply it blindly[16]). As Maj also notes, a number of factors favor being mindful of identifying "presumed" triggering events: for instance, "… the presence itself of a

---

[16]Though I will not argue for this, I think that part of what lead to the elimination of the bereavement exclusion clause is linked with the fear of false negatives (i.e. the fear of overlooking people who are really suffering from major depression and who might need treatment or might commit suicide). It is disputable that the elimination of the clause was really the solution to that problem or even if there was a problem in the first place with the clause as such (by contrast as with the use of the clause by psychiatrists; see on this Wakefield and First 2012; Wakefield and Schmitz 2014).

depressive state may affect the individual's accuracy in reporting life events" (2012, 222). Finally, as it became clear in recent debate about the validity of the bereavement exclusion for a diagnosis of major depression, patients with different levels of psychosocial adversity experienced prior to the episode of depression do not differ significantly on several variables (Lamb et al. 2010, 22; for critical comments on the Lamb et al. paper, see Wakefield and First 2012), and their response to antidepressants is unrelated to the presence or absence of such an event (so much the worse, then, for proportionality as an important factor to identify pathological depression).

Where proportionality might not be a good indicator of depression, some have argued that phenomenology might be a better indicator of differences in underlying mental conditions (Maj 2012). It is believed that the phenomenology of "ordinary sadness" and depression are quite different (Lamb et al. 2010; it seems that this was recognized by the DSM in its bereavement exclusion clause which mentioned that the sadness experienced after the death of a loved one does not have all the features of major depression; for instance, it has no severe psychomotor retardation, no morbid preoccupation with his or her worthlessness, no impairment in overall function, etc.). In ordinary sadness related to death, the emotional connection with significant others is not severed as it is in depression; dysphoria is experienced in waves rather than being omnipresent; self-esteem and personal potency are not affected, etc.

One might argue that the distinctive phenomenological experiences of normal sadness and depression are caused by different underlying neural mechanisms. If such is the case, it is not at all clear that the two are related. In depression, motivational mechanisms might be impeded, where in normal sadness they are not – it is just the case that one simply does not know what to do.

3. The problem with the idea that neuroscience neglects the role of life events: Contrary to what Nesse says about neuroscience, it is untrue that "it neglects the role of life events and other causal factors that interact with brain variation to cause most depression" (2009, 22). True, neuroscientists have not been interested in providing a precise description of the nature of events that trigger depression[17] as they have tried to provide an explanation in molecular and neural terms of "how adversity gets under the skin" (to use the title of Steven Hyman's 2009 paper). But, as epidemiologic studies have shown, genes alone are insufficient for depression, and environment in one form or another has to play a role (Caspi et al. 2003; Kendler et al. 2005; Hariri et al. 2005).

Nesse is also wrong to suggest that adopting a brain perspective "encourages studying major depression as if it is one condition with one etiology" (2009, 22). A quick glance at the literature on depression in neuroscience provides reasons to reject Nesse's statement. For instance, one of the primary investigators in the

---

[17] What counts as a stressors is often undefined, though not always, see, Hill et al. 2001; Goodman et al. 2011.

Research Domain Criteria of the NIMH, Bruce Cuthbert, says that "... the problem with the DSM disorders is that they are very heterogeneous and may involve multiple brain systems." (quoted by Miller 2010, 1437). Similarly, Krishnan and Nestler conclude their review paper by stating "[...] researchers and clinicians must embrace the polysyndromic nature of depression and use a multidisciplinary approach to explore the neurobiological bases for depression's many subtypes" (Krishnan and Nestler 2008, 901). Lee and colleagues (2010) explain the absence of a simple relationship between biogenic amines and depression by saying that "... depression is a group of disorders with several underlying pathologies" (1); while Lilienfeld reminds neuroscientists that "they are not dealing with one disorder, but with multiple phenocopies that stem from diverse causes" (2007, 268). In light of this, Nesse's suggestion appears to mischaracterize neuroscientists' attitudes toward depression.

However, what Nesse is right about is that neuroscience does not typically consider the possibility that people with genetic or brain variations might actually be advantaged in certain environments – in other words, that variation itself might be adaptative, or that it may reflect a frequence-dependent adaptation. Such a possibility is considered by Nettle (2004) who proposes that increasing neuroticism (a personality factor linked with increased chance of depression) might have been selected for its beneficial effects. Nesse might also be right about the fact that the focus on depression as a pathological state has taken attention away from studying the function of low mood (this is a sociological and historical claim that could be studied empirically), and from considering some individuals who present behavioral or physiological symptoms of depression as healthy.

4. The problem with the symptoms left unexplained: As mentioned at the beginning of this section, one constraint that satisfying evolutionary explanations should meet is that they should explain how a condition's symptoms are responses to particular problems. It should not select only certain symptoms that it can explain well and leave unexplained certain central symptoms of a condition. Unfortunately, this is what happens in Nesse's case.

Many symptoms of major depression are left unexplained by Nesse's theory: sexual dysfunction, physical pain, sleep issues, and increased suicide risk are hardly addressed (Varga 2012, 49). Moreover, Nesse's explanation of certain symptoms is not at all obvious. For example, as Murphy (2006) remarks, why should the breakdown of the low mood mechanism generate loss of sleep or inability to make decisions or concentrate? Further, why is the disengagement mechanism not accompanied by a positive affect or a motivational structure of some sort that would cause behavior to change? This idea has precedent in the literature: for instance, animals experiencing severe food restriction will increase – not decrease – their energy expenditure and increase risk-taking behavior. In a recent paper, Nettle (2009) used optimal-foraging models and suggested that Nesse is at least partially correct: "when things are going quite badly, it is not time to take risks, but as things improve, greater experimentation is warranted" (3). However, the models also predicts that "... there comes a dire point beyond which it is maladaptative to avoid risks and conserve energy: the situation is already too dangerous for that. Instead, the individual should be highly motivated to take risks and try new solutions; to do anything that has any chance of returning her to the acceptable range of states" (ibid., 3). Nettle notes that this state might be found in patients classified as depressive because of their negative affective tone, but whose symptoms include locomotor acceleration and restlessness, and a feeling of speeding and a desire to follow risky, pleasurable impulses (perhaps thought of as a form of "dysphoric mania"). What Nettle proposes is a further refinement of functional theories of the kind defended by Nesse. According to Nettle, adaptative responses in the case of loss of resources would be different as a function of the individual's evaluation of the condition's severity. As he states, "[t]he mood responses to different types of situations will show different suites of design features that represent adaptative strategies in that context [...] Thus, a mood representing a response to dire circumstances could involve simultaneous activation of negative emotion systems [...] and behavior approach systems. Such a mood state would be like depression, in its negativity, but also like positive mood, in its energy and risk-proneness". (ibid., 4)

5. The problem with the lack of consistency with other findings from basic sciences: Andrews and Thomson's theory fares better in terms of the first constraint because it tries to incorporate all features associated with depression and explain that they are part of coordinated responses to a specific kind of problem.[18] Their notion that features of rumination might be adaptive, and their notion that cognitive resource allocation to social problems might impede non-relevant laboratory tasks are both worth exploring. Yet Andrews and Thomson don't fare as well with the second constraint.

Firstly, it is unclear that the rumination of depressive individuals targets the resolution of a problem. Repeatedly thinking: "I am worthless", "I am a failure", "nobody really likes me", etc. hardly seems like problem-solving. Moreover, studies on depressive subjects show that "rumination prompts them to appraise their problems as overwhelming and unsolvable and to fail to come up with effective problem solutions" (Nolen-Hoeksema et al. 2008, 400–1). Secondly, rumination is thought to help solve the problems that triggered the depressive episode, but, as Varga (2012) points out, there is not much support for this notion. Instead, the evidence points to the idea that rumination enhances the effects of depressed mood on thinking. Indeed, Andrews and Thomson's support for their idea comes from a study from Hayes and colleagues (2005) which, as Varga observes, concludes something different, which is that the "important tasks in treating depression are *to reduce patterns of avoidance and rumination* and to facilitate processing" (my emphasis; 112, quoted by Varga 2012, 49). Thirdly, Andrews and Thomson also argue that the depressed have cognitive features that facilitate the resolution of social problems. However, it is not at all obvious that more rapid or more rational (from a game-theoretical perspective) solutions to social dilemma help to resolve social problems, rather than generating more of them. Moreover, as Nettle (2004) points out, the

---

[18] Though I have not presented it in section "Andrews and Thomson: Rumination and motivation", their theory also explains why (and predicts in which situations, see 2009, 645) people will attempt to escape pain generated by depression or try to commit suicide, for example.

depressed also have cognitive features that might handicap them in this task: they are slower and less accurate than control subjects at reading non-verbal social cues; they show impaired social skills; they seem more realistic than others only when the normal population is unrealistically positive (and depressive individuals are unrealistic when the normal population is reasonably accurate) and "… depressives perform worse than controls on tasks designed to tap inter-personal problem solving skills" (96).[19] Finally, it is not at all clear that rumination enables individuals to escape their condition, or that it helps them gather social support. In regards to the former, Varga notes: "Because the ruminating person will be focused on her depressive symptoms, which typically involves negative self-ascriptions, the conclusion will often be that he/she lacks the capacity to engage in constructive activities. Ruminating depressives will lack confidence in their solutions that might be the reason why they often do not pursue them … Studies reveal that even if the ruminator acknowledges that a certain activity would have an effect, they have trouble in motivating themselves to actually engage in these activities" (2012, 49).[20] With regard to the latter, if it is true that ruminators are more likely to look for social support and sometimes receive it, they also are more prone to aggressive behavior and are often criticized for their inability to cope, as others become frustrated with their continued need to discuss their loss or problems (Nolen-Hoeksema et al. 2008, 403 and 408; see also Coyne 1976).

Another issue with Andrews and Thomson's proposal is that they assume that depression triggers are social or predominantly social in nature. Here, one wonders about the direction of causality: is depression caused by social problems or are social problems caused by depression? Depression can cause marital problems, lack of social support, or the defection of social partners – all of which are also identified as factors in depression. And if depression is caused by social problems, does it allow people suffering from it to acquire more support or new deals with cooperative partners? Hagen has provided data for PPD, but no such data are available for depression in general.

Moreover, if depression is adaptative and is designed to solve social problems, why is it that Keller et al. (1992) found 70 % of those who suffer major depression will have at least one other episode and 20 % will develop it as a chronic condition (rate of continuous freedom from illness is very low – 11 % over 25 years; Nettle 2004, 95)? What these numbers suggest is, as Murphy notes, "if depression is an adaptation designed to make them [the depressive] function better in society, it is not working" (295). Indeed, once depression has achieved its function, should it not

---

[19] As Allen and Badcock observe: "… although some recent studies have shown that mild depressed states facilitate both social reasoning and performance on theory of mind tasks, other studies using the same assessment procedures have found that in clinical populations, these advantages are absent or even reversed" (2006, 822).

[20] As Nolen-Hoeksema and colleagues note "… rumination leads people to see obstacles to the implementation of solutions, to be less willing to commit to implementing the solutions they generate, and to be more likely to disengage from real-life problems than to continue trying to solve them " (2008, 408).

disappear? Why, then, does it become chronic in 20 % of cases?[21] If one accepts Andrews and Thomson's theory, this means that for some individuals, having an episode of depression makes them more likely to reencounter a similar kind of problem – this is hardly progress![22]

One last problem with their account is, as Nettle points out, if "all normal human beings have the capacity to feel physical pain … there is no evidence that all individuals have the capacity to become clinically depressed. Rather, it seems likely that most depression is the result of an inherited diathesis borne by a minority of the population" (2004, 93). Indeed, according to him, there is no support for the idea that depression is a universal adaptation.[23]

6. The problem of comorbidity: It is widely known that there is an important comorbidity between anxiety and depression. For instance, among patients in the general population who meet criteria for major depression, approximately 50 % also suffer from anxiety disorder (Hirschfeld 2001; Sandi and Richter-Levin 2009). An evolutionary explanation of depression should be able to explain why this is the case. Nesse (2009) explains this by positing that the problems that trigger depression sometimes also demand greater vigilance, thus also triggers threat systems. The question then becomes "Why do these two systems break down, and why do they so often break down together?" Nesse has no response to this question. Likewise, Andrews and Thomson do not provide an explanation of the

---

[21] Worse, as Nettle (2004) and Nesse (2000) observe, as depressive episodes continue (for third and subsequent episodes of endogeneous depression), the triggers required to produce depression become smaller and less related to life events.

[22] As an editor of this volume observed, "design does not imply success": for instance, the evolutionary function of spermatozoids is to fertilized egg cells, even if most of them will never achieved this feat. There are two problems with this remark in the context of the discussion of Andrews and Thomson's theory. First, remember that they claim that "performance on the triggering problem [should be considered] as a crucial metric for evaluating depressive cognition" (2009, 637). If most depressions fail to solve triggering problems and are followed by other episodes of depression, then depressive cognition does not seem to be very efficient at this task. Second, if most cases of depression are not adaptive (that is, they failed to provide a solution to the problem that triggered them), the usefulness of an evolutionary theory of depression for psychiatry is questionable. We are left with people who suffer, who have problems that they cannot solve themselves: knowing that their problems are the result of an evolutionary mechanism which failed to accomplish its function is not of a great practical help. As to recurrence, it is possible that the initial loss that provoked the depression is typically followed later by other losses. The problem would be with the life of the depressives, not with the depressives themselves. I do not want to deny this possibility, but it seems to me that more empirical works need to be done on this: first, to substantiate the claim; and second, to show that these losses are not caused by the very mechanism that is supposed to fix the situation, i.e. depression.

[23] This last point has been contested lately. Some authors (Moffit et al. 2010; Rohde et al. 2013) have been arguing that the low rate of depression found in epidemiological survey is an artifact of the retrospective method used in those surveys (in which respondents are asked to retrospect over the past years to recall episode of depression). The use of a prospective method (basically, longitudinal studies) gives much higher rates of depression in the general population (with rates of 40–50 % of the sample having had an experience of depression compared to 12–17 % with retrospective studies).

comorbidity of anxiety and depression, nor for that matter, of the comorbidity of depression and hypomania.

Neuroscience seems better equipped to explain such comorbidity. According to Sandi and Richter-Levin (2009), there is good reason to think that high-anxiety traits (or neuroticism) play a crucial role in explanation of depression. In their paper, they describe "the dysfunctional neurocognitive cascade" that leads individuals with hyperactive amygdala to develop depression. A hyper-reactivity of the amygdala, coupled with impaired prefrontal cortex ability to control the activation of the amygdala, makes individuals more prone to experience fear and stress. This leads to an enhanced activation of the HPA axis, which is known to increase the activation of neurons in the basolateral amygdala, which activate the production and release of CRF (corticotropin-releasing factor) in the central nucleus of the amygdala and prefrontal cortex. Higher activity of the amygdala combined with phasic release of CRF produce emotional potentiation for memory ("increased storage of both fear association and of negative emotional episodic memory" (2009, 316) and impair memory retrieval and working memory. The resulting system is, as Sandi and Richter-Levin put it, a "sensitized systems" with an exaggerated focus on the negative side of events. Confrontation with stressful events will increase amygdala and HPA axis activation, which translates into greater attention to negative events, and recall of negative memory. It will also translate into further dysfunction (and structural changes) to the hippocampus and prefrontal cortex, which will render individuals ineffective at certain cognitive tasks, which in turn will increase their feelings of hopelessness. Thus here, one is tempted to say that, contrary to Nesse's claim, "evolutionary theory is not enough, neuroscience is essential".

7. The problem with the interpretation of treatment efficacy: The last point is related to the previous two points, and relates to the remission of symptoms. In his "Reconstructing the Evolution of the Mind is Depressingly Difficult", Andrews claims that one way to identify the problems that depression has evolved to solve is by assessing treatment efficacy. As he puts it: "Although antidepressants alleviate acute depression, they do not prevent relapse, whereas talking therapies do. Moreover, talking therapies that attempt to address social problems [...] are often the most effective. Because treating the cause should be more effective than treating the symptom, the fact that social interventions are better than medications at preventing relapse suggests that the cause of depression resides more in the social environment than in a malfunctioning nervous system" (2007, 49). As was shown earlier, one consequence of Andrews and Thompson's theory is that only therapies encouraging rumination should have long-lasting effects.

There are many problems with this view, of which I will only address two. As was emphasized by Adolph Grünbaum (1984), the success of a therapy does not constitute proof of truth of the principles it postulates as causally efficacious. Antidepressants might not be a very effective cure for depression (Andrews et al. 2011), or they may even be harmful (Andrews et al. 2012), but because some kind of cure is working does not mean that it works as a result of its having identified the true causes of depression. However, for our present purposes, let's pretend it does. Let's pretend that the causes of depression are indeed social, and that we have to treat them in order to get better. Even if such is the case, it is not clear that therapies permitting rumination would work better than others that do not. Nolen-Hoeksema and her colleagues argue that

> Inducing dysphoric or depressed participants to distract from their moods and ruminations for just 8 min leads them to generate solutions to problems that are just as effective as non-depressed participants' solutions and significantly more effective than those generated by dysphoric participants induced to ruminate. The short distraction induction also leads dysphoric and depressed participants to express more control and self-efficacy, to appraise the causes of problems more optimistically, and to have more confidence in their ability to overcome their problems than do dysphoric people induced to ruminate [...] These results suggest that attempts to resolve self-discrepancies will be more successful and less likely to devolve into perseverations about problems if individuals are either in a neutral or positive mood or if they first use neutral or positive distractions to lift their moods and interrupt ongoing rumination (Nolen-Hoeksema et al. 2008, 415).

This brings me to the second problem, which is related to the first. Contrary to depression therapies based on content (for instance, Beck's cognitive therapy or CT[24]), Bar (2009) proposes a "content-less" therapy. Like Andrews and Thomson, he focuses on one symptomatic characteristic of depressive individuals, their tendency for rumination. For Bar, rumination implicates the fact that thinking revolves around the same negative ideas. Rumination can be opposed to broad associative thinking, i.e. thinking which involves thought processes that advance smoothly from one context to the other. Bar's rather bold hypothesis rests on the observation that positive mood promotes associative thinking (an idea developed and explored by Isen et al., 1985), and inversely, that associative thinking promotes positive mood. Observing that the contextual associations network in the brain functions abnormally in depressive subjects, and that chemical and electrical stimulation therapies work on parts of the contextual associative network, Bar suggests that rumination might be caused by over-inhibition of MTL (medial temporal lobe) by MPFC (medial prefrontal cortex) and neighboring anterior cingulated cortex. Given the link between association and positive mood, Bar then proposes that therapies should promote the "acquisition of mental habits of broad associative activation and a cognitive-driven reconstruction of the underlying cortical network" (2009, 460). This is how Hayes et al. are interpreting the success of their writing therapy: it works by avoiding patterns of rumination and facilitates processing.

If Andrews and Thomson's theory is right, this would suggest that Bar's proposals about using associations to create good mood would produce long-term detri-

---

[24] Beck's CT is "... a structured, skill-based psychotherapy that focuses on modifying the faulty thoughts, evaluations, attributions, beliefs and processing biases that characterized anxiety and depression. It is assumed that CT results in significant reduction of symptoms by weakening or deactivating disorder-related maladaptive schemas and strengthening alternative, more positive modes of thinking. Patients are taught to identify their maladaptive thinking, evaluate its accuracy, generate more adaptive and realistic perspectives and test-out the utility of their new perspective through structured behavioural homework assignments" (Clark and Beck 2009, 420). Note that this kind of therapy, which is known to be quite successful, seems to be focused on getting rid of the cognitive features that are deemed to be essential by Andrews and Thomson to solve the depressives' problems.

mental effects and would likely create further depressive states. The latter requires testing. For the moment, Bar's explanation is more consistent with the reason why deep electric stimulation and other means to cure depression are working.

## Conclusion

My conclusion is concise: this paper examined two recent proposals from leading evolutionary psychiatrists concerning depression. I have shown that these proposals have different, important problems: they either leave aside (unexplained) certain central and costly traits of depression, or they are inconsistent with current established knowledge about depression. As such, one should not forget the status of these proposals – they are speculations. For this reason, one should not base actions (for instance, therapy) on them yet (which is not to say that we should reject all evolutionary explanations of depression. I have been pointing to the weaknesses of current evolutionary explanations of depression; I did not formulate an overall argument against them!).

I opened this paper by rehashing evolutionary psychiatrists' positions concerning the potential role of evolutionary considerations in psychiatry. It is clear that at this time (and for years to come), the momentum of depression research comes from genetics, genomics, or the brain sciences. This is clearly where institutions such as the NIMH are putting their money, with projects like RDoC initiative (for a description and criticism of that very project, see Faucher and Goyer 2015). Even if I have been very critical of evolutionary approaches to different mental disorders and to psychiatry in general (see for instance, Faucher 2012; Faucher and Blanchette 2011), I do not think it should be completely ignored either – even if it might not deserve the status of "basic science" for psychiatry that Nesse advocates. At present, evolutionary psychiatrists can't offer well-confirmed theories; they might never be able to produce such theories. Yet, their proposals can play a heuristic function by changing the focus of current brain sciences, and questioning traditional positions in this field (for instance, trying to explain the depression epidemic by the fact that current diagnostic criteria capture natural reactions to losses). If only for those reasons, we should keep an attentive – yet critical – ear to what evolutionary psychiatrists have to say.

## References

Akil, H., Brenner, S., Kandel, E., Kendler, K. S., King, M. C., et al. (2010). The future of psychiatric research: Genomes and neural circuits. *Science, 327*, 1580–1581.

Allen, N. B., & Badcock, P. (2006). Darwinian models of depression: A review of evolutionary accounts of mood and mood disorders. *Progress in Neuro-Psychopharmacology and Biological Psychiatry, 30*, 815–826.

Andreasen, N. C. (1997). Linking mind and brain in the study of mental illnesses: A project for a scientific psychopathology. *Science, 275*, 1586–1593.

Andrews, P. W. (2007). Reconstructing the evolution of the mind is depressingly difficult. In S. Gangestad & J. A. Simpson (Eds.), *The evolution of mind: Fundamental questions and controversies* (pp. 53–59). Oxford: Oxford University Press.

Andrews, P. W., & Thomson, J. A. (2009). The bright side of being blue: Depression as an adaptation for analyzing complex problems. *Psychological Review, 116*(3), 620–654.

Andrews, P. W., & Thomson, J. A. (2010). Depression's evolutionary roots. *Scientific American Mind, 20,* 57–61.

Andrews, P. W. & Thomson, J. A. (2011, January 10). Coyne battles Darwin, many other evolutionary biologists—and himself. *Psychiatric Times.* http://www.psychiatrictimes.com/coyne-battles-darwin-many-other-evolutionarybiologists%E2%80%94and-himself.

Andrews, P. W., Kornstein, S. G., Halberstadt, L. J., Gardner, C. O., & Neale, M. C. (2011). Blue again: Perturbational effects of antidepressants suggest monoaminergic homeostasis in major depression. *Frontiers in Psychology, 2,* 159. http://dx.doi.org/10.3389/fpsyg.2011.00159

Andrews, P. W., Thomson, J. A., Amstadter, A., & Neale, M. C. (2012). Primum non nocere: An evolutionary analysis of whether antidepressants do more harm than good. *Frontiers in Psychology, 3,* 117. doi:10.3389/fpsyg.2012.00117.

Bar, M. (2009). A cognitive neuroscience hypothesis of mood and depression. *Trends in Cognitive Sciences, 13*(11), 456–463.

Burns, J. K. (2004). An evolutionary theory of schizophrenia: Cortical connectivity, metarepresentation, and the social brain. *Behavioral and Brain Sciences, 27,* 831–885.

Caspi, A., Sugden, K., Moffitt, T. E., et al. (2003). Influence of life stress on depression: Moderation by polymorphism of 5-HTT gene. *Science, 301,* 386–389.

Clark, D. A., & Beck, A. T. (2009). Cognitive theory and therapy of anxiety and depression: Convergence with neurobiological findings. *Trends in Cognitive Sciences, 14*(9), 418–424.

Cooper, R. (2004). What is wrong with the DSM. *History of Psychiatry, 15,* 5–25.

Coyne, J. C. (1976). Depression and the response of others. *Journal of Abnormal psychology, 85*(2), 186–193.

Durrant, R., & Heig, B. D. (2001). How to pursue the adaptationist program in psychology. *Philosophical Psychology, 14*(4), 357–380.

Faucher, L. (2012). Evolutionary psychiatry and nosology: Prospects and limitations. In M. Bishop (Ed.), *The Baltic yearbook of cognition, logic and communication* (Vol. 7, pp. 1–64).

Faucher, L., & Blanchette, I. (2011). Fearing new dangers: Phobias and the complexity of human emotions. In A. De Block & P. Adriaens (Eds.), *Maladapting minds: Philosophy, psychiatry and evolutionary theory* (pp. 34–64). New York, Oxford University Press.

Faucher, L., & Goyer, S. (2015). RDoC: Thinking outside the DSM box without falling into reductionist trap. In S. Demazeux & P. Singy (Eds.), *The DSM-5 in perspective: Philosophical reflections on the psychiatric Babel* (pp. 199–224). Dordrecht: Springer.

Frances, A. (2009). Whither DSM-V? *British Journal of Psychiatry, 195,* 391–392.

Frances, A., & Widiger, T. (2012). Psychiatric diagnosis: Lessons from the DSM-IV past and cautions for the DSM-5 future. *Annual Review of Clinical Psychology, 8,* 109–130.

Galatzer-Levy, I. R., & Galatzer-Levy, R. M. (2007). The revolution in psychiatric diagnosis: Problems at the foundations. *Perspectives in Biology and Medicine, 50*(2), 161–180.

Gilbert, P. (2006). Evolution and depression: Issues and implications. *Psychological Medicine, 36,* 287–297.

Goodman, S., Rouse, M. H., Connell, A. M., Broth, M. R., Hall, C. M., & Heyward, D. (2011). Maternal depression and child psychopathology: A meta-analytic review. *Clinical Child and Family Psychology Review, 14,* 1–27.

Grünbaum, A. (1984). *The foundations of psychoanalysis: A philosophical critique.* Berkeley: University of California Press.

Guze, S. (1992). *Why psychiatry is a branch of medicine.* Oxford: Oxford University Press.

Hagen, E. H. (1999). The functions of postpartum depression. *Evolution and Human Behavior, 23,* 323–336.

Hagen, E. H. (2002). Depression as bargaining: The case of postpartum. *Evolution and Human Behavior, 23,* 323–336.

Hagen, E. H. (2003). The bargaining model of depression. In P. Hammerstein (Ed.), *Genetic and cultural evolution of cooperation* (pp. 95–123). Cambridge, MA: MIT Press.

Hagen, E. H. (2011). Evolutionary theories of depression: A critical review. *Canadian Journal of Psychiatry, 56*(12), 716–726.

Hagen, E. H., & Barrett, C. (2007). Perinatal sadness among Shuar women. *Medical Anthropology Quarterly, 21*(1), 22–40.

Hariri, A. R., Drabant, E. M., Munoz, K. E., et al. (2005). A susceptibility gene for affective disorders and the response of the human amygdala. *Archives of General Psychiatry, 62*, 146–152.

Hayes, A. M., Beevers, C. G., Feldman, G. C., Laurenceau, J. P., & Perlman, C. (2005). Avoidance and processing as predictors of symptom change and positive growth in an integrative therapy for depression. *Internal Journal of Behavioral Medicine, 12*(2), 111–122.

Hill, J., Pickles, A., Burnside, E., Byatt, M., Rollinson, L., Davis, R., & Harvey, K. (2001). Child abuse, poor parental care and adult depression: Evidence for different mechanisms. *British Journal of Psychiatry, 179*, 104–109.

Hirschfeld, R. (2001). The comorbidity of major depression and anxiety disorders: Recognition and management in primary care. *Primary Care Companion of the Journal of Clinical Psychiatry, 3*(6), 244–254.

Horwitz, A. W. (2011). Creating an age of depression: The social construction and consequences of the major depression disorder. *Society and Mental Health, 1*(1), 41–54.

Horwitz, A. W., & Wakefield, J. (2007). *The loss of sadness: How psychiatry transformed normal sorrow into depressive disorder*. Oxford: Oxford University Press.

Hyman, S. E. (2009). How adversity gets under the skin. *Nature Neuroscience, 12*(3), 241–243.

Hyman, S. E. (2010). The diagnosis of mental disorders: The problem of reification. *Annual Review of Clinical Psychology, 6*, 155–179.

Insel, T., Cuthbert, B., et al. (2010). Research domain criteria (RDoC): Toward a New classification framework for research on mental disorders. *American Journal of Psychiatry, 167*(7), 748–751.

Isen, A. M., Johnson, M. M., Mertz, E., & Robinson, G. F. (1985). The influence of positive affect on the unusualness of word associations. *Journal of Personality and Social Psychology, 48*(6), 1413–1426.

Kandel, E. R. (1998). A New intellectual framework for psychiatry. *American Journal of Psychiatry, 155*, 457–469.

Keller, M. C., & Miller, G. (2006). Resolving the paradox of common, harmful, heritable mental disorders: Which evolutionary genetic models work best? *Behavioral and Brain Sciences, 29*, 385–452.

Keller, M. C., & Nesse, R. (2005). Is Low mood an adaptation? Evidence for subtypes with symptoms that match precipitants. *Journal of Affective Disorders, 86*, 27–35.

Keller, M. C., & Nesse, R. M. (2006). The evolutionary significance of depressive symptoms: Different adverse situations lead to different depressive symptom patterns. *Journal of Personality and Social Psychology, 91*(2), 316–330.

Keller, M. C., Neale, M. C., & Kendler, K. S. (2007). Association of different adverse life events with distinct patterns of depressive symptoms. *American Journal of Psychiatry, 164*, 1521–1529.

Keller, M. B., Lavori, P. W., Mueller, T. I., Endicott, J., Coryell, W., Hirschfeld, R. M., et al. (1992). Time to recovery, chronicity, and levels of psychopathology in major depression. A 5-year prospective follow-up of 431 subjects. *Archives of General Psychiatry, 49*(10), 809–816.

Kendler, K. S., Kuhn, J., Vittum, J. W., et al. (2005). The interaction of stressful events and a serotonin transporter polymorphism in the prediction of episodes of major depression: A replication. *Archives of General Psychiatry, 62*, 529–535.

Kendler, K. S., Gardner, C. O., & Prescott, C. A. (2006). Toward a comprehensive developmental model for major depression in men. *American Journal of Psychiatry, 163*, 115–124.

Kendler, K. S., Fiske, A., Gardner, C. O., & Gatz, M. (2009). Delineation of two genetic pathways to major depression. *Biological Psychiatry, 65*, 808–811.

Kennair, L. E. O. (2003). Evolutionary psychology and psychopathology. *Current Opinion in Psychiatry, 16*, 691–699.

Kirk, S. A., & Kutchins, H. (1992). *The selling of DSM: The rhetoric of science in psychiatry*. The Hague: Adeline De Gruyter.

Klinger, E. (1975). Consequences of commitment to and disengagement from incentives. *Psychological Review, 82*, 1–25.

Krishnan, V., & Nestler, E. J. (2008). The molecular neurobiology of depression. *Nature, 455*(16), 894–902.

Lamb, K., Pies, R., & Zisook, S. (2010). The bereavement exclusion for the diagnosis of major depression: To be, or not to be. *Psychiatry, 7*(7), 19–25.

Lee, S., Jeong, J., Kwak, Y., & Park, S. K. (2010). Depression research: Where are we now? *Molecular Brain, 3*, 8. doi:10.1186/1756-6606-3-8.

Lilienfeld, S. O. (2007). Cognitive neuroscience and depression: Legitimate versus illegitimate reductionism and five challenges. *Cognitive Therapy and Research, 31*, 263–272.

Maj, M. (2012). When does depression become a mental disorder? In K. S. Kendler & J. Parnas (Eds.), *Philosophical issues in psychiatry II* (pp. 221–228). New York: Oxford University Press.

Mayes, R., & Horwitz, A. V. (2005). DSM-III and the revolution in the classification of mental illness. *Journal of History of the Behavioral Sciences, 41*(3), 249–267.

McGuire, M., Troisi, A., & Raleigh, M. (1997). Depression in evolutionary context. In S. Baron Cohen (Ed.), *The maladapted mind: Classic readings in evolutionary psychopathology* (pp. 255–282). Hove: Psychology Press.

McReynolds, W. T. (1979). DSM-III and the future of applied social science. *Professional Psychology, 10*(1), 123–132.

Miller, G. (2010, March 19). Beyond DSM: Seeking a brain-based classification of mental illness. *Science, 327*, 1437.

Mineka, S., & Öhman, A. (2002). Phobias and preparedness: The selective, automatic, and encapsulated nature of fear. *Biological Psychiatry, 52*(10), 927–937.

Moffit, T. E., Caspi, A., Taylor, A., Kokaua, J., Milne, B. J., Polancyk, G., & Poulton, R. (2010). How common are common mental disorders? Evidence that lifetime prevalence rates are doubled by prospective *versus* retrospective ascertainment. *Psychological Medicine, 40*, 899–909.

Morris, S. E., & Cuthbert, B. N. (2012). Research domain criteria: Cognitive systems, neural circuits, and dimensions of behavior. *Dialogues in Clinical Neurosciences, 14*, 29–37.

Mulder, R. T. (2008). An epidemic of depression or the medicalization of distress. *Perspectives in Biology and Medicine, 51*(2), 238–250.

Murphy, D. (2006). *Psychiatry in the scientific image*. Cambridge, MA: MIT Press.

Murphy, D. (2009). Psychiatry and the concept of disease as pathology. In M. Broome & L. Bortolotti (Eds.), *Psychiatry as cognitive neuroscience* (pp. 103–117). Oxford: Oxford University Press.

Nesse, R. (1990). Evolutionary explanations of emotions. *Human Nature, 1*, 261–289.

Nesse, R. (2000). Is depression an adaptation? *Archives of General Psychiatry, 57*, 14–20.

Nesse, R. (2002). Evolutionary biology: A basic science for psychiatry. *World Psychiatry, 1*(1), 7–9.

Nesse, R. (2005). Twelve crucial points about emotions, evolution and mental disorders. *Psychological Review, 11*(4), 12–14.

Nesse, R. (2006). Evolutionary explanations for mood and mood disorders. In D. Stein, D. Kupfur, & A. Schatzberg (Eds.), *Textbook of mood disorders* (pp. 159–175). Washington, DC: American Psychiatric Publishing.

Nesse, R. (2009). Explaining depression: Neuroscience is not enough, evolution is essential. In C. M. Pariante, R. Nesse, R. Nutt, & D. Wolpert (Eds.), *Understanding depression: A translational approach* (pp. 17–35). Oxford: Oxford University Press.

Nesse, R., & Berrige, K. C. (1997). Psychoactive drug use in evolutionary perspective. *Science, 278*, 63–66.

Nesse, R., & Ellsworth, P. C. (2009). Evolution, emotions, and emotional disorders. *American Psychologist, 64*(2), 129–139.

Nesse, R., & Jackson, E. D. (2011). Evolutionary foundations for psychiatric diagnosis: Making the DSM-V valid. In P. R. Adriaens & A. De Block (Eds.), *Maladapting minds* (pp. 173–197). New York: Oxford University Press.

Nesse, R., & Stein, D. (2012). Towards a genuinely medical model for psychiatric nosology. *BMC Medicine, 10*(5), 1–9.

Nesse, R., & Williams, G. C. (1995). *Why we get sick: The new science of Darwinian medicine.* New York: Times Books.

Nesse, R., & Williams, G. (1997). Are mental disorders diseases? In S. Baron Cohen (Ed.), *The maladapted mind: Classic readings in evolutionary psychopathology* (pp. 1–22). Hove: Psychology Press.

Nettle, D. (2004). Evolutionary origins of depression: A review and reformulation. *Journal of Affective Disorders, 81*, 91–102.

Nettle, D. (2009). An evolutionary model of low mood states. *Journal of Theoretical Biology, 257*(1), 100–103.

Nolen-Hoeksema, S., Wisco, B. E., & Lyubomirky, S. (2008). Rethinking rumination. *Perspectives on Psychological Science, 3*(5), 400–424.

Pariante, C., & Lightman, S. L. (2008). The HPA axis in major depression: Classical theories and new developments. *Trends in Neurosciences, 31*, 9.

Parker, G. (2005). Beyond major depression. *Psychological Medicine, 35*, 467–474.

Ploeger, A., & Galis, F. (2011). Evolutionary approaches to autism. *McGill Journal of Medicine, 13*(2), 38–43.

Price, J. S., Sloman, L., Gardner, R., Jr., Gilbert, P., & Rohde, P. (1997). The social competition hypothesis of depression. In S. Baron Cohen (Ed.), *The maladapted mind: Classic readings in evolutionary psychopathology* (pp. 241–254). Hove: Psychology Press.

Price, J. S., Gardner, R., Wilson, D., Sloman, L., Rohde, P., & Erickson, M. (2007). Territory, rank and mental health: The history of an idea. *Evolutionary Psychology, 5*(3), 531–554.

Rohde, P., Lewinsohn, P. M., Klein, D. N., Seeley, J. R., & Gau, J. M. (2013). Key characteristics of major depressive disorder occurring in childhood, adolescence, early adulthood and adulthood. *Clinical Psychological Science, 1*(1), 30–40.

Sandi, C., & Richter-Levin, G. (2009). From high anxiety trait to depression: A neurocognitive hypothesis. *Trends in Neurosciences, 32*(6), 312–320.

Sloman, L. (2008). A new comprehensive evolutionary model of depression and anxiety. *Journal of Affective Disorders, 106*, 219–228.

Stein, D. J., Newman, T. K., Avitz, J., & Ramesar, R. (2006). Warriors versus worriers: The role of COMT gene variants. *CNS Spectrums, 11*(10), 745–748.

Tsou, J. Y. (2011). The importance of history for philosophy of psychiatry: The case of DSM and psychiatric classification. *Journal of the Philosophy of History, 5*, 446–470.

Varga, S. (2012). Evolutionary psychiatry and depression: Testing two hypotheses. *Medicine, Health Care and Philosophy, 15*, 41–52.

Wakefield, J. C., & First, M. B. (2012). Validity of the bereavement exclusion to major depression: Does the empirical evidence support the proposal to eliminate the exclusion in DSM-5? *World Psychiatry, 11*, 3–10.

Wakefield, J. C., & Schmitz, M. F. (2014). Uncomplicated depression, suicide attempt, and the DSM-5 bereavement exclusion debate: An empirical evaluation. *Research on Social Work Practice, 24*(1), 37–49.

Wakefield, J. C., Schmitz, M. F., First, M. B., & Horwitz, A. V. (2007). Extending the bereavement exclusion for major depression to other losses. *Archives of General Psychiatry, 64*, 433–440.

Watson, P. J., & Andrews, P. W. (2002). Toward a revised evolutionary adaptationist analysis of depression: The social navigation hypothesis. *Journal of Affective Disorders, 72*, 1–14.

Widiger, T. A. (2011). A shaky future for personality disorders. *Personality Disorders: Theory, Research, and Treatment, 2*, 54–67.

Widiger, T. A., & Sankis, L. M. (2000). Adult psychopathology: Issues and controversies. *Annual Review of Psychology, 51*, 377–404.

# Is an Anatomy of Melancholia Possible? Brain Processes, Depression, and Mood Regulation

Denis Forest

**Abstract** Neurobiological models of depression aim to explain its conditions through a description of the underlying neurocircuitry. The present paper analyses the skeptical doubts that may be raised in response to neurobiological accounts of depression and the conditions under which these models may shed some light on the corresponding phenomena. Far from excluding other kinds of enquiries, neurobiological models may greatly benefit from a philosophical enquiry on our affective life, and especially from closer attention paid to ill-defined phenomena like moods. I suggest that what is crucial to depression is defective affective regulation, and that it is with this perspective that we may make sense of neurophysiological data.

## Introduction

The central problem of a philosophy of psychiatry today is not difficult to grasp: everything is plausible and you can argue in favor of almost anything. What I mean is that there is no conception of mental disorders that cannot be defended. The risk, then, is that any attempt to argue in favor of a thesis may lead us in a circle: first, you pick up your favorite view of the world; then, you spend enough time to find in the available literature innumerable reasons to believe it is true; lastly, you are even more convinced that your first intuitions were sound.

Take, for instance, depression. If you favor naturalism, you will find what you are looking for in the expanding body of discoveries concerning the neural correlates of depressive states (Drevets 1998; Fitzgerald et al. 2008), in the development of animal models of mood disorders (Overstreet 2012), and in a wide range of specula-

I would like to thank Jerome Wakefield and Steeves Demazeux for their feedback on the draft of this paper, Samuel Lepine for his comments on an earlier version, and Larry Dewaële for his careful reading of the final version.

D. Forest (✉)
Department of Philosophy, Université Paris Ouest Nanterre, Nanterre, France

Institute d'Histoire et de Philosophie des sciences et des techniques, Paris, France
e-mail: denis.forest@u-paris10.fr

© Springer Science+Business Media Dordrecht 2016
J.C. Wakefield, S. Demazeux (eds.), *Sadness or Depression?*
History, Philosophy and Theory of the Life Sciences 15,
DOI 10.1007/978-94-017-7423-9_7

tions about the evolutionary history of affective mechanisms (Nettle 2004). You will end up with the very biological view of depression that was your starting point. However, the philosopher who has little sympathy for a naturalistic ontology, or for evolutionary explanations of our mental features, will remain remarkably unimpressed. Thinking that depressive states are the states of the mind of a person, and not of his or her brain, he has at his disposal causal models of depression as they have been formulated by sociologists (Brown and Harris 1978), ethnographic enquiries offering evidence that culture and context matter in the development and symptomatology of mental disorders in general (Kleinman 1988) and of depression in particular (Kleinman 1986; Kitanaka 2011, 2016), and analysis of the consequences of a shift from a professional culture of responsibility to a culture of initiative and performance (Ehrenberg 2009, 2016). If he has a constructivist or a Foucauldian turn of mind, and if he is ready to challenge psychiatry as a form of so-called "bio-power" and as an agent of normalization of conducts, the philosopher also may also take advantage of the growing literature about what is now called the medicalization of ordinary life (Conrad 2007), a chief example of which is the unmotivated diagnosis of depression (Horwitz and Wakefield 2007). All of this may lead to endless clashes, to a pessimistic, Weberian view of the disunity of knowledge, where differences of methodology and perspective lead to attitudes that cannot be reconciled. It may result in awkward attempts of reconciliation, or more radically, in a robust form of skepticism for which no treatment is currently available.

In the present article, I shall review first the reasons why a neuroscientific approach of depression may be judged unsatisfactory and then consider how we could defend it. What I call a neuroscientific approach is a view in which depression is seen as an impairment of the joint activity of crucial brain regions, as the product of a "depressive neural network". This view can be understood as a development of the neuroscientific tradition of symptom localization (Mayberg 2009) and of the mechanistic decomposition of the mind-brain in key processes and components (Bechtel and Richardson 2010). It is worth noting that this view may be challenged on grounds other than an anti-naturalistic stance: in particular, the idea that some kind of chemical imbalance is the origin of depression (for an historical perspective: see Healy 1997, Chapter 5) may suit advocates of reductionism (Bickle 2003), according to whom we should focus directly on the lower-level components and activities that are studied by molecular neuroscience, such as serotonin reuptake. But even if we leave aside theoretical alternatives to a reductionist view of explanation in neuroscience (Craver 2007), it is striking that progress in antidepressant pharmacological treatment is often judged "limited" (Holtzheimer and Mayberg 2011). Moreover, depressive relapse following the end of such treatment along with the high number of patients who do not respond to antidepressant drugs remain major medical problems. In this context, it is no coincidence that new neurobiological models of depression with innovative therapeutic implications are proposed (Mayberg 1997; Drevets et al. 2008) and updated (Mayberg 2009). My own view will be, first, that these recent circuit models of depression are not idle theoretical constructs, but that their significance depends ultimately on a correct understanding of what corresponding physiological mechanisms are for. Second, I shall argue that to develop a neurobiology of depression, a prior analysis of mood and affective states may be useful where we try to identify which questions are worth asking. Consequently, I suggest that philosophy of psychiatry and philosophy of mind become closely related.

The title of this paper is intended as a reference to the 1621 classic work by Burton, *The Anatomy of melancholy* (Burton 1621), but also to the title of the pioneering PET scan study of Bench and colleagues "The anatomy of melancholia: focal abnormalities of cerebral blood flow in major depression" (Bench et al. 1992) and to the subtitle of an article by Wayne C. Drevets, who has made a significant contribution to the development of fMRI studies of depression: "Functional Neuroimaging studies of depression: the anatomy of melancholia" (Drevets 1998). Melancholia is here seen as the affective side of depressive disorders in general, not as a distinct clinical entity. The debate about whether or not we should consider melancholia (or 'endogenous depression') as a mood disorder distinct from major depression has not been settled yet and has even become more intense during the preparation of the DSM-5 (Parker et al. 2010; Healy 2013). The present paper does not take sides in this controversy. The key issue here is not classification based on clinical and biological features. It is how (and under which conditions) neuroscience fits in the broad explanatory project of psychiatry. In this case, the target of the explanation is the pattern of recurrent, harmful disturbances of affective life that is typically shared by depressive disorders.

## Depression and the Brain: The Skeptical View

There are at least three kinds of reasons why findings about the brains of patients suffering from depression could be welcomed with caution. The first kind has to do with the central role of neuroimaging methods in investigations that focus on the depressive brain (Gotlib and Hamilton 2008). The conclusions of these investigations have suggested crucial roles for structures like the amygdala, parts of the anterior cingulate cortex and dorsolateral prefrontal cortex. Meanwhile, working models like the model of limbic-cortical dysregulation (Mayberg 1997), where increased subgenual cingulate activity and decreased dorsolateral prefrontal activity are correlated, have been proposed. We could, for one, remain skeptical about the significance of neuroimaging studies of depression, as they have been conducted since the 1990s, on general methodological grounds. As they reveal differences in regional blood flow related to neural activity, and not neural activity itself, it may be that imaging techniques do not provide us with a picture of regional brain activity as accurate as it is supposed to be. Stressing that this point does not imply, in itself, that depression has no biological dimension, or that research about brain states in the context of depression, is by itself misguided. Pointing out that we don't know enough about x because of the intrinsic limitations of a given technique (which is supposed to give us access to x) is not claiming that x does not exist or that x has no intrinsic significance. But it is clear that there is an ongoing debate about brain imaging techniques (Logothetis 2008; Roskies 2008; Forest 2014). In principle, one may believe that depression has a biological nature and hold, however, that to get a picture of a given pattern of regional blood flow is far from enough to understand the corresponding brain activity (Hardcastle and Stewart 2002). Secondly, we can also doubt that images of the brain are by themselves revelatory in the context of depression because of the ambiguous relation between what is shown by a given picture of the brain and the corresponding depressive state. According to Kessler and his colleagues (Kessler et al. 2011), images do reveal differences between the brain of patients suffering from depression and the brain of control subjects, but the special features of the depressed brain may be understood (a) as neural predispositions (non sufficient conditions), (b) as genuine etiological factors, (c) as mere consequences of episodes of depression, or (d) as compensatory brain mechanisms. Reduction of hippocampal volume, for instance, may be a consequence of depression, and decreased amygdala-frontal connectivity, a factor of susceptibility. As a consequence, it is not impossible that explanatory models of depression based on fMRI studies often count as genuine etiological factors that should be considered as predispositions, mere consequences of depression or byproducts of the disorder with or without a compensatory role. Accordingly, it is plausible that many neural correlates of depression have no explanatory relevance (Craver 2007) because they have no causal role in the production of a given psychological or behavioral feature of depression. It is legitimate to question our current ability to disentangle these different factors.

The second kind of reason has to do with the relation between psychological and neurobiological levels of analysis. In standard medical practice, the presence of depression is defined by diagnostic criteria, and it may be tempting to think that we could substitute a brain-based approach for this symptom-based approach. If depression is a well-defined medical category, and if neuroscience is able to identify the neural signature of depression (or what the philosopher Robert C. Roberts would call its "neurological map"), one can think that brain research will be able to address two key issues: knowing what depression is, and knowing who is (really) depressed. Knowledge of deep neurobiological causes would supersede knowledge of mere psychological epiphenomena. But this is also dubious. The first observation we could make is that neurobiological mechanisms involved in depression may be mechanisms that are not unique to it; as a consequence, a different basis for diagnosis does not mean that we shall be on firmer ground when we speak of depression, but rather that we may adopt a revisionary attitude where the very existence of depression as a legitimate medical entity would be challenged. A new entity would be, for instance, disorders of the neurobiological system that has the function to mediate and regulate negative affects. As parts of the medial prefrontal cortex are components of such a system, and as the altered functioning of these parts has been implicated both in depression (Drevets 2000) and post-traumatic stress disorder (Shin et al. 2005), we would have reason to revise or eliminate usual diagnostic categories, rather than reason to give them a neurobiological basis (Meier, in Forgeard et al. 2011). What should be noted, however, is that in this case, nothing tells us that it will be easier to agree on "natural" categories if we try to define them in terms of neurobiological systems rather than constellations of symptoms: because of the many causal roles that may be ascribed to the same brain regions, because of ubiquitous mutual and reentrant connections in the brain, because of the many criteria we could use to define a given neural system, because of the lack of correspondence of such systems with traditional, gross anatomical divisions, we could end up with as many disputes about the boundaries of a given system (and its pathologies) as about our current clinical entities.

The second observation we could make is that, whether or not the neurobiological enquiry takes this dramatic, revisionary turn, it could be that there is no neurobiological knowledge of depression that is not only related to, but also dependent on, clinical knowledge and psychological analysis. According to Robert C. Roberts (Roberts 2003), the neurological analysis of emotions is to its conceptual analysis what a physical analysis of sound patterns are to the corresponding musical analysis of a work of music. Just as it is only if he has some kind of understanding of musical concepts that an expert acoustician will be able to make sense of a physical account of a symphonic piece, it is only because he has an understanding of the psychological significance of given neural events that a neuroscientist will be able to make sense of his discoveries about, for instance, the amygdala. One description is no substitute for the other, and that would hold for brain knowledge of mood disorders as well. The psychological lexicon of ordinary descriptions of negative moods, as well as familiar, narrative explanations of why they occur would be ineliminable: they would possess, in particular, both the relevant conceptual framework and the appropriate level of generality.

The third source of reservation about the alleged benefits of the ongoing neurobiological enquiry would come from the problem of the boundaries of depression. Heated recent debates about false positives due to over-inclusive diagnostic criteria, and about the potential consequences of the removal of the bereavement exclusion clause in the DSM-5 (Wakefield and First 2012), are testimony enough that this is not a purely academic and theoretical debate. In their influential book, Horwitz and Wakefield have argued that symptomatology alone is unable to distinguish between normal sadness as it is motivated by a loss and depression as a mental disorder (Horwitz and Wakefield 2007). It is very doubtful, with the current state of our knowledge of the depressive brain, that pointing to intrinsic neurobiological differences is in itself sufficient to settle the issue. As it is plausible that brain correlates of sadness and brain correlates of depression will have much in common (for the corresponding evidence, see Mayberg et al. 1999), we may have to deal with two kinds of undesirable but plausible cases. First, if some pattern, which we will refer to as P1, is understood as suggesting depression, then some may argue that P1 includes only non-essential differences from normal brain functioning. Second, if another pattern, P2, is understood as suggesting normal sadness, it is also possible that others will claim that it is only because, for instance, the level of activation in key region R that is considered sufficient to reveal some dysregulation is far too high; the consequence being that P2 is in fact the sign of a marked disruption of affective brain systems that remains ignored because of a flawed interpretation of data. Brain science, then, if symptomatology is ambiguous, may fail to effectively solve the demarcation problem. In these dubious cases, even equipped with the most-advanced technology, we would be back to the solution of Horwitz and Wakefield: only the context of the emergence of symptoms, and how they evolve with time, will allow us to make a well-motivated distinction between normal sadness and depression.

## Beyond Mere Correlates

Confronted with the results of fMRI studies of depression, the skeptic is ready to point out (a) that there is only a "limited overlap" between regions that have been identified by different neuroimaging studies of depression (Fitzgerald et al. 2008), and (b) that the status of these alleged "neural correlates" of the disorder remains ambiguous. However, differences in experimental techniques and populations of patients may explain why only a few regions are consistently identified by different types of studies. Second, conclusions of such studies should not be considered apart from evidence coming from other kinds of research. Moreover, it would be unfair to judge the evidential base of brain-working models of depression on the conclusions of PET and fMRI studies alone. Let's consider, for instance, reports made about the consequences of brain lesions. Neuroimaging studies have suggested that abnormal patterns of activation of parts of the prefrontal cortex (PFC) play a role in the pathogenesis of depression. To support the view that ventromedial PFC hyperactivity and dorsolateral PFC hypoactivity do play such a role, it is possible to consider the consequences of strokes and injuries that impair the functioning of these regions. A study by Koenigs and colleagues (Koenigs 2008) suggests that bilateral lesions in the dorsolateral PFC cortex confer increased vulnerability to depression, while bilateral lesions in the ventromedial PFC are associated with low levels of depression. Even if inferences from local lesions to functional specialization are always dubious because of the complexity of the functional architecture of the brain (Sporns et al. 2000), this kind of study adds support to causal interpretations of fMRI results, if we adopt a view of causal relations where A is causally related to B if and only if an intervention on A modifies B (Woodward 2003). Local lesions play the role of "natural interventions" and even if we take into account possible side effects of focal lesions, it is reasonable to think that this kind of study may help disambiguate fMRI results.

Even more interesting are the reasons offered by Mayberg (Mayberg 2009) to ascribe a critical role to a specific brain component, the subcallosal cingulate gyrus (SCC, Brodmann area 25, with parts of areas 24 and 32) in the complex neural network involved in depression.

1. SCC activity has been repeatedly observed as a correlate of acute negative affective states;
2. SCC is one of the regions where metabolic effects can be identified in a context of clinical improvement due to antidepressant treatment, while hyperactivity in SCC is characteristic of treatment-resistant patients;

3. Cellular abnormalities have been observed in the subgenual region in patients suffering from mood disorders: in particular, a reduced number of glial cells, which are cells that play a crucial role in physiological processes essential to normal neural activity (Ongür et al. 1998);
4. There are efferent and afferent connexions of the SCC with regions like the insula, brainstem and hypothalamus, suggesting a regulatory role for SCC in physiological activities responsible for circadian rhythm and appetite;
5. Deep brain stimulation targeting directly the SCC has yielded marked effects, in contrast with regions that are anatomically close to it.

Ascribing a crucial role to the SCC region in an extended neural network, then, is trying to make sense of a large body of data, as much as it is a part of a therapeutic strategy. Making sense of a large body of data aims in particular at finding a solution to the problem of the co-occurrence of apparently unrelated symptoms. This is an intended, general benefit of working models: for instance, on the one hand, the association between sad moods and impaired attention is well documented in the clinical literature; on the other hand, the increased activity in depression of the sub-genual cingulate region, characteristic of the experience of sadness, seems to deactivate regions known for their involvement in attentional processes (Mayberg et al. 1999). A functional model, then, has two closely related motivations: explaining why we have a given clinical profile, and making sense of the corresponding pattern of brain activation.

In a sense, a "circuit model" of depression is parasitic on a model of corresponding physiological functioning, as, for instance, it is only because SCC is connected to regions already known for their involvement in mood monitoring and mood regulation that we can expect, or understand why, its stimulation may have distinctive effects in these domains. But as it is in the context of research on depression that the physiological meaning of the SCC region begins to be understood, models of depression, in turn, help us to update and complete the description of mechanisms involved in the genesis and regulation of affective states. Accordingly, in agreement with what has been suggested by Moghaddam-Taaheri through her "broken-normal view" (Moghaddam-Taaheri 2011), progress in our understanding of pathological mechanisms of depression and of affective mechanisms are tightly linked. And to use a notion introduced by Kitcher (Kitcher 2003), as the research is moved by both epistemic and practical interests, the discovery of the role of the SCC region gets its "scientific significance" from both kinds of context.

## On Moods and Mood Regulation

Problems of the second and the third kind listed above (the relation between symptoms and brain mechanisms, the role of brain knowledge in the definition of the disorder) are probably deeper and more specific to depression research. The second suggestion I want to make is that recognizing the importance of the neuroscientific view of depression does not preclude that we need not only a psychological investigation, but also a prior conceptual analysis of affective states. I would even suggest that it is only if we have a better understanding of what affective states are that we can hope to shed some light on neural mechanisms that play a role in depression, and on the proper domain of affective disorders.

Oddly, philosophy of psychiatry is often divorced from the literature in philosophy of mind and moral philosophy about emotional states. However, it seems difficult to consider "emotion", "sadness", or "depression" as unproblematic terms associated with notions that would not be worth enquiring about. For instance, central to Horwitz and Wakelfield's view of depression is a certain idea of what sadness is as an emotion. The depressed individual would be depressed because what he experiences is similar to a normal (or proportionate) response to circumstances that usually yield sadness and grief, although his experience is due to the internal failure of the corresponding affective mechanisms. In this case, being authentically sad is being in a state (a) that has the appropriate relation to circumstances that justify it (the individual has reasons to be sad); (b) that is the product of affective mechanisms that have the function to detect negative events and to adjust one's emotional response to them. The understanding of depression, then, is subordinate to an understanding of emotional life.[1] But we should note several things. First, depression is usually considered a mood disorder, rather than an emotional disorder. When a Capgras patient is not emotionally aroused by the presence of a person he is close to, one can think that there is some kind of underlying disturbance of emotional mechanisms: the symptoms have to do with the appraisal of a given, specific situation, while depression has an intrinsic dimension of generality. Moreover, direct lesions to brain parts that are essential to emotional mechanisms do not typically lead to depressive states (Mayberg 2003). Perhaps, then, sadness and emotional responses to specific events are not the most appropriate starting point when we consider depression as affective state, whereof we would like to give a proper and independent description.

Second, philosophers have made efforts to distinguish moods from emotions by using criteria that are less trivial and vague than duration. One of them is that emotions have a given intentional dimension, a proper object, while the same is not obviously true or paradigmatically true of moods. This has led to several suggestions: moods are objectless, they are identified by the way we feel, not by reference to a specific object or collection of objects (Armon-Jones 1991); moods are there to tell us about our situation in general, rather than to detect a given change in our environment, as it is the case with emotions (Prinz 2004); when depression is an

---

[1] To say that depression should not be confused with experiences of intense sadness (due for instance, to a loss) does not mean that the fact that MDD is usually adversity-triggered is ignored. As Jerome Wakefield has convincingly shown (Wakefield 2015), in no way does the "bereavement exclusion" necessitate that grieving people cannot be diagnosed with depression. But to define tests in order to draw the line correctly between normal sadness and depression may be problematic: for instance, impairment in role functioning or even a feeling of worthlessness, if temporary, may not be a clear sign of a depressive, pathological state. This is why, to define depression, we may focus on the recurrence of the symptoms rather than on their specificity.

emotion, rather than a mere mood, it has something to do with the way we view our own future, being linked to "poor prospects" (Roberts 2003). Another distinction would be that emotions have reasons while moods may have mere causes (Roberts 2003): X may view his future in terms of poor prospects because he is tired, or because he is already in a melancholy mood, and he may rationalize his mood in terms of upcoming failure while the view of an upcoming failure is a mere consequence of his internal disposition, not a cause for it. Being in a negative affective state without a proper reason is no sign of disorder by itself, as it may be a consequence of the normal variability of our affective dispositions, and a sign of our sensitivity to external events, like bad weather, internal events, and exhaustion. Starting with an analysis of mood, rather than a reference to sadness, could lead us to a different view of depression.

Another interesting feature of moods is that they have the ability to alter one's disposition and one's answer to external events. This is what Griffiths has expressed in asserting "they cause global changes in propensities to occupy other states and to respond to stimuli" (Griffiths 1997); this could be understood, at the neurobiological level, in terms of modification of the "the probability of transitions between a given input, internal states, and output" (ibid., p. 255). Moods usually persist, pervade our mental life, and have non-specific causal powers such as when they modulate our emotional response to environmental changes. For instance, were I not in the mood in which I am now, I would not respond to somebody's demand as I do (Roberts 2003, pp. 114–115). The association of negative moods with mood-congruent representations in working-memory is a phenomenon well known to psychologists (Siemer 2005). To sum up, I would define melancholy as the combination of two features: it is a state of mind with a character similar to sadness that may persist without reason, and it is a kind of disposition to negative appraisals of events and stimuli.

One source of confusion in the literature is that depression, as we have just seen, may be considered in some cases as an emotion, rather than a mood; and second, that usually philosophers of mind are not concerned with the question of what is pathological and what is not when they deal with emotions and moods. But these confusions are not inevitable. We can distinguish between (a) depression as an emotional state, the consequence of the negative appraisal of a given event to which I am not indifferent (I am depressed about something and I have good reasons to be so), (b) melancholy, as the mood that we have defined above, with no intrinsic pathological character, and (c) melancholia as the harmful propensity to remain in such a mood or to return to it, a propensity that is typical of depressive disorders. This would be, I think, in full agreement with the recent proposal of Holtzheimer and Mayberg: "We [...] propose that the primary abnormality of depression is not the depressive state itself, but rather the inability to appropriately regulate that state" (Holtzheimer and Mayberg 2011). The dimension of disorder does not come, then, from an additional qualitative character of symptoms, or from a lack of reasons to be sad. It comes from a "recycling" of negative thought in rumination, rather than from the negative content per se. In line with Griffiths' suggestion, this can be understood as a modified probability of transition between states, where the individual becomes unable to alter his mood, to regain his concentration or his appetite, or to escape anhedonia and find new sources of pleasure. The failure of many antidepressant treatments would come from the fact that they are able to "shift a patient out of the depressive state without preventing reentry into that state" (Holtzheimer and Mayberg 2011). But then we need to know much more about what affective regulation consists in and how we could analyze it in cognitive terms. If (or when) inhibition of irrelevant processes and contents is crucial, depression may be understood in reference to executive (dys)function, and disorders of selective attention. If (or when) depression results from diminished reappraisal of negative emotions, this may be conceived in reference to metacognition (X is unable to form second-order thoughts about his negative feelings that would help him to regulate his mood), and therapies aiming at the development of metacognitive abilities of patients may be promising (Segal et al. 2006). It is possible that there is some room for variability here, and that, if affective regulation may follow more than one path, this could lead to different styles of depressive thought.

Moreover, this analysis of moods and mood regulation may suggest interesting questions for neuroscience, or help us to select the most interesting studies or the most promising lines of research from the trove of current literature. Instead of looking for neural correlates of intense sadness, or dark moods, or specific symptoms, we may look for neural systems involved in affect regulation, reappraisal, selective attention, and inhibition of negative thoughts. For instance, why we have reasons to care about the neural correlates of the inhibition of negative stimuli, like the increased activation of the rostral anterior cingulate cortex –rACC, in depressive patients (Eugène et al. 2010), is because psychological investigation suggests that what is essential to depression in many cases is not an initial orientation towards negative stimuli, but the difficulty to disengage one's attention from them (Joormann and Gotlib 2010).

Conceptual analysis, then, may help us determine relevant questions neuroscience can address and how we should characterize the corresponding mechanisms. Neural correlates of depression are only intelligible if they are the harmful alteration of mechanisms of which we understand the usual output and purpose; and there is no interesting characterization of such an output that is not at least compatible, if not derived from, our understanding of our emotional life. If depression is a vicious circle, it is not emotion, but reappraisal, not mood itself, but affective regulation, of which it is important to discover and understand the specific neural conditions. The idea would be of a mutual benefit: on the one hand, conceptual analysis of our mental life may help us to single out the most interesting questions – what is worth being investigated, like reappraisal and affect regulation – and on the other hand, finding which neural circuits are involved in the pathogenesis of depression will constrain our analysis of what goes wrong in depression at a psychological level.

Lastly, it may be possible to articulate different kinds of explanations: for instance, social sciences may identify environmental conditions that heighten the frequency of melancholy moods; moral philosophy can add to our understanding of the link between our moods and our concerns or prospects; and the most decisive contribution of neuroscience would be to explain how these moods supersede other kinds of affective states and where the powerlessness of the individual (in terms of mood regulation) may come from. Social sciences would deal with kinds of risk exposure, moral philosophy with the relations between self-perception and affective life, neurobiology with the vicious circle in which the individual is trapped in depression.

## Conclusion: Acoustics and Musical Thought

A neuroscientific model of depression like the one offered by Mayberg may appear unappealing, or irrelevant, for two main reasons. The first is that depression is no ordinary pathology: there is something deeply unbelievable, or even offensive, in the idea that things as intimate as negative mood and anhedonia may have something to do with the relations between the anterior insula, the dorsomedial thalamus and the midbrain ventral tegmental area, as they are pictured on a diagram: in these matters, detail, and neuroscientific jargon seem only to make things worse. As a patient says (quoted by Kleinman 1988, 87): "Depression may be the disease, but it's not the problem. The problem is my life". However, when a life is plagued by depression, it may be because of a downward spiral whereof a neuroscientific description may be both relevant and useful. The second reason is that for a philosopher it may seem reasonable to think that either neuroscience is an optional complement to our understanding of affective life, or if it has to be taken more seriously, it is only in the context of a kind of radical eliminativism where hard science will supersede the concepts of folk psychology. But, to use Roberts' metaphor already mentioned above, if the science of acoustics does not eliminate musical aesthetics, it does not mean that the two have to remain forever on two different levels, that the science of sounds does not contribute anything substantial to music as an art. Recent history tells us that composers who have learned about the properties of sound waves are able to rethink musical composition and conceive new kinds of musical patterns, as has been the case with spectral music. In a similar way, it is not impossible that, in addition to its current and future therapeutic applications, a neuroscientific account of depression may stimulate philosophical thought about our affective life and expand our understanding of ourselves.

## References

Armon-Jones, C. (1991). *Varieties of affect.* Toronto/Buffalo: University of Toronto Press.
Bechtel, W., & Richardson, R. (2010). *Discovering complexity. Decomposition and localization as strategies in scientific research* (2nd ed.). Cambridge, MA: MIT Press/Bradford Books.
Bench, C. J., et al. (1992). The anatomy of melancholia: Focal abnormalities of cerebral blood flow in major depression. *Psychological Medicine, 22*(3), 607–615.
Bickle, J. (2003). *Philosophy and neuroscience: A ruthlessly reductionistic account.* Dordrecht: Kluwer.

Brown, G. W., & Harris, T. (1978). *Social origins of depression. A study of psychiatric disorders of women*. New York: The free press.

Burton, R. (1621/1989). *The anatomy of melancholy. What it is, what it is, with all the kinds, causes, symptomes, prognostickes and severall cures of it*. Oxford: Clarendon Press.

Conrad, P. (2007). *The medicalization of society*. Baltimore: Johns Hopkins University Press.

Craver, C. (2007). *Explaining the brain*. Oxford: University press.

Drevets, W. C. (1998). Functional neuroimaging of depression: The anatomy of melancholia. *Annual Review of Medicine, 49*, 341–361.

Drevets, W. C. (2000). Neuroimaging studies of mood disorders. *Biological Psychiatry, 48*, 813–829.

Drevets, W. C., Price, J. L., & Furey, M. L. (2008). Brain structural and functional abnormalities in mood disorders: Implications for neurocircuitry models of depression. *Brain Structure and Function, 213*, 93–118.

Ehrenberg, A. (2009). *The weariness of the self. Diagnosing the history of depression in the contemporary age*. Montreal: McGill Queen University Press.

Ehrenberg, A. (2016). Beyond depression: personal equation from the guilty to the capable individual (chap. 3). In J. C. Wakefield, & S. Demazeux (Eds.), *Sadness or depression? International perspectives on the depression epidemic and its meaning*. Dordrecht: Springer.

Eugène, F., et al. (2010). Neural correlates of inhibitory deficits in depression. *Psychiatry Research, 181*(1), 30–35.

Fitzgerald, P. B., et al. (2008). A meta-analytic study of changes in brain activation in depression. *Human Brain Mapping, 29*(6), 683–695.

Forest, D. (2014). *Neuroscepticisme. Les sciences du cerveau sous le scalpel de l'épistémologue*. Paris: Ithaque.

Forgeard, M., et al. (2011). Beyond depression. *Clinical Psychology, 18*(4), 275–299.

Gotlib, I. H., & Hamilton, J. P. (2008). Neuroimaging and depression. Current status and unresolved issues. *Current Directions in Psychological Science, 17*(2), 159–163.

Griffiths, P. (1997). *What emotions really are*. Chicago: University of Chicago Press.

Hardcastle, V. G., & Stewart, C. M. (2002). What do brain data really show? *Philosophy of Science, 69*(3), 572–582.

Healy, D. (1997). *The anti depressant era*. Cambridge: Harvard University Press.

Healy, D. (2013). Melancholia: Past and present. *Canadian Journal of Psychiatry, 58*(4), 190–194.

Holtzheimer, P. H., & Mayberg, H. (2011). Stuck in a rut: Rethinking depression and its treatment. *Trends in Neuroscience, 34*(1), 1–9.

Horwitz, A. V., & Wakefield, J. C. (2007). *The loss of sadness. How psychiatry transformed normal sorrow into depressive disorder*. Oxford/New York: Oxford University Press.

Joormann, J., & Gotlib, I. H. (2010). Emotion regulation in depression: Relation to cognitive inhibition. *Cognition and Emotion, 24*(2), 281–298.

Kessler, H., Traue, H., & Wiswede, D. (2011). Why we still don't understand the depressed brain – not going beyond snapshots. *GMS Psycho-Social-Medicine, 8*, 1–6.

Kitanaka, J. (2011). *Depression in Japan: Psychiatric cures for a society in distress*. Princeton: Princeton University Press.

Kitanaka J. (2016). Depression as a problem of labor: Japanese debates about work, stress, and a new therapeutic ethos. In J. C. Wakefield, & S. Demazeux (Eds.), *Sadness or depression? International perspectives on the depression epidemic and its meaning*. Dordrecht: Springer.

Kitcher, P. (2003). *Science, truth and democracy*. Oxford: Oxford University Press.

Kleinman, A. (1986). *Social origins of distress and disease, depression, neurasthenia and pain in modern China*. New Haven: Yale.

Kleinman, A. (1988). *Rethinking psychiatry. From cultural category to personal experience*. New York: The Free Press.

Koenigs, M. (2008). Distinct regions of prefrontal cortex mediate resistance and vulnerability to depression. *The Journal of Neuroscience, 28*(47), 12341–12348.

Logothetis, N. (2008). What we can do and what we cannot do with fMRI. *Nature, 453*, 869–878.

Mayberg, H. (1997). Limbic-cortical dysregulation: A proposed model of depression. *Journal of Neuropsychiatry and Clinical Neurosciences, 9*, 471–481.

Mayberg, H. (2003). Modulating dysfunctional limbic-cortical circuits in depression: Towards development of brain-based algorithms for diagnosis and optimised treatment. *British Medical Bulletin, 65*, 196–207.

Mayberg, H. (2009). Targeted electrode-based modulation of neural circuits for depression. *The Journal of Clinical Investigation, 119*, 717–725.

Mayberg, H., Liotti, M., Brannan, S. K., McGinnis, S., Mahurin, R. K., Jerabek, P. A., Silva, J. A., Tekell, J. L., Martin, C. C., Lancaster, J. L., & Fox, P. T. (1999). Reciprocal limbic-cortical function and negative mood: Converging PET findings in depression and normal sadness. *American Journal of Psychiatry, 156*(5), 675–682.

Moghaddam-Taaheri, S. (2011). Understanding pathology in the context of physiological mechanisms: The practicality of a broken-normal view. *Biology and Philosophy, 26*, 603–611.

Nettle, D. (2004). Evolutionary origins of depression: A review and reformulation. *Journal of Affective Disorders, 81*, 91–102.

Ongür, D., Drevets, W., & Price, J. (1998). Glial reduction in the subgenual prefrontal cortex in mood disorders. *Proceedings of the National Academy of Science of the USA, 95*, 13290–13295.

Overstreet, D. H. (2012). Modeling depression in animal models. *Methods in Molecular Biology, 829*, 125–144.

Parker, G., Fink, M., Shorter, E., Taylor, M. A., Akiskl, A., Berrios, G., Bolwig, T., Brown, W., Carroll, B., Healy, D., Klein, D. F., Koukopoulos, A., Michels, R., Paris, J., Rubin, R. T., Spitzer, R., & Swartz, C. (2010). Whither melancholia? The case for its classification as a distinct mood disorder. *American Journal of Psychiatry, 167*(7), 745–747.

Prinz, J. (2004). *Gut reactions. A perceptual theory of emotions.* New York: Oxford University Press.

Roberts, R. C. (2003). *Emotions: An essay in aid of moral psychology.* Cambridge: Cambridge University Press.

Roskies, A. (2008). Neuroimaging and inferential distance. *Neuroethics, 1*, 19–30.

Segal, Z. V., et al. (2006). Cognitive reactivity to sad mood provocation and the prediction of depressive relapse. *Archive of General Psychiatry, 6*, 749–755.

Shin, L. M., et al. (2005). A functional magnetic resonance imaging study of amygdala and medial prefrontal cortex responses to overtly presented fearful faces in posttraumatic stress disorder. *Archives of General Psychiatry, 62*(3), 273–281.

Siemer, M. (2005). Mood-congruent cognitions constitute mood experience. *Emotion, 5*, 296–308.

Sporns, O., Tononi, G., & Edelman, G. M. (2000). Connectivity and complexity: The relationship between neuroanatomy and brain dynamics. *Neural Networks, 13*, 909–922.

Wakefield, J. C. (2015). The loss of grief: Science and pseudoscience in the debate over DSM-5's elimination of the bereavement exclusion. In S. Demazeux & P. Singy (Eds.), *The DSM-5 in Perspective: Philosophical Reflections on the Psychiatric Babel* (pp. 157–178). Dordrecht: Springer.

Wakefield, J., & First, M. B. (2012). Validity of the bereavement exclusion to major depression: does the empirical evidence support the proposal to eliminate the exclusion in DSM-5? *World Psychiatry, 11*, 3–10.

Woodward, J. (2003). *Making things happen.* Oxford: Oxford University Press.

# Loss, Bereavement, Mourning, and Melancholia: A Conceptual Sketch, in Defence of Some Psychoanalytic Views

Pierre-Henri Castel

**Abstract** Today, arguing in favor of the psychoanalytic view of depressive states is likely to be hopeless, not so much for epistemological reasons, but because most contemporary clinicians (including many psychodynamically-oriented therapists) have lost sight of the intuitions at the core of the Freudian and post-Freudian visions of mourning and bereavement. This paper, through a close reading of one of Henry James's most praised short stories, almost a contemporary of Freud's work on melancholia, offers a detour back to the origin of this misunderstanding. It is a plea for the aesthetic, philosophical, and anthropological re-education of therapists, upstream from the conceptual quandaries that have plagued an ill-founded refutation of psychoanalytic views on depression.

When it comes to defending psychoanalytic views, the danger of misunderstanding is always great. But it does not so much arise because of their conceptual articulation, or of their empirical content; rather, it originates from the unavailability, for contemporary clinicians, of the "form of life," as Wittgenstein would have put it, within which the psychoanalytically relevant grammatical rules and factual regularities are smoothly interwoven, and provide a type of emotional and linguistic evidence which cannot be reached otherwise. So it should not come as a surprise if my point of departure is a literary one. For in what kind of world could Freudian views be better appraised than in the very world, and at the very time, they were designed and offered to the general debate?

In one of his most praised short stories, first published in 1895, "The Altar of the Dead," Henry James (1895/1984) presents two strikingly evocative characters. Stransom has lost his spouse-to-be, Mary Antrim, an undetermined number of years

I am especially grateful to Louis A. Sass, who revised the first draft of this paper, and helped me to overcome my reluctance to write about psychoanalysis in English. I also thank Steeves Demazeux and Jerry Wakefield for their precious comments.

P.-H. Castel (✉)
Centre National de la Recherche Scientifique (CNRS), Ecole des Hautes Etudes en Sciences Sociales (EHESS), Paris, France
e-mail: pierrehenri.castel@free.fr

© Springer Science+Business Media Dordrecht 2016
J.C. Wakefield, S. Demazeux (eds.), *Sadness or Depression?*
History, Philosophy and Theory of the Life Sciences 15,
DOI 10.1007/978-94-017-7423-9_8

before the plot unfolds. To the disconsolate memory of her, and for the needs of his private cult, he erects a magnificent shrine of light and tapers, in a church lost in a remote London neighbourhood: the altar of the Dead. There, one sad and gloomy evening, he meets a "nameless lady," not too much younger than himself, and "in mourning unrelieved," as James depicts her. The reader is at first struck by the close analogy of their predicaments, both spiritual and physical. Both exhibit the same moral pain in their bereavement, including enduring and pervasive sadness and world-weariness; both are bereft of all intimacy with friends and family; they show the same fidelity to their dear lost ones; they follow the same rites of mourning, speaking half-jokingly about their odd "community of service"; and they both inexorably age, barely coping with the dark prospect of their own termination.

The plot thickens as they unexpectedly realize, after years spent in prayer at the altar of the Dead, that one and only one man is the shared object of their most poignant ambivalence. His name is Acton Hague. A friend of Stransom, turned secret foe for reasons James artfully keeps in a hazy background, he appears to have been the mourning niece's lover, and the most distressful deception of her life—once again, we do not know why. As this paper is not intended to be a spoiler, I will say no more. Suffice it to say that François Truffaut made use of James' short story for the scenario of his 1978 film, *The Green Chamber*, and that Stransom comes to a tragic end, in an arch-typical melancholic abandonment of his own life, at the very minute the mourning niece finds her final relief, and opens her heart again, though rather unconsciously, to the possibility of life.

Here is the typically psychoanalytic question I will now try to articulate: why do most human beings, when bereaved, *painfully learn to live with their loss*, whereas a few others, who display the same behaviour, and who ache from the same depressive mood, *slowly die with their dead*?

A brief observation, made in passing in "The Altar of the Dead," will be my thread. Uncovering the abyss of their mutual misunderstanding, the mourning niece ponders: "We simply had different intentions". In other words, whatever may be the behavioural similarities, and the purely quantitative variations between depressive states lumped together for statistical purposes, we are still in need of an explanation for such dissimilar outcomes in bereavement. The underlying *intentional* structure of loss and bereavement endows them with an unmistakable clinical specificity. And this structure likely accounts for the *subjective* fate, in the long run, of these painful experiences. My first endeavour will be to make a bit more explicit what such an intentional analysis of loss and bereavement might be. For it somehow blurs the alleged clinical differences between "normal" and "pathological mourning," or between "major depressive disorder" with or without "psychotic features" and "melancholic features"—all classifications that take into account only observable and behavioural characteristics of depressive states. Conversely, such an intentional analysis of loss and bereavement might establish the grounds for a more psychologically significant difference between all these conditions.

The two fates of Stransom and "the mourning niece" are but an introduction to Freud's "Mourning and melancholia". Actually, I aim to show that some Freudian and post-Freudian views on these two conditions are best understood in the light of an intentional analysis of loss and bereavement. This entails a number of consequences, not for the pharmacological management of depressive states (once more, their purely behavioural components are similar all along), but for its relational and inter-subjective dimensions.

So which are the grounds for an intentional description of depressive states in psychoanalysis?

## Abraham's 1912 View on Melancholia

There is a constant that runs through all psychoanalytic theories of depression: depression is seen as a form of (forbidden) hate towards some external object, which backfires onto the self in a punitive way. I contend that this process makes sense only if its inherent intentionality is taken into account. Intentionality, here, does not refer to "intending to do something," wilfully, and with a goal; rather, it is the more abstract and more mental "aboutness" we find in the relation of a mind to its objects.

Karl Abraham's 1912 framing of that idea was the following (Abraham 1953): Melancholics cannot repress their hostile impulses, so projection is their last line of defence. But they cannot keep their hate at bay through projection—that is, fix it for good in the external world, according to the classic paranoid pattern of persecutors, who, however, usually guess as if "from within" what the patient is about to do in order to escape the persecutors' evil intents. That is the reason why these aggressive motions backfire onto the self, inducing the typical feeling of being justly punished even for non-existent or trivial misdeeds. In this way, Abraham envisioned melancholia as paranoia in reverse, as a self-persecution. And melancholics do look oddly shameless in their self-reproach—until you realize *who else* they are actually attacking under the cover of self-accusation. But why such a reversal of paranoia? Because the roots of melancholia are to be found in the subject's "ambivalence". The hated object is also (and remains) a loved object. Hence, the weight of hatred must ultimately fall back upon that loving self, who cannot cope with the negative side of his or her ambivalence through repression, and who must therefore be punished for it. This is just what happens to Stransom with respect to his former friend Hague.

## Grammatical and Psychological Coordinates of Intentionality

Beyond the literary or clinical context, the idea that depressive feelings are but "inverted" aggressive impulses emerges in various ways. Both in French and in English, one can provide good examples of this reversal. For example, the English "grief", means "grievance" in French.

This is not a mere coincidence. To borrow philosopher John L. Austin's distinction, the illocutionary content of aggressive utterances is usually replete with perlocutionary effects of the depressive kind, and vice versa. For, whatever we intend to convey, the very fact of saying "You make me sad" to somebody often expresses not so much sadness as anger and resentment. Reciprocally, we may cry out of moral pain when shouting, "I hate you so much" to a loved one. From a more psychological standpoint, sadness is often consciously experienced as an inward rage barred from public display; anger, similarly, when not fully acted out, commonly reverts to grief and feelings of helplessness. Finally, children (and dominated people as well) appear to be highly sensitive to the actual possibility of openly displaying either their resentment or their moral pain. The opposition of inward *vs.* outward feelings will often reflect socially coded constraints on the legitimacy of the public exhibition of affective states. Agitated and violent children may actually be sad, while passive or submissive women, internally consummated with rage.

But there is more to the matter, as Abraham suggested. And this will help us to understand the intentional aspect of this projective reversal of aggression into self-aggression (with depression as self-punishment). In fact, this reversal does not imply a fuzzy affective transmutation of outward hate into inner depressive feelings, but, rather, two distinct processes:

1. A semantic reversal of "to love" into "to hate"
2. A grammatical permutation of the subject and the object of the verb.

In this process, "I love you" first turns into "I hate you" (ambivalence), and then (via projection), "I hate you" turns into "You hate me" (and hence, I feel dejected, valueless, saddened, and the like).

But what exactly is this double process meant to explain? Following Abraham, it explains why self-persecution is so intense and perspicuous in melancholia. The subject "knows" all too well which secret aggressive impulses he or she should not have even conceived of, which were addressed to whom, and why they were ultimately returned upon him. Even if he is not conscious of all this, the stringent, inescapable, and torturing directedness of self-reproach makes it unmistakable in itself.

To this extent, the biology of mood disorders cannot be the end of the story. If, on the one hand, we suspect a grammatically ordered transformation of sadness into aggression, and, on the other hand, have some ground to connect it to the social context of our moral life, we need nothing more to suggest the possibility that our affective states may well follow some intentional patterns as well as causal neurobiological laws.

## Affective vs. Epistemic Intentionality

But what kind of "aboutness" is this? Or, in philosophical parlance, what kind of object-directedness or intentionality does it demonstrate?

Certainly not epistemic intentionality, such as the one linking, for instance, a belief to the state of affairs being believed. In epistemic intentionality, the object must precede the intention directed to it. One cannot believe in a state of affairs one knows for sure to be false. To believe something is to believe that something is true—objectively true. The intentionality I am referring to, by contrast, is an *affective* intentionality. But as we know, being desirable, lovable, hateful, is neither an intrinsic nor an objective property of anything. Desirability originates from the subjective desire that aims at or targets the desired thing. So when one considers whether one "truly" wishes anything, one does not look at the desired object, but at oneself. By contrast, when one checks whether one "truly" believes in something or not, one pays attention to its objective properties. Thus, if holding-for-true requires objective grounds, holding-for-good originates from our subjective intent.

More: our wish to believe usually prevails over belief. This is wishful thinking: if we cannot believe in something because it is false or because it does not exist, we hallucinate it. We just create out of nothing, or rather, out of ourselves (projectively), the missing content of a representation, and this plays the same role in our thinking processes that a well-grounded referential picture of reality would normally play.

## Freud: A Two-Level Model of the Mourning Self

Here enters the bizarre and seductive idea put forth both by Freud and Abraham: not only do we hallucinate what we wish to believe, but, through projection, we even substitute ourselves for the non-existent object of our projection. The hallucinating subject, at the culmination of the projective process, somehow becomes the hallucinated object. And the less we have on the object's side, the more the subject is doomed to provide of its own substance as a compensation for the non-existence, or paucity, of its objective counterpart. In other words, as soon as we accept the ultimate affective privacy of bereavement, there is no limit to the inner closeness of the lost loved object we wishfully hope to still exist. That is, when the object is forever lost, we tend to identify ourselves with it, and we incorporate it so as to make it live and exist out of our own flesh and blood. But this implies that there will always be a slippery slope from:

1. Becoming in the name of love the lost object, in order to keep it within us and;
2. Losing ourselves within the lost object, out of love for it.

Once again, such formulas ought not to be taken as the descriptions of a psychological mechanism—even though Abraham drew a nightmarish picture of such a mechanism, in which the mourner "eats" its object, or, conversely, is "eaten" by it, and feels himself "excreted" by it (or dejected). More simply, the formulas specify within which logical boundaries affective states can transform into each other. They preserve the aboutness of these transformations (the specificity of their intentional objects) even as the mode (with what sort of mental attitude or direction of relationship the objects are related to) changes. And finally, they capture some poignant elements apropos of what we feel in grief, with a quite interesting nuance: if losing ourselves in merger with the lost object is an intrinsic possibility of our life, then, beyond sadness, a deep-seated anxiety also looms on the outer limits of true bereavement.

Freud's "Mourning and Melancholia" (1915–1917/1957) takes for granted:

1. Abraham's grammatical analysis of projection;
2. The parallel between mourning and melancholia, with two caveats, (a) the idea that in usual mourning, what we lost is obvious whereas outbreaks of melancholia are much more enigmatic, and (b) the fact that melancholia, unlike mourning, implies a strong ambivalence to the lost object;
3. Melancholia as paranoia in reverse.

But Freud goes much deeper than Abraham when he brings in his notion of narcissism, for he implies *two distinct levels of subject-object intentional relationship*. At the first level, the ego of the mourner develops its identification with the lost object—tainted with hallucinatory elements, of course, but still preserving a clear distinction between the ego and its loved object. The point is that, in Freud's view, the desperate need to save, at all cost, one's relationship to the love object, entails trespassing the clear distinction between the bereaved subject and its object. At some point, both collapse into one subject-object ("The *shadow* of the *object* fell upon the ego"). That new subject-object becomes, in turn, at the second level, the object of a certain valuation from another instance: the one responsible for moral conscience in everyday life, and which is in clinical accounts of guilt nothing but the super-ego.

Freud is eager to improve the plausibility of his view with a clinical parallel. He insists that in obsessional neurosis, the super-ego makes itself felt as the moral agent judging and condemning the relations between the subject and its desired objects, and calling for their repression. Here, the super-ego no longer condemns a *relationship*. It targets the very *identity* of the subject to its (lost) object, or the product of the so-called "narcissistic identification" of the mourner with its object. Consequently, when its dejection has reached its climax, the self really ejects itself as "one" (ego and super-ego together) in a frightening acting out. This ejection is often to be taken literally (think of the typical suicide of melancholics jumping out of a window without warning). In James' short story, Stransom identifies with the "one" taper missing from the array of the altar of the Dead, the one that could have stood for Hague. It would have been the only one taper meaningful to his fellow mourner. But so far, he had always denied it to her. Surrendering at last, he instantly follows Hague into death, to the niece's disbelief.

Hence Freud's construct makes room for a more complex view of depressive states than does the strictly behavioural approach. Depressive states may not differ merely in degree of intensity, for there may be qualitative and structural differences between major depressive states, and melancholia proper. Freud's construct also leaves open the question as to what exactly "self-esteem" and its loss in depression consist in. In my loss of self-esteem, do I mourn some obscure ideal trait of the lost love object I identified with? Or, rather, do I despise myself, and feel radically ashamed of the very fact of remaining still alive, whilst other valued people have died? Of course, we cannot answer such questions with a scale of psychomotor retardation; or by objectively assessing whether the supposed closeness of the lost object was delusional or not. We have to pay attention to the intentionality of loss. This is the rule of thumb of clinical sense and sensibility, and the only alternative to the "flight to objectivity" in mental matters.

## Melanie Klein's Critique of Freud

Freud's sketch also drew a set of critics from other psychoanalysts. Perhaps most prominent in this regard is Melanie Klein, with her reappraisal of Freudian mourning, through her use of her notion of the "depressive position" (Klein 1940; Leader 2008). Because of her idea of a "depressive position", which is in fact no pathology, but, on the contrary, a necessary step in all psycho-therapeutic transformation, Melanie Klein remains, without doubt, the most influential writer in the field of depression and psychoanalysis. Let me list a few of her objections to Freud:

1. Freud himself acknowledges that normal mourners always "rebel" against the mourning process. It is, after all, a highly paradoxical process, that must achieve detachment and renunciation to the lost object through a systematic and exhaustive re-investment of past memories (usually through idealization) in the process of their ultimate "de-cathexis". Yet, the more we think of our lost love ones, the less we want to let them part from us! Or, maybe, we just wish, at times, that we could expel the dead from our living mind. This is hard to see as a mere instance of a conflict between reality-testing and wishful thinking. Ambivalence obviously exists not only in melancholia, but in normal mourning as well. In James's story, the niece is clearly "ambivalent" with respect to her lost lover, Hague.
2. Is it so clear that in mourning, we know what we have lost, whereas in melancholia, the triggering factors remain hidden? Freud himself was not so sure. For it is unclear what exactly we mourn when we mourn somebody; at the same time, many melancholia outbreaks are easy to trace back to some manifest disillusion or moral wound.
3. Finally, Freud was compelled to admit to a *normal* form of "narcissistic identification". Before reaching the developmental level at which the ego enjoys a full-fledged capacity for loss, identifying with the lost object (orally absorbing it, in dream-like parlance) was, in fact, its only available coping mechanism. But this implies that what can be deemed a "regression" in melancholia was once a necessary ingredient of our psychic growth. And as infants, we had no other option.

The fruitful way to proceed is to envision the Kleinian development as a conceptual extension of Freud's ideas. In this respect, Melanie Klein put forward a number of important aspects, not previously mentioned by Freud, of bereavement and mourning:

1. First, she clearly envisioned that the template of "moral conscience" upon which Freud devised his version of the super-ego falls short of what his concept of narcissistic identification should have hinted to him. For if we are such stuff as narcissistic identifications are made on, our super-ego is formed much earlier than any moral conscience. The instance that either lauds or deprecates the mourning ego is nothing but the memory of past and insurmountable identifications with our first love objects (namely, the Oedipal ones, particularly for our arch-object, the first care-giver, the Mother).

2. This implies that, instead of one moral conscience, we have a whole internal
   world of past identifications and fantasied objects that serve as the very ideals for
   narcissistic identifications. This, of course, is but James's altar of the Dead itself:
   a beautiful presentation of all our lost "Others", as he literally puts it. But what
   does this imply? Mourning is no longer, as in Freud, a desperately private trial.
   Confronting our losses, we call out for help to our Oedipal figures, who mourn
   with us and within us. Our fantasized parents share our burden of grief, and they
   recall their past love to our bereaved self. Note that the dream language in which
   all this is expressed now incorporates the reassuring voice and the amicable gaze
   of our first love objects. At the climax of the short story, and before its final tragic
   turn, Mary Antrim's uncanny descent, as a radiant ghost, almost saved Stransom.
   But he could not take hold of this motherly and celestial hand, and instead
   slipped into death.

Losing someone, to sum up, is no longer a private experience turned in upon
itself. It conjures up an "inner world" of identifications, or of fantasied lost love
objects that have silently become parts of our selves, but which emerge and speak
out when we are torn apart in bereavement. More precisely, the feeling of being
locked into one's grief, as a desperately lonely mourner, is true melancholia. Normal
mourning implies just the opposite: recalling a host of vivid self-memories. This is
why Melanie Klein reads Freud's famous motto, "in mourning, the world is empty,
in melancholia, the ego itself is deserted", precisely the other way round. "In melancholia", Melanie Klein might suggest, "our inner world shrinks down like a
shagreen (think of the French "peau de chagrin", and of Balzac's 1831 short story),
while in normal mourning, the ego copes with the loss of its object thanks to the
strength and vividness of its deeper narcissistic base".

One crucial consequence is the following: depressive states are to be evaluated in
light of their intentional content (*what* is lost *to whom*?). But they are also endowed
with an intrinsic therapeutic quality. For depression goes with integration, and
detachment from love objects with new narcissistic layers of our affective self,
much deeper than what our ego is aware of. So loss in the outer realm implies re-
creation within the inner self. The "depressive position" is born out of this dynamic
process. It follows that the true *psychotic* depression which melancholia is can be
defined not as the failure of ordinary mourning, but as the failure to process our
ambivalence (or our anxiety about attacking the good object), through what Melanie
Klein called the "depressive position".

## Lacan and Anxiety in Mourning

One psychoanalyst specifically emphasized the role of anxiety in mourning: Lacan
(1962–1963/2004).

His starting point is the claim that mourning is not only the loss of a love object,
but the loss of someone *to whom* we were, or fantasized ourselves to be (no difference, here), a love object. As Stransom put it: "Mine are only the Dead who died

possessed *of* me" [my emphasis]. Mourning reveals the true dependence of human beings on each other: our love objects are subjects, and those whom we miss are themselves subjects whom we experience as missing us. It is important to recognize the reciprocity of loss. For among the torturing questions we raise in mourning are surely these: "What would the dead person have thought of this? What would he or she have liked me to do?" What we were *for* the dead, and the plain fact that such a question is now forever without an answer, instills anxiety in mourning. Conversely, a sign that mourning is over, and loss consummated, is the moment when we realize how strange, and even how alien *to us*, was the very person we loved, and whom we thought of as loving us. We lived by him or her, and we never understood how poorly we knew him, what he actually wanted of us. At this turning point, we know that we have parted from that person for good. Sadness is gone, and with it, all the anxiety attached to what the lost person may have thought and wished about us, and which could have been a source of guilt and resentment towards him. The niece's salvation relies upon this, in James' tale. At the very last, she sees that Hague was not the "One" she must love better than her own living love. Freed of anxiety to disappoint her lost lover, she breathes again, alas, at the very moment Stransom succumbs to what Henry James calls his "malady of life."

Being a human being and living in a symbolic order, Lacan suggests, means that we cannot separate what the "Others", be they dead or alive, are *to us*, from what we are *to them*. Hence, our Oedipal identifications depend on kinship, and on what it prescribes, both emotionally and in terms of social subordination. What may seem an oddity, the bi-directionality of loss in mourning, actually manifests the way the individual's mental and affective life is woven into social networks that extend far beyond what we are consciously aware of. This is why, to our amazement, we may feel *more anxious than sad* in mourning. And it may even be the case, even more counter-intuitively, when the lost person is *not* one we loved, but one whose putative desires and expectations were much more meaningful to us than what we ever thought.

Lacan's view of anxiety in mourning, to this extent, radicalizes the Kleinian stance. For the Kleinian "inner world" of past projective/narcissistic identifications is better understood as a "symbolic world", a world of enduring social re-creation of what we mean to each other. Going all the way through the paradoxical mourning process, namely, painfully re-investing all our memories of the lost object so that at the end we can detach ourselves from it, finally turns up as a cultural task. We must erect an "altar" in our memory, a monument that both enshrines the lost object as "good", and forgiven, and that marks an impassable frontier between it and us, a line which prevents it from eliciting our regrets any further. Our individualistic societies are perhaps not the best place to understand this, for we usually collapse the time for private grief and mourning, and the time for the collective rites of funerals. But what are funerals in societies that celebrate them at a distinct moment of time, namely, as a closing chapter of the mourning period? It is the time when the Dead are ascribed to their symbolic place, whence they shall never return. Thus funerals are intended to soothe not grief, but *anxiety* about intentions of the Dead. They relieve the haunted mourner, not his sadness. And this, once again, is a social process. It is not the kind of process Freud or Melanie Klein would have conceived of, but only

Lacan, who regarded the Unconscious as the "Other's discourse" rather that existing within a private psyche, and who thought of symbols as elements of language and shared collective representations to which, as subjects, we are all "subjected".

## Concluding Remarks

Let me sum up my argument about the irreducibility of intentionality in mourning and in melancholia, for it epitomizes the contribution of psychoanalysis to the issue of depression.

1. If we rely on solely behavioural criteria, there is no way to make the crucial distinction between two distinct meanings and psychological experiences of depressive states: one which is t*o painfully learn to live with our loss* (normal mourning), and the other, which is *to let oneself die with the dead* (melancholia as psychosis). Henry James's Stransom, on the one hand, and the "unnamed lady", on the other hand, typify both the behavioral indiscernibility of these two conditions, and their dramatically divergent outcomes.
2. Not only do we have to read loss as an *intentional* concept (focusing on its "aboutness"), as a loss "of x", as a loss "for me", but even as a loss of "the X (a subject) who lacks me". I suggest that a logico-grammatical analysis of loss and bereavement coincides, at least to some extent, with certain psychological traits of mourning (e.g. to its paradoxical process, its possible derailment in psychosis, its link to anxiety beyond sadness).

The Freudian challenge to contemporary treatments of depression (namely, cognitive-behavioral therapies) should now appear self-evident:

1. Psychoanalysis implies that there cannot be any "mourning work" in a melancholic patient; indeed, the impossibility of it is what rigorously defines this condition. This is paradoxical, for it is not literally Freudian, but rather Kleinian and Lacanian. Prodding such a patient into remembering his loss, with the goal of his finally overcoming it, will ultimately fail because such a patient lacks the full ability to maintain *within himself* what James called the "altar of the Dead". Any such reinforcement of his memories will entice him all the more into following his lost object into death—far from helping him to identify with the many affective links which connected him to it, as is the case with a maturing sense of self in normal mourning.
2. Instead of indiscriminately addressing "negative cognitions" and an oversimplified "loss of self-esteem", therapists should pay attention to their design. For instance, I would consider it significant to scrutinize the exact nature of negative cognitions *about* one's own negative cognitions. *Which self*, moreover, identified to what kind of inner objects, and sustained by which past narcissistic identifications, do we suppose in the background of the mourning process?
3. Far from regarding the culture of mourner as peripheral information, therapists should recognize that to mourn is an attempt to re-create a livable *symbolic*

world, a world that must survive the disappearance of an object intimately connected to a host of other lost emotional objects. It is not a brain-centered, nor an individual-centered process. For we are "ritual animals", as Wittgenstein aptly remarked, and we must be treated as such.

4. Last but not least, we should learn from the melancholy geniuses of art what the consummation of loss actually consists in. Neither in the vanishing of sadness nor in its forceful voiding, but rather in the artful creation of an intrinsically artificial device: a *symbolic hole* within which a *whole world* can be both lost, and yet, somehow, survive.

# References

Abraham, K. (1912/1953). Notes on the psychoanalytical investigation and treatment of manic–depressive insanity and allied conditions. In *Selected papers on psychoanalysis* (Vol. I, pp. 137–156). New York: Basic Books.

Freud, S. (1915–1917/1957). Mourning and melancholia. In *The standard edition of the complete psychological works of Sigmund Freud* (Vol. XIV). London: Hogarth Press.

James, H. (1895/1984). The altar of the dead. In E. Wagenknecht (Ed.), *The tales of Henry James*. New York: Frederick Ungar Publishing Company.

Klein, M. (1940). Mourning and its relation to manic-depressive states. *International Journal of Psychoanalysis, 21*, 125–153.

Lacan, J. (1962–1963/2004). *Le Séminaire, livre X: L'angoisse*. Paris: Seuil. English edition: Lacan, J. (2014). *Anxiety: The seminar of Jacques Lacan, book X* (C. Gallagher, Trans.). Oxford: Polity.

Leader, D. (2008). *The new black: Mourning, melancholia, and depression*. London: Hamish Hamilton.

# Suffering, Meaning and Hope: Shifting the Focus from Depression in Primary Care

Christopher Dowrick

**Abstract** The diagnosis of depression is not fit for the purposes of primary care. It is inherently problematic, with regard to both validity and utility, and can be challenged on ethical and evolutionary grounds. It has iatrogenic effects, including reducing the sense of personal agency. These effects are exacerbated by GPs' deterministic explanatory metaphors, and aggravated in cross-cultural consultations which attempt to integrate experiences of traumatized self-identity within routine technical practices.

We need a theory of the person based not on medical assumptions of passivity but on awareness of personal agency. Two key concepts are coherence and engagement. Coherence involves an understanding of ourselves as consistent beings, persons with the capacity to lead our own lives. We make sense of ourselves in terms of our engagement with the world around us: this is crucial in creating and sustaining our sense of identity and well-being.

To provide high quality primary care for depressive feelings, we cannot limit ourselves to individualized biomedical perspectives. In our clinical encounters we do well to see depressive feelings through our patients' eyes. We should acknowledge suffering, explore meaning and offer hope. We need to incorporate concepts of agency and coherence within our dialogues with patients, expand social understandings of distress and encourage engagement at the community level.

## The Problem of Depression

Depression is commonly diagnosed in primary care. In a major international study on mental illness in general health care involving 15 centres across the world, the overall prevalence of current depression, using criteria of ICD-10, was estimated to be 10.4 % (Goldberg and Lecrubier 1995). In a study of general practice attenders in Montpellier, in France, 16.5 % met DSM-IV criteria for depressive disorders (Norton et al. 2009). Compared with standardised diagnostic criteria such as these,

C. Dowrick, M.D., FRCGP (✉)
University of Liverpool, Liverpool, UK
e-mail: cfd@liverpool.ac.uk

© Springer Science+Business Media Dordrecht 2016
J.C. Wakefield, S. Demazeux (eds.), *Sadness or Depression?*
History, Philosophy and Theory of the Life Sciences 15,
DOI 10.1007/978-94-017-7423-9_9

general practitioners (GPs) are more likely to over-diagnose than under-diagnose depression: for every 100 unselected cases seen in primary care, a meta-analysis of reported studies (Mitchell et al. 2009) estimates that GPs make 15 false positives diagnoses, miss 10 cases and identify 10 cases of depression.

There are apparent benefits in making the diagnosis of depression in primary care. Its existence enables researchers to generate epidemiological information about the prevalence and trajectory of the disorder. It provides clinicians with a basis for discriminating between different treatment options, and hence generating guidelines regarding clinical care (NICE 2009). It offers distressed people the possibility of exculpation, insofar as the diagnosis of a disease implies that symptoms are not the fault of the person suffering from them; and carries with it the implication that the medical profession will take responsibility for providing treatment and care (Killingsworth et al. 2010).

But the diagnosis of depression is inherently problematic with regard both to its validity, the extent to which it can be seen as a discrete entity with natural boundaries, and utility, the extent to which it reliably informs treatment decisions (Kendell and Jablensky 2003). It can be challenged on ethical and evolutionary grounds, and has potentially noxious effects.

## Problems of Validity

### Genetic Bases

The validity of the diagnosis cannot be predicated on a firm genetic basis, since evidence in this field is equivocal. While numerous studies indicate an interaction between genes (most commonly the 5-HTT gene) and environment in increasing the risk of depressive disorders (Caspi et al. 2003; Uher and McGuffin 2008), there is a need for caution in interpreting these findings (Munafò et al. 2009). Only a handful of specific genes have been identified, and further advances will require the analysis of hundreds of affected individuals and their families (Cowan et al. 2002). The effects of the 5-HTT gene are far from clear. Positive linkage of effects tends to be over-reported in small samples, and the combined analyses of multiple datasets, including a larger number of candidate genes and polymorphisms, will be necessary for an adequate assessment of the presence and impact of depression susceptibility genes (Levinson 2006). Genetic studies have not yet proved useful as a basis for disease biomarkers or approved diagnostic tests (Miller and O'Callaghan 2013).

Genetic variations are more related to generic than specific vulnerability. Associations have been found, for example, between short variations of the 5-HTT gene and predisposition to alcohol disorders (Pinto et al. 2008) and schizophrenia (Sáiz et al. 2007), while there is accumulating evidence for an overlap in genetic susceptibility across the traditional classification systems that divide schizophrenia from mood disorders (Craddock and Forty 2006).

All we can safely say at present is that there is some evidence to support the hypothesis that certain genetic and early environmental factors may predispose certain people to react more adversely than others to stressful experiences later in life. This does not give genetic support for a specific diagnosis of depressive disorder.

## Border Disputes

The current received wisdom that depression is a unitary concept derives from the position adopted by Akiskal and McKinney (1975). In a seminal paper they proposed that a large number of disparate conceptual models should be integrated within a unified framework, with the depressive syndrome 'conceived as the psychobiological final common pathway'.

However there are at least three current border disputes involving the diagnostic category of depression. In *Beyond Depression* (Dowrick 2009) I have characterised these as anti-imperialist, integrationist and fundamentalist. For the anti-imperialists, the borders between depression and other mental states are unclear. In consequence other diagnoses such as adjustment disorder are in serious danger of annexation or obliteration (Casey et al. 2001). Integrationists see depression's current borders as too small, narrow and rigid. They advocate diagnostic amalgamation with other mental states, arguing for overlap of depressive symptoms with normality, with anxiety (Shorter and Tyrer 2003), or with the symptoms of physical conditions. Fundamentalists take the opposite view. For them the state of depression is too large and unwieldy to be adequately defended. They advocate withdrawal to a safer, central heartland and provide evidence for discrete sub-sets of the depressive condition (Parker 2007a, b).

My own position is closest to the fundamentalists. I see the homogenisation of depression as a mistake (Dowrick and Frances 2013). I would resurrect the term *melancholia* to distinguish rarer and more severe forms of depression from the increasingly common diagnoses related to reactive distress: not least as an antidote to DSM-5's toxic expansion of depressive diagnoses to include grief reactions (Parker 2013).

## *Problems of Utility*

The utility of the diagnosis is also under threat, with expanding evidence of a substantial placebo effect of antidepressant medication.

Although published pharmaceutical drug trials usually indicate benefit of active drug over placebo (Gibbons et al. 2012), we cannot always have confidence in these data. Turner et al. (2008) found evidence of selective publication bias of clinical trials submitted to the United States' Food and Drug Administration (FDA). Trials which showed positive effects of antidepressants compared with placebo were much more likely to be published than trials showing negative or questionable effects. Thirty seven studies viewed by the FDA as having positive results were published, and only one study viewed as positive was not published. In contrast 36 studies viewed by the FDA as having negative or questionable results were either not published at all or else published in a way that conveyed a positive outcome. The difference in apparent effect size of antidepressants between FDA and published data was 32 % in favour of the published data. Similarly, the balance of risks and benefits of antidepressants for children looks very different when unpublished data from pharmaceutical research are added to results published in peer-reviewed journals (Whittington et al. 2004).

Kirsch and colleagues have undertaken detailed analyses of the antidepressant medication data submitted to the FDA. Using Hamilton's depression rating scale as their benchmark, they found that the mean overall difference between responses to antidepressant drugs and placebo in this database was only two points (Kirsch et al. 2002), well below accepted levels of clinical significance (Löwe et al. 2004). They subsequently found that drug-placebo differences increase in relation to initial severity. There is virtually no difference at moderate levels of initial depression and a relatively small difference for patients with severe depression. Conventional criteria for clinical significance are reached only for patients at the upper end of the very severely depressed category (Kirsch et al. 2008). The lack of evidence for the effectiveness of antidepressant medication for milder depressive diagnoses has been confirmed by Fournier et al. (2010) and Barbui et al. (2011) amongst others.

The proportion of people responding to placebo appears to be increasing over time (Walsh et al. 2002). As treatments for depression have become more widely available and socially acceptable, it has become easier to recruit members of the general public to take part in clinical trials, rather than relying on patients referred from other clinicians. As a result, it is possible that clinically important characteristics of patients taking part in treatment studies may have altered. For example, people coming forward from the general public may have less chronic types of depression, or experience fewer contributory life difficulties, than those recruited through hospital clinics. There are also some methodological changes in the studies themselves. The main difference is that the average length of the trials increased significantly during the 20 years under review. This would give more time for the cumulative effects of non-specific interventions which are inherent and inevitable in clinical trials, and – importantly – provides a longer period during which spontaneous recovery could be observed.

The evidence for efficacy of psychological interventions such as cognitive behaviour therapy is open to equal or even stronger challenge, on the grounds that their precise modes of action have not been adequately tested. Contextual factors such as the impact of hope generated by an apparently scientific approach to treatment, the effects of therapist personality, or the benefits of time spent with a sympathetic professional may be equally if not more important than the specific formal components of a given therapeutic approach (Parker 2007a, b).

## *Ethical and Evolutionary Perspectives*

Jerome Wakefield has offered a conceptual rationale for the decision to award some negative emotional experiences the status of an illness, by defining them in terms of *harmful dysfunction* of our biological mechanisms for responding to loss (Wakefield 1992a, b; Horwitz and Wakefield 2007).

According to Wakefield, *harmful* is a value term based on social norms. It refers to something which causes disbenefit under present environmental standards, and which is socially disvalued according to the standards of a given culture. One example would be extreme male aggression, which had Darwinian survival value but is not seen as useful or generally acceptable in modern western societies. Wakefield sees *dysfunction* as a factual, scientific term, referring to the failure of an internal mechanism to perform a natural function for which it was designed by evolution. Function is based on natural selection, and has at its root the ability to ensure reproductive success (Wakefield 1992b). He draws explicit parallels between organs such as the heart and artefacts such as a chair. These have specific functions, and can be defined as dysfunctional if they cannot perform as they are supposed to perform. In the same way he argues that mental mechanisms can be seen to either to function effectively, or not. Both parts of the concept are needed for the definition of disorder.

On this basis Wakefield argues that much of the current conceptualization of depression as a disorder is invalid, and that the diagnosis should be reserved only for those relatively few cases where harm and dysfunction are beyond doubt (Wakefield and Schmitz 2013).

This position is supported within the parameters of evolutionary biology, where theorists have postulated the functionality of many depressive symptoms in minimising harm in situations where biological fitness is threatened, including social losses and failure to reach personal goals (Keller and Nesse 2005). In relation to social competition, depression may be effective as a strategy enabling the individual to accept defeat in antagonistic encounters and accommodate to what would otherwise be unacceptably low social rank (Price et al. 1994; Faucher 2016). It may also be useful as a means of enhancing analytic abilities and encouraging reluctant social partners to provide help (Watson and Andrews 2002).

More generally, we may not believe that the experiences which form the core of the depressive syndrome, or their corollaries in terms of action failure, should be negatively evaluated at all. To an orthodox Buddhist, a description of the core of depressive disorder as the generalisation of hopelessness is strongly reminiscent of the fundamental concept of *dukkha*. The experience of this emotion or mental state, for a Buddhist, is not necessarily a symptom of a common mental illness: it may simply be an accurate understanding of the world as it is (Obeyesekere 1985). Then we have Eric Wilson's passionate essay *Against Happiness*, based on his fear that its overemphasis 'might be dangerous, a wanton forgetting of an essential part of a full life' (Wilson 2008), and his case for the generative power and deep heart of melancholia, enabling Keats to appreciate how beauty is enriched by our awareness of life's transience:

in the very temple of Delight
Veil'd Melancholy has her sovran shrine.

## *Iatrogenic Effects*

Although some of the more extreme depressive experiences do warrant the label of a disorder, reaching for a diagnosis of depression can all too often lead to the medicalisation of experiences of distress and suffering, which may better be seen as normal, unavoidable, sometimes even necessary facets of human experience (Dowrick and Frances 2013).

The diagnosis of depression may simply be unnecessary. For example, Brown and Harris (1978) have developed a highly sophisticated and influential life span model of depression, involving a complex interaction of adversity, support and self-esteem. Although they predicate this on an assumption of depression as a biologically rooted psychiatric condition, what would happen to the model if the concept of depression were removed from it? Clearly it would raise some practical difficulties in pursuing a research programme since there would no longer be any specific criteria by which to judge who should be recruited to their studies. But the key elements of their model – the range of social and individual factors which predict whether or not we feel life is going well – would survive quite happily on their own. These factors and their interactions are a useful guide to all of us in understanding how our lives are going, regardless of whether or not we consider ourselves to be depressed.

Diagnosing depression can also have harmful consequences. As Horwitz and Wakefield (2007) argues, the introduction of routine depression screening in places like New York represents 'a new form of social penetration of our private emotions', affecting our view of the abnormality of distressing feelings and enhancing the apparent legitimacy of psychiatric interventions.

Diagnosis can mould the perceptions of doctors and their patients, who come to see themselves as 'depressed' people and are encouraged to take on this mantle when they next encounter social stresses or emotional difficulties. Ian Hacking uses the concept of classificatory looping to describe how our methods of classifying people interact with the people being classified, and ultimately change the nature of these people. People are aware of being classified, in contrast to quarks, chemical elements or rock formations. People tend to 'act under a description': that is to say their ways of being 'are by no means independent of the available descriptions under which they may act' (Hacking 1999). Thus when individuals are aware of the classification they have been awarded, the way they experience themselves changes. Their feelings and behaviours may evolve because they are so classified. Alternatively, they may attempt to rid themselves of the classificatory system by altering their behaviour and feelings. At the same time, those around the classified individual – members of their immediate family, the wider community and those professionals and institutions dealing with them – may also react and behave differently to the individual as a consequence of the classification.

More specifically, while people may value antidepressants insofar as they enable them to return to normal functioning by reducing symptoms, they may also lose their sense of being normal, precisely because they are having to rely on external agents. They may wish to stop taking medication when they feel better, but fear the consequences of so doing and hence decide to play safe and continue to take them (Verbeek-Heida and Mathot 2006). If antidepressants are not as useful as is commonly supposed, then such loss of personal agency or increase in fearfulness become important iatrogenic effects.

## Negotiating Distress

These iatrogenic tendencies are unwittingly exacerbated by the prevalent metaphors employed by GPs. We tend to use mechanical metaphors to explain diseases. We consider patient's problems as puzzles, and cast ourselves on the role of problem solvers and controllers of disease. We talk about the body as a system. When talking about psychological unease, we use words based on the physical metaphors of tension and relaxation, and speak about ways in which medication such as tranquillisers may 'affect what is a finely balanced system' (Skelton et al. 2002). Our explanatory practices have a strong orientation towards determinism, which is of limited utility in an arena like depression, where in reality doctors have few answers.

These problems are further aggravated when we attempt to introduce the diagnosis of depression within cross-cultural perspectives (see also Kitanaka 2016).

The Cross-Cultural RE-ORDER study is part of a large mixed-method longitudinal study of depression in primary care in Melbourne, Australia. It involved semi-structured and interpreted interviews with 24 people from Vietnamese and East Timorese communities, and five GPs (Kokanovic et al. 2010). This study posed a central dilemma: how to integrate experiences grounded in one social context into the matrices provided by another? We identified a *tremendous collision* between migrants, whose experience was framed by patterns of alienation, traumatized self-identity, and GPs, for whom cultural differences were seen as technical problems of practice.

Migrants saw their distress as related to housing and finance, familial disintegration, marital breakdown, intergenerational conflict, immigration issues and cultural distance:

> Oh, my first impression was that it was so cold... It was cold. From Malaysia where it was hot, we had on only light clothing. So it was terribly cold. It was on a Saturday that we arrived; there was no one in the city. ... I thought how come there were no people in this country. The streets were deserted. I thought now I was in another country, and I did not know English, I did not know how I would start a new life. That was my continuing worry.

The GP perspectives focused on patients' need for pragmatic assistance with practical life problems:

> They quite often present distress in terms of pragmatic issues that are going on like a son is causing trouble in the family [...] or it's housing problem, or trouble with visa, or some relational difficulty... They seem to want a pragmatic sort of help... like offering some help with housing or an offer to see the offending member of the family.

Our interpretation is that the diagnosis of depression here is not a clinical entity, but a mechanism of decoupling: it replaces loss with illness, and individualizes previously social problems.


## Changing Discourse

Medicine needs a new perspective, a theory of the person based not on passivity but on agency and creative capacity. Human beings need a sense of meaning, of purpose, an understanding of the ends of life, a belief in ourselves as valuable and valued persons. These may be construed by some in lofty, noble and universal terms, and by others as immediate, pragmatic, and highly personal.

Developing a conceptual framework within which to make sense of what we know about depression, in *Beyond Depression* (Dowrick 2009) I propose two principal components:

- An understanding of ourselves as *coherent* beings, neither wholly individualised on the one hand, nor illusory, fragmented, or role-playing on the other; and within this, an understanding of ourselves as persons with the capacity to lead our own lives;
- A belief that we make sense of ourselves in terms of our *engagement* with the world around us: the context of the history, place or 'practices' within which we find ourselves, and which we have the ability to modify; and within this, a belief that such engagement – whether construed in political, social or personal terms – is crucial in creating and sustaining our sense of identity and well-being.[1]

Within this framework we can begin to think of patients not as passive victims of circumstance, whether that circumstance be genetic or social, but as persons with the capacity to lead purposeful lives.


## *Coherence*

The concept of coherence is predicated on the belief that human life has an essential unity throughout its whole extent. We are fundamentally real and intrinsically valuable beings, who have the capacity to change and progress. We are predetermined neither by our biology nor by our social roles. Coherence contains elements of desire, memory, imagination and curiosity.

My understanding of desire derives from Spinoza's *conatus:* "the endeavour by which each thing endeavours to preserve in its being is nothing other than the actual essence of the thing" (Spinoza 2000). It is apparent in literature with the '*life hungry*

---

[1] Although developed independently, these concepts of coherence and engagement have strong resonance with two bases of personality health - *identity cohesion* and *interpersonal functioning* – in DSM-5's alternative dimensional approach to personality disorder (American Psychiatric Association 2013).

*stupidity'* of Pi, when faced with the prospect of sharing a lifeboat with a Royal Bengal tiger (Martel 2002); and in life, with Joe Simpson's response to falling onto a precarious ice bridge inside a vast Andean crevasse (Simpson 1997). The *conatus* provides a basis for articulating our determination to survive, come what may.

Memories are the principle means by which we can demonstrate our sense of continuity to ourselves, linking cognition and emotions in a way that produces a sense of self-coherence (Wollheim 1984). They can be turned into a source of energy, either by drawing new implications from old memories or else by expansion, incorporating the experiences of others (Zeldin 1994).

Curiosity refers to our eagerness to find out about new things, our inquisitiveness, our sense of excitement at finding the unexpected. In 350 BC Aristotle introduced his Metaphysics with the statement 'All men by nature desire to know' (Ross 1953). Descartes (1649/1967) agrees: our innate curiosity is an essential means of increasing knowledge. Zeldin takes this argument a stage further. Reflecting on the life of Alexander von Humboldt, he concludes that curiosity can be a successful remedy against sadness and fear. If we use our personal worries as stimuli to explore the general mystery of the universe 'the limits of curiosity are at the frontiers of despair' (Zeldin 1994).

Imagination is the ability to produce ideas or images of what is not present or has not been experienced, and the ability to deal resourcefully with unexpected or unusual problems. The enhancement of memory by imagination can help us 'through the traffic jams of the brain' (Zeldin 1994). However imagination is only liberating when it is constructive, arranging fertile marriages between images and sensations, recombining obstacles to make them useful, spotting what is both unique and universal in them.

Our health is related to our sense of coherence (Antonovsky 1987). A strong sense of coherence has been directly correlated with self-rated health (Eriksson et al. 2007), while a weak sense of coherence is significantly predictive of the onset of depressive disorders (Lehtinen et al. 2005) and the onset of diabetes (Kouvonen et al. 2008). Importantly, our sense of coherence is not a static set of personal attributes. It can change over time, or as the result of therapeutic interventions such as mind-body therapies (Fernros et al. 2008), and salutogenic group therapy with focus on personal narratives, health promoting factors and active adaptation (Langeland et al. 2006).

## Engagement

Our sense of identity has important social dimensions. Language and culture are important in defining and shaping our understanding of emotional states. They are also highly relevant to understanding ourselves. As the Hegelian French philosopher Paul Ricoeur puts it, our desire has an 'intersubjective structure'. Our engagement with the world around us is both profound and crucial. We make sense of ourselves in terms of our engagement with the world around us: the context of the history, place or 'practices' within which we find ourselves, and which we have the ability to modify. Such engagement – whether construed in political, social or personal terms – is crucial in creating and sustaining our sense of identity and well-being.

Engagement may take the form of participation in practices and moral communities, in 'coherent and socially established cooperative human activity' with inherent standards of excellence (MacIntyre 1984). Practices involve the use of a set of skills in a systematic way, with the intention of enriching our lives and the lives of those around us. They may be self-contained, such as chess, music or sport; or purposive, such as law and politics.

Engagement more often takes the simpler form, proposed by Charles Taylor, of the affirmation of ordinary life through investment in our 'webs of interlocution':

> in the family tree, in social space, in the geography of social statuses and functions, in my intimate relations to the ones I love, and also crucially in the space of moral and spiritual orientation within which my most important defining relations are lived out' (Taylor 1984).

Or it may take the form of engagement with the circumstances in which we find ourselves, whether they involve cultural alienation or physical illness, and – with Camus' Sysiphus, endlessly rolling his rock up the mountain – our determination to make of them the best we can:

> 'La lutte elle-même vers les sommets suffit à remplir un cœur d'homme. Il faut imaginer Sisyphe heureux'.[2] (Camus 1942)

Engagement is good for us. Absorption in pursuits and activities beyond oneself are central to proposals for a psychology of positive emotions, aimed at understanding and building on our virtues and strengths. Identifying our signature strengths and using them in new ways can increase our happiness and reduce depressive symptoms for at least 6 months (Seligman et al. 2005). A sense of engagement also reduces the likelihood that low income will lead to the development of diabetes (Tsenkova et al. 2007).

The combination of a sense of personal coherence and an engagement with the world around us enhances our sense of personal resilience, the capacity to maintain or regain well-being in the face of adversity (Ryff 2014). Adopting strategies to enhance personal resilience improves outcomes for people diagnosed with depressive disorders in primary care (Griffiths et al. 2015).

## Implications

What we clinicians should do, in our encounters with patients whom we think may be depressed, is to help generate meaning and purpose out of suffering and distress. This is the essence of healing.

Scott and colleagues (2008) provide persuasive qualitative evidence that high quality primary care consultations can enable meaning-making. Trust, hope, and a

---

[2] *The struggle itself towards the heights is enough to fill a man's heart. We should imagine that Sisyphus is happy.*

sense of being known, can be fostered within the clinical encounter, especially if we value and create a non-judgmental emotional bond with the patient, manage our power in ways that provide most benefit for the patient, and display a commitment to caring over time. We are more likely to achieve this if we have self-confidence, emotional self-management, mindfulness, and knowledge.

At the heart of the healing process lie two assumptions. The first assumption is that the emergence of meaning, order or form is therapeutic in itself, particularly for people who are feeling lost, alone, frightened or misunderstood (Gask et al. 2003). The second assumption is that such emergence is most effective if it is mutual, if we find ways of engaging with our patient's conceptual worlds, if understanding of problems and their solutions are negotiated and agreed by both sides, not just imposed arbitrarily by the doctor.

The emergence of meaning is an imaginative construction, built by processes which take the event of a life and mould them into a coherent narrative. The doctor must be able to use their imagination empathically and thereby enter the patient's world. The solution comes in seeking more detail, however small, in the reality of the patient's life. Each detail triggers new scope for the imagination, a renewed possibility of empathy and a much increased chance of the patient feeling heard. Heath (1999) reminds us that as doctors we have a 'responsibility to locate hope through the glimpse of an alternative'.

The diagnosis of depression, as currently deployed, is too rigid and restrictive to be useful in primary care. We do better with less diagnosis and more understanding, with fewer prescriptions and more listening; and with a view of our patients not as machines in need of an overhaul, but as persons leading their lives. We should see the experience of illness through the patient's eyes (McWhinney 2000), and focus with patients on enhancing a sense of coherence and engagement with social roles. We can usefully build on two key elements of the medical encounter: the acknowledgment of suffering, and the offer of hope.

The adjectives *depressing* and *depressed* are generally safer than the noun *depression*. Adjectives by definition must be related to a subject other than themselves, whereas a noun assumes an independent state, a thing in itself. Saying to someone 'you must have found that really depressing' is powerful for two reasons: it offers the possibilities of empathy, and indicates that the core problem is outside – not inside – that person. As a clinician, I am relatively comfortable talking with patients about 'feeling depressed', or 'having depressed thoughts' since these phrases refer to specific sensations and experiences and are not defining of the patient as a whole. The statement 'I think you are depressed' is more troublesome. Although it allows for several possible interpretations, it is explicitly making a globally defining statement about the other person, and when made by a doctor to a patient it is more likely than not to be understood as conferring formal clinical status on their problems.

To provide high quality care we need to work across biomedical and social perspectives, and engage at both individual and community levels (Furler et al. 2010). We should pay careful attention to our patients' perspectives on what may be causing their problems, not least because these may be radically different from our own. We should be sensitive when elucidating their health beliefs, when enquiring about the ways in which they make sense of their experiences. Although patients may sometimes have clear and consistent explanatory models, they often hold beliefs about the cause of their problems which are tentative and fluid, sometimes internally contradictory, and characterised by uncertainty (Kokanovic et al. 2013).

We should look carefully at the ways in which general practice delivers mental health care, and how this may impact on patients' illness experience. Many people with high levels of mental distress are currently disadvantaged: either because they are unable to access care, or because when they do have access to care it does not address their needs (Dowrick et al. 2009). We have demonstrated the benefits of a new multi-faceted model of care with three principal components: increasing community aweareness that primary care can provide help for common mental health problems; increasing the competence of primary care teams in understanding and responding to the differing ways in which people present suffering; and tailoring psychosocial interventions to meet the needs of people from under-served groups (Dowrick et al. 2013).

We need to reorient our assumptions about the nature and purpose of the consultation, and revise our understanding of our patients: not as passive victims of disease or circumstance but as active agents, experts in leading their lives, who occasionally need some help, some new ways of looking at old ideas, and perhaps an instillation of hope.

We need to acknowledge and take seriously the misery, suffering, loss and grief that they bring with them into the consulting room. Empathy is crucial: even in settings of high social deprivation, it increases patients' sense of enablement and predicts change in their feeling of well-being (Mercer et al. 2008). So is our ability to listen, and then listen even more. Ronald Epstein (1999) encourages clinicians to expand our attentiveness, curiosity and presence. He argues that we should cultivate habits of mind such as experiencing information as novel, thinking of "facts" as conditional, seeing situations from multiple perspectives, suspending categorization and judgment and engaging in self-questioning. Mindful practice is not easy: it requires mentorship and guidance. But its goal of 'compassionate informed action in the world' is of high intrinsic and instrumental value.

# References

Akiskal, H. S., & McKinney, W. T. (1975). Overview of recent research in depression: Integration of ten conceptual models into a comprehensive clinical frame. *Archives of General Psychiatry, 32*, 285–305.

American Psychiatric Association. (2013). *Diagnostic and statistical manual of mental disorders* (5th ed.). Arlington: American Psychiatric Publishing.

Antonovsky, A. (1987). *Unravelling the mystery of health: How people manage stress and stay well.* San Francisco: Jossey-Bass.

Barbui, C., Cipriani, A., Patel, V., Ayuso-Mateos, J. L., & van Ommeren, M. (2011). Efficacy of antidepressants and benzodiazepines in minor depression: Systematic review and meta-analysis. *British Journal of Psychiatry, 198*, 11–16.

Brown, G. W., & Harris, T. (1978). *Social origins of depression.* New York: Free Press.

Camus, A. (1942). *Le Mythe de Sisyphe*. Paris: Gallimard.

Casey, P., Dowrick, C., & Wilkinson, G. (2001). Adjustment disorders: Fault line in the psychiatric glossary. *British Journal of Psychiatry, 179*, 479–480.

Caspi, A., Sugden, K., Moffitt, T. E., Taylor, A., Craig, I. W., Harrington, H., McClay, J., Mill, J., Martin, J., Braithwaite, A., & Poulton, R. (2003). Influence of life stress on depression: Moderation by a polymorphism in the 5-HTT gene. *Science, 301*, 386–389.

Cowan, W. M., Kopnisky, K. L., & Hyman, S. E. (2002). The human genome project and its impact on psychiatry. *Annual Review of Neuroscience, 25*, 1–50.

Craddock, N., & Forty, L. (2006). Genetics of affective mood disorders. *European Journal of Human Genetics, 14*, 660–668.

Descartes, R. (1649/1967). Treatise on the passions of the soul. In E. S. Halden & G. R. T. Ross (Trans.), *Philosophical works of Descartes*. Cambridge: Cambridge University Press

Dowrick, C. (2009). *Beyond depression* (2nd ed.). Oxford: Oxford University Press.

Dowrick, C., & Frances, A. (2013). Medicalising unhappiness: New classification of depression risks more patients being put on drug treatment from which they will not benefit. *BMJ, 347*, f7140.

Dowrick, C., Gask, L., Edwards, S., Aseem, S., Bower, P., Burroughs, H., Catlin, A., Chew-Graham, C., Clarke, P., Gabbay, M., Gowers, S., Hibbert, D., Kovandzic, M., Lamb, J., Lovell, K., Rogers, A., Lloyd-Williams, M., Waheed, W., & AMP Group. (2009). Researching the mental health needs of hard-to-reach groups: Managing multiple sources of evidence. *BMC Health Services Research, 9*, 226.

Dowrick, C., Chew-Graham, C., Lovell, K., Lamb, J., Aseem, A., Beatty, S., Bower, P., Burroughs, H., Clarke, P., Edwards, S., Gabbay, M., Gravenhorst, K., Hammond, J., Hibbert, D., Kovandžić, M., Lloyd-Williams, M., Waheed, W., & Gask, L. (2013). Increasing equity of access to high quality mental health services in primary care: A mixed-methods study. *Programme Grants for Applied Research, 1*(2), 1–184.

Epstein, R. M. (1999). Mindful practice. *JAMA, 282*, 833–839.

Eriksson, M., Lindström, B., & Lilja, J. (2007). A sense of coherence and health. Salutogenesis in a societal context: Aland, a special case? *Journal of Epidemiology and Community Health, 61*, 684–688.

Faucher, L. (2016). Darwinian blues: Evolutionary psychiatry and depression. In J. C. Wakefield & S. Demazeux (Eds.), *Sadness or depression? International perspectives on the depression epidemic and its meaning*. Dordrecht: Springer.

Fernros, L., Furhoff, A. K., & Wändell, P. E. (2008). Improving quality of life using compound mind-body therapies: Evaluation of a course intervention with body movement and breath therapy, guided imagery, chakra experiencing and mindfulness meditation. *Quality of Life Research, 17*, 367–376.

Fournier, J. C., DeRubeis, R. J., Hollon, S. D., Dimidjian, S., Amsterdam, J. D., Shelton, R. C., & Fawcett, J. (2010). Antidepressant drug effects and depression severity: A patient-level meta-analysis. *JAMA, 303*, 47–53.

Furler, J., Kokanovic, R., Dowrick, C., Newton, D., Gunn, J., & May, C. (2010). Managing depression among ethnic communities: A qualitative study. *Annals of Family Medicine, 8*, 231–236.

Gask, L., Rogers, A., Oliver, D., May, C., & Roland, M. (2003). Qualitative study of patients' perceptions of the quality of care in general practice. *British Journal of General Practice, 53*, 278–283.

Gibbons, R. D., Hur, K., Brown, C. H., David, J. M., & Mann, J. J. (2012). Benefits from antidepressants: Synthesis of 6-week patient-level outcomes from double-blind placebo-controlled randomized trials of fluoxetine and venlafaxine. *Archives of General Psychiatry, 69*, 572–579.

Goldberg, D., & Lecrubier, Y. (1995). Form and frequency of mental disorders across centres. In T. B. Üstün & N. Sartorius (Eds.), *Mental illness in general health care: An international study*. Chichester: Wiley, on behalf of the World Health Organisation.

Griffiths, F., Boardman, F., Chondros, P., Dowrick, C., Densley, K., Hegarty, K., Gunn, J. (2015). The effect of strategies of personal resilience on depression recovery in an Australian cohort: A mixed methods study. *Health, 19*(1), 86–106.

Hacking, I. (1999). *The social construction of what?* Cambridge, MA: Harvard University Press.

Heath, I. (1999). 'Uncertain clarity': Contradiction, meaning and hope. *British Journal of General Practice, 49*, 651–657.

Horwitz, A. V., & Wakefield, J. C. (2007). *The loss of sadness: How psychiatry transformed normal sorrow into depressive disorder*. New York: Oxford University Press.

Keller, M. C., & Nesse, R. M. (2005). Is low mood an adaptation? Evidence for subtypes with symptoms that match precipitants. *Journal of Affective Disorders, 6*, 27–35.

Kendell, R., & Jablensky, A. (2003). Distinguishing between the validity and utility of psychiatric diagnoses. *The American Journal of Psychiatry, 160*, 4–12.

Killingsworth, B., Kokanovic, R., Tran, H., & Dowrick, C. (2010). A care-full diagnosis: Three Vietnamese Australian women and their accounts of becoming "mentally ill". *Medical Anthropology Quarterly, 24*, 108–123.

Kirsch, I., Moore, T. J., Scoboria, A., & Nicholls, S. (2002). The emperor's new drugs: An analysis of antidepressant medication data submitted to the US Food and Drug Administration. *Prevention and Treatment, 5*, Article 23.

Kirsch, I., Deacon, B. J., Huedo-Medina, T. B., Scoboria, A., Moore, T. J., & Johnson, B. T. (2008). Initial severity and antidepressant benefits: A meta-analysis of data submitted to the food and drug administration. *PLoS Medicine, 5*, e45.

Kitanaka, J. (2016). Depression as a problem of labor: Japanese debates about work, stress, and a new therapeutic ethos. In J. C. Wakefield & S. Demazeux (Eds.), *Sadness or depression? International perspectives on the depression epidemic and its meaning*. Dordrecht: Springer.

Kokanovic, R., May, C., Dowrick, C., Furler, J., Newton, D., & Gunn, J. (2010). Negotiations of distress between East Timorese and Vietnamese refugees and their family doctors in Melbourne. *Sociology of Health & Illness, 32*, 511–527.

Kokanovic, R., Butler, E., Halilovich, H., Palmer, V., Griffiths, F., Dowrick, C., & Gunn, J. (2013). Maps, models and narratives: The ways people talk about depression. *Qualitative Health Research, 23*, 114–125.

Kouvonen, A. M., Väänänen, A., Woods, S. A., Heponiemi, T., Koskinen, A., & Toppinen-Tanner, S. (2008). Sense of coherence and diabetes: A prospective occupational cohort study. *BMC Public Health, 6*, 46.

Langeland, E., Riise, T., Hanestad, B. R., Nortvedt, M. W., Kristoffersen, K., & Wahl, A. K. (2006). The effect of salutogenic treatment principles on coping with mental health problems: A randomised controlled trial. *Patient Education and Counseling, 62*, 212–219.

Lehtinen, V., Sohlman, B., Nummelin, T., Salomaa, M., Ayuso-Mateos, J. L., & Dowrick, C. (2005). The estimated incidence of depressive disorder and its determinants in the Finnish ODIN sample. *Social Psychiatry and Psychiatric Epidemiology, 40*, 778–784.

Levinson, D. F. (2006). The genetics of depression: A review. *Biological Psychiatry, 60*, 84–92.

Löwe, B., Unützer, J., Callahan, C. M., Perkins, A. J., & Kroenke, K. (2004). Monitoring depression treatment outcomes with the PHQ-9. *Medical Care, 42*, 1194–1201.

MacIntyre, A. (1984). *After virtue* (2nd ed.). Notre Dame: University of Notre Dame Press.

Martel, Y. (2002). *Life of pi*. Edinburgh: Canongate.

McWhinney, I. (2000). Being a general practitioner: What it means. *The European Journal of General Practice, 6*, 135–139.

Mercer, S. W., Neumann, M., Wirtz, M., Fitzpatrick, B., & Vojt, G. (2008). General practitioner empathy, patient enablement, and patient-reported outcomes in primary care in an area of high socio-economic deprivation in Scotland: A pilot prospective study using structural equation modeling. *Patient Education and Counseling, 73*, 240–245.

Miller, D. B., & O'Callaghan, J. P. (2013). Personalized medicine in major depressive disorder – Opportunities and pitfalls. *Metabolism, S1*, S34–S39.

Mitchell, A. J., Vaze, A., & Rao, S. (2009). Clinical diagnosis of depression in primary care: A meta-analysis. *Lancet, 374*, 609–619.

Munafò, M. R., Durrant, C., Lewis, G., & Flint, J. (2009). Gene X environment interactions at the serotonin transporter locus. *Biological Psychiatry, 65*, 211–219.

NICE. (2009). *Treatment and management of adults with depression (update), CG 90*. London: National Institute for Health and Clinical Excellence.

Norton, J., de Roquefeuil, G., David, M., Boulenger, J. P., Ritchie, K., & Mann, A. (2009). Prevalence of psychiatric disorders in French general practice using the patient health questionnaire: Comparison with GP case-recognition and psychotropic medication prescription. *Encephale, 35*, 560–569.

Obeyesekere, G. (1985). Depression, Buddhism, and the work of culture in Sri Lanka. In A. Kleinman & B. Good (Eds.), *Culture and depression: Studies in the anthropology and cross-cultural psychiatry of affect and disorder* (pp. p134–p152). Berkeley: University of California Press.

Parker, G. (2007a). Defining melancholia: The primacy of psychomotor disturbance. *Acta Psychiatrica Scandinavica, S433*, 21–30.

Parker, G. (2007b). What is the place of psychological treatments in mood disorders? *International Journal of Neuropsychopharmacology, 10*, 137–145.

Parker, G. (2013). Opening Pandora's box: How DSM-5 is coming to grief. *Acta Psychiatrica Scandinavica, 128*, 88–91.

Pinto, E., Reggers, J., Gorwood, P., Boni, C., Scantamburlo, G., Pitchot, W., & Ansseau, M. (2008). The short allele of the serotonin transporter promoter polymorphism influences relapse in alcohol dependence. *Alcohol and Alcoholism, 43*, 398–400.

Price, J., Sloman, L., Gardner, R., Gilbert, P., & Rhode, P. (1994). The social competition hypothesis of depression. *British Journal of Psychiatry, 164*, 309–315.

Ross, W. D. (1953). *Aristotle's metaphysics*. Oxford: Clarendon.

Ryff, C. D. (2014). Psychological well-being revisited: Advances in the science and practice of eudaimonia. *Psychotherapy and Psychosomatics, 83*, 10–28.

Sáiz, P. A., García-Portilla, M. P., Arango, C., Morales, B., Alvarez, V., Coto, E., Fernández, J. M., Bascarán, M. T., Bousoño, M., & Bobes, J. (2007). Association study of serotonin 2A receptor (5-HT2A) and serotonin transporter (5-HTT) gene polymorphisms with schizophrenia. *Progress in Neuropsychopharmacology and Biological Psychiatry, 31*, 741–745.

Scott, J. G., Cohen, D., Dicicco-Bloom, B., Miller, W. L., Stange, K. C., & Crabtree, B. F. (2008). Understanding healing relationships in primary care. *Annals of Family Medicine, 6*, 315–322.

Seligman, M. E., Steen, T. A., Park, N., & Peterson, C. (2005). Positive psychology progress: Empirical validation of interventions. *American Psychologist, 60*, 410–421.

Shorter, E., & Tyrer, A. (2003). Separation of anxiety and depressive disorders: Blind alley in psychopharmacology and classification of disease. *BMJ, 327*, 158–160.

Simpson, J. (1997). *Touching the void*. London: Vintage.

Skelton, J., Wearn, A., & Hobbs, F. (2002). A concordance-based study of metaphoric expressions used by general practitioners and patients in consultation. *The British Journal of General Practice, 52*, 114–118.

Spinoza, B. (2000). *Ethics* (G. Parkinson, Ed. & Trans.). Oxford: Oxford University Press.

Taylor, C. (1984). *Sources of the self*. Cambridge: Cambridge University Press.

Tsenkova, V. K., Love, G. D., Singer, B. H., & Ryff, C. D. (2007). Socioeconomic status and psychological well-being predict cross-time change in glycosylated hemoglobin in older women without diabetes. *Psychosomatic Medicine, 69*, 777–784.

Turner, E. H., Matthews, A. M., Linardatos, E., Tell, R. A., & Rosenthal, R. (2008). Selective publication of antidepressant trials and its influence on apparent efficacy. *New England Journal of Medicine, 358*, 252–260.

Uher, R., & McGuffin, P. (2008). The moderation by the serotonin transporter gene of environmental adversity in the aetiology of mental illness: Review and methodological analysis. *Molecular Psychiatry, 13*, 131–146.

Verbeek-Heida, P. M., & Mathot, E. F. (2006). Better safe than sorry--why patients prefer to stop using selective serotonin reuptake inhibitor (SSRI) antidepressants but are afraid to do so: Results of a qualitative study. *Chronic Illness, 2*, 133–142.

Wakefield, J. C. (1992a). Disorder as harmful dysfunction: A conceptual critique of DSM-III-R's definition of mental disorder. *Psychological Review, 99*, 232–247.

Wakefield, J. C. (1992b). The concept of mental disorder: On the boundary between biological facts and social values. *American Psychologist, 47*, 373–388.

Wakefield, J. C., & Schmitz, M. F. (2013). When does depression become a disorder? Using recurrence rates to evaluate the validity of proposed changes in major depression diagnostic thresholds. *World Psychiatry, 12*, 44–52.

Walsh, B. T., Seidman, S. N., Sysko, R., & Gould, M. (2002). Placebo response in studies of major depression: Variable, substantial, and growing. *JAMA, 287*, 1840–1847.

Watson, P. J., & Andrews, P. W. (2002). Towards a revised evolutionary adaptationist analysis of depression: The social navigation hypothesis. *Journal of Affective Disorders, 72*, 1–14.

Whittington, C. J., Kendall, T., Fonagy, P., Cottrell, D., Cotgrove, A., & Boddington, E. (2004). Selective serotonin reuptake inhibitors in childhood depression: Systematic review of published versus unpublished data. *Lancet, 363*, 1341–1345.

Wilson, E. G. (2008). *Against happiness: In praise of melancholy*. New York: Sarah Crichton Books.

Wollheim, R. (1984). *The thread of life*. Cambridge: Cambridge University Press.

Zeldin, T. (1994). *An intimate history of humanity*. London: Sinclair-Stevenson.

# An Insider View on the Making of the First French National Information Campaign About Depression

**Xavier Briffault**

**Abstract** The first national public health information campaign on depression – *"Depression, know more about it to get out of it"* – was implemented in France in 2007, nearly 20 years after the first campaign on this topic was initiated in the United States by the NIMH. The chapter is based on an observant participation by the author, who has been involved in the making of the campaign at all stages and levels of its design and implementation; it will present the multiple logics that occurred in shaping the campaign messages for the general public and health professionals.

The chapter will examine the exchanges and documents (e-mails, meetings, forums, successive versions of the final documents…) produced by and between the various stakeholders involved in the design of the campaign during the entire process (experts from different backgrounds, professional associations, government agencies, institutes of quantitative and qualitative surveys, user groups, communication departments and agencies, designers, health professionals of various types, depressed people, general public…) and their contributions to the making of the final content of the campaign.

We will particularly highlight how conflicts are negotiated between apparently irreconcilable positions of actors whose ideological presuppositions, professional interests, working methods, and categories of analysis diverge, within a EBM framework strictly imposed by the public health agency supporting the campaign, and the constraints that this whole system imposed on the answer that could be proposed to the original question: "Depression, how to get out of it?".

X. Briffault (✉)
French National Scientific Research Center, Cermes3 (Centre de recherche, médecine, sciences, santé, santé mentale, société), Paris, France
e-mail: briffault.xavier@wanadoo.fr

© Springer Science+Business Media Dordrecht 2016
J.C. Wakefield, S. Demazeux (eds.), *Sadness or Depression?*
History, Philosophy and Theory of the Life Sciences 15,
DOI 10.1007/978-94-017-7423-9_10

## Introduction

Information campaigns on public health are not restricted to physical illness or usual hygienist recommendations (tobacco, alcohol, nutrition, sexual health...). They also extend to mental health issues. Many public health institutions, including the WHO, recommend the use of information campaigns in the field of mental disorders, particularly depression (Dumesnil and Verger 2009).

The first French national public health information campaign on depression, "*La dépression, en savoir plus pour en sortir*",[1] was implemented in 2007, nearly 20 years after the first campaign on this topic was initiated in the United States by the NIMH (the DART[2] and the NDSD[3] projects – see below). This chapter is based on the author's participant observation; he was involved in the making of this campaign at all stages and levels of design and implementation (Briffault et al. 2008; 2010a, b, c; Briffault and Beck 2009; Beck et al. 2009a, b). This privileged access to internal communications (minutes of meetings, emails, comments on documents...) allows for the analysis of the multiple logics involved in shaping the messages of the campaign for the general public as well as for health professionals. For ethical reasons, only data directly involved in the production of content for the campaign are used here, and all content is presented anonymously, as well as the name of the public health organization supporting the campaign (replaced with "the Agency").

This chapter will specifically focus on how conflicts were negotiated between apparently irreconcilable positions of actors whose ideological presuppositions, professional interests, working methods, and categories of analysis were divergent. These conflicts occurred in an Evidence-Based Medicine (EBM) framework strictly imposed by the public body supporting the campaign, and within the constraints imposed on the whole system by the intention to respond to the initial question: "depression, how to get out of it?"

## A Brief History of Information Campaigns About Depression

Since the first national information campaign on depression for the general public, called the "Depression Awareness, Recognition and Treatment" – DART, USA (Regier et al. 1988), many others followed in different countries: in 1991, still in the U.S., the "National Depression Screening Day" (NDSD) – which from this time became a recurring event (Magruder et al. 1995; Greenfield et al. 1997, 2000); in 1992, in the United Kingdom, the "Defeat Depression Campaign" (Baldwin et al. 1996; Priest et al. 1996; Paykel et al. 1997, 1998; Moncrieff and Moncrieff 1999; Rix et al. 1999; Paton et al. 2001); in 1997, still in the UK, the campaign *Changing Minds* (Crisp et al. 2000, 2005; Benbow 2007); in 2000, in Australia, the campaign

---

[1] Depression, knowing more about it to get out of it.

[2] Depression Awareness, Recognition and Treatment.

[3] National Depression Screening Day.

*Beyond Blue* (Ellis and Smith 2002; Parslow and Jorm 2002; Jorm et al. 2005, 2006; Highet et al. 2006); in 2001, the campaign NAAD (*Nuremberg Alliance Against Depression*) (Althaus and Hegerl 2003), followed by the campaign EAAD (*European Alliance Against Depression*) (Hegerl et al. 2006, 2007); in 2003, in the United States, a campaign targeted at men, *Real Men, Real Depression* (Rochlen et al. 2005, 2006); in Scotland in 2005, the campaign *Doing Well* (McCollam et al. 2006); and finally, in 2007 in France, the campaign of the Agency *"La dépression, en savoir plus pour en sortir"* (Briffault et al. 2007); for a more detailed review see (Dumesnil and Verger 2009), and (Quinn et al. 2013) (Kravitz et al. 2013) (Lanfredi et al. 2013) for the many other campaigns that continued to flourish after 2007.

## Internationalized Rhetoric and Categories

Information campaigns on public health are presented as vectors of public information on disorders and their treatment and claim to be based on scientific data. However, these campaigns do not only provide the population supposedly "neutral" information originating from scientific research; they make choices based on their objectives, the strategies used to achieve them, the scientific paradigms on which they are based and the influences of various social actors involved in the design of messages. In addition, the scientific foundations on which they are based, for example the chosen nosographic options, do themselves carry specific orientations that shape the content that can be produced from the initial rational and axiomatic (Horwitz and Wakefield 2007; Kirk and Kutchins 1992).

In this, the messages broadcast by the national campaigns are not only informative, but also, to speak like the philosopher J.L. Austin, "performative": they establish, through the legitimacy and communication power of the institutions that support them, a definition of mental disorders, mental health, and psyche, and they carry a specific anthropology. If this performative dimension does exist in each kind of public health communication, it is especially operative in the case of mental problems. These do indeed rely little or not at all on any identified pathophysiology, and their definitions – which are not at all consensual – set the boundaries of normal and pathological as well as (see Horwitz and Wakefield, this volume) or even more than, they describe them (Kendell and Jablensky 2003). Public communication provides terms and meaning of terms, conceptual organizations, relational grammars, forms of organization of social relations (role of patient, role of peers...) that participate in the social definition of disorders (Ehrenberg 2006a, 2004b; Jorm 2006).

Initiated by the National Institute For Mental Health (NIMH), the first information program on depression in the world, DART, and its successor, NDSD, implemented a rhetorical structure and content that flourished in subsequent campaigns; these are found almost identically in subsequent campaigns in other countries, as well as in the French campaign that we are considering here. This rhetorical structure takes the following form (the details of this analysis are developed in [Briffault et al. 2010a]): (1) there exists an observable, isolable and characterizable entity, namely depression; (2) this entity has serious individual and collective consequences; (3) those who are affected are stigmatized, despite the fact that; (4) depression is a disease; (5) that is very common and can affect anyone at any time; (6) for which affected people are not responsible; (7) this disease is complex, poorly understood, and has multifactorial origins, without any specific cause that can be identified; (8) however, there exist effective treatments, pharmacological and psychotherapeutic; (9) but they are too scarcely used or are too often misused; (10) and the disease is often incorrectly identified/diagnosed or diagnosed only with difficulty; finally, (11) the use of services provided by competent professionals capable of delivering these treatments is too low. To address these shortcomings, (12) professional and general public information about depression is necessary.

How does this rhetorical structure, based on a set of implicit and explicit set of theoretical assumptions, happen to be used in the French campaign, and how do the various stakeholders involved in the design of the campaign fit into it? This what we will describe in examining from the inside the vicissitudes of the central question of the definition of depression, its treatment, and its relations to the various professional jurisdictions (Abbott 1988).

## The Institutional Order and How the Campaign Is Made

The report of the first meeting of the group of experts convened by the Agency (2005b) states that "an information program to inform the general public and general practitioners about depressive disorders and possibilities of treatment is in preparation by the Agency since the spring of 2004". The "strategic orientation of the information campaign" has been defined as "a first working group consisting of the main departments of the Ministry of Health and Solidarity (DGS,[4] DGAS,[5] DHOS,[6] DREES[7]), HAS,[8] AFSSAPS[9] and INSERM[10] [that] met from September 2004 to May 2005". This group has produced a draft document: "Depressive disorders: definition and management. Summary of French Recommendations" (Agency 2005e). This campaign is part of the "no. 1 strategic axis of the mental health program of the Agency: to inform the general public about depressive disorders, treatment options and care pathways in France" (Agency 2005d), which is stated to derive from the objective n°60 of the Law n°2004-806 of 9 August 2004 on public health policy, which is formulated as follows:

---

[4] Direction Générale de la Santé.

[5] Direction Générale de l'Action Sociale.

[6] Direction de l'Hospitalisation et de l'Organisation des Soins.

[7] Direction de la Recherche, des Etudes, de l'Evaluation et des Statistiques.

[8] Haute Autorité de Santé.

[9] Agence Française de Sécurité Sanitaire des Produits de Santé.

[10] Institut National de la Santé et des Recherches Médicales.

> Bipolar, depressive and neurotic disorder: increase by 20 % the number of people suffering from bipolar, depressive, neurotic and anxious disorders that are treated in accordance with good practice recommendations. Prior goal: Develop and validate screening instruments. Indicators: Number of people suffering from depressive, neurotic or anxious disorders that are treated in accordance with good practice recommendations (Française 2004).

This n°60 objective, as specified for example in the explanations given to communication agencies in charge of the media campaign (TV, radio) (Agency 2005a), comes from:

> The axis 1.1 of the "Psychiatry and Mental Health" plan (2005–2008) of the Ministry of Health: "Better inform and prevent" which plans to implement several large public communication campaigns between 2006 and 2009 in order to "let the public know main diseases, their causes, symptoms and treatments, in order to change perceptions and improve in the long term medical monitoring of people with mental disorders" (santé 2004).

It is specified in the plan that "the content of the information will be drawn from the collective expertise of INSERM, the national and international best practice recommendations and the latest scientific data in the field" and that "the messages will be declined in one or more media tailored to different audiences".

The plan also states that "recommendations have been made by various national and international organizations including WHO (OMS 2001) *and the "International Consensus Group on Depression and Anxiety"*" (Ballenger et al. 2001) and that "a number of countries and international organizations have already implemented such actions (United Kingdom, Canada, USA)".

It is also asserted, without any bibliographical reference, that "the scientific evaluation of these campaigns showed that they had a positive impact on knowledge and attitudes of people in terms of mental health and care, and that they could also encourage the use of services". The work program of the Agency states that "the information [will be developed according to the guidelines of the plan] and will be studied with working groups involving the DGS and other departments concerned (DHOS, DGAS...), different agencies and health institutes (ANAES, AFSSAPS, Inserm...), professional associations and mental health users and professionals".

The budget forwarded by the plan for the campaign is € 7 million. The main tool of the campaign is a paper information booklet (88 pages), of which the campaign distributed nearly one million copies, accompanied by a website[11] that contains content in a form suitable for use online, and by a major media campaign (TV, radio).

## A Redaction Group Mainly Composed of Medically Oriented Experts

The group of experts involved in the design of the information campaign includes a sub-group dedicated to the drafting of the final information booklet (Agency 2007) and presented as "authors," and a second sub-group dedicated to reviewing and

---

[11] http://www.info-depression.fr/

control, presented under the heading "This guide has been produced with the assistance of …".

The first sub-group of authors includes 7 people: a psychologist heading the "Maison des usagers"[12] at Sainte-Anne Hospital (Paris); a representative of the National Federation of Former Psychiatric Patients (FNAP-PSY); a physician representing the national health insurance; a psychiatrist from the hospital of Saint-Antoine (Paris); a psychiatrist specialized in suicide from the hospital of Lyon I; a representative of the France Depression Association[13]; and a social scientist specialized in mental health (the author of this chapter). These authors do act *intuitu personae* as experts of their respective fields, although the two representatives of associations also act as representatives of their users and their interests.

The second sub-group – reviewing and control – includes, in addition to the previous people, some fifteen people: a representative of the French Federation of Psychiatry (FFP)[14]; a representative of the general practitioners; a representative of the French Federation of Psychologists (FFPP)[15]; a representative of the French Federation of Psychotherapy (FF2P)[16]; a representative of the School for Parents and Educators[17]; a representative of the National Union for Suicide Prevention[18]; a representative of the National Union of Families and Friends of Mentally Ill Persons (UNAFAM)[19]; a representative from the collective expertise center of INSERM[20] and some representatives of AFSSAPS[21] and HAS.[22] These experts act as representatives of their respective professional groups.

## The DSM, the Inescapable Frontier between Normal and Pathological

The design of the campaign takes place in a difficult French context, which differs from the context encountered in Britain or the United States. The French context is marked by various controversies occurring in the field of mental health, especially regarding the effortful development of legislation on the use of the title of psychotherapist and the publication by INSERM of two controversial reports (INSERM

---

[12] http://www.ch-sainte-anne.fr/site/centrhosp/usagers/maison.html

[13] http://www.france-depression.org/

[14] http://psydoc-fr.broca.inserm.fr/

[15] http://www.psychologues-psychologie.net/

[16] http://www.ff2p.fr/

[17] http://www.ecoledesparents.org/

[18] http://www.infosuicide.org/

[19] http://www.unafam.org/

[20] http://www.inserm.fr/qu-est-ce-que-l-inserm/missions-de-l-institut/mission-expertise

[21] http://ansm.sante.fr/

[22] http://www.has-sante.fr

2004, 2005) that generated important ideological conflicts (Briffault 2009; Thurin and Briffault 2006; Ehrenberg 2004c, 2006b, 2007; CCNE 2006). In this context, one of the central concerns of the Agency and group of experts is to avoid raising new controversies. In particular, great care is taken not to excessively "medicalize" depressive states, not to suggest that more and more "existential anxiety" will be included in the jurisdiction of psychiatry, and in particular, not to overly promote psychopharmacology and give the impression that the pharmaceutical industry is covertly influencing the campaign. It is thus stated in the literature review given to the experts by the Agency that:

> Mental and behavior disorders are not just variations within the limits of "normal", but are clearly abnormal or pathological phenomena. To be considered as such, the anomalies should be permanent or repeated, and cause distress or disability in one or more than one areas of everyday life" (WHO, 2001). Periods of sadness, depression or discouragement are part of the normal human feelings and experiences. These are common reactions encountered in face of various difficulties of life. They can be linked with personal, relational or social difficulties or appear without real cause. To talk about depression in terms of pathology, it is necessary that a number of criteria (symptoms, severity, duration, psychological distress, social disabilities) be present (Agency 2005e).

This laudable attempt to not let "normal sadness" (Horwitz and Wakefield 2007) be lumped into the jurisdiction (Abbott 1988) of psychiatric depressive disorders, however, faces a problem: as the problem has been formulated in the initial institutional order and review of the literature that has resulted, the reference to the international DSM and ICD psychiatric nosology for the definition of these pathological criteria cannot be avoided, since it is explicitly stated that:

> These criteria are defined in the manuals of psychiatric diagnoses. The Diagnostic and Statistical Manual of Mental Disorders (DSM-IV) and the International Classification of Mental and Behavioural Disorders (ICD-10) present the totality of mental disorders and behaviors. They list the pathologies, define the various disorders and their symptoms and enable to formulate psychiatric diagnosis.

Since the campaign is being conducted by a governmental agency of a country (France) affiliated to the WHO (OMS 1986, 1998, 2005), the reference to the worldwide organization is mandatory, as well as the use of its particular conception of mental disorders and their diagnosis:

> WHO (2001) states that "the symptoms and signs have been defined with precision to ensure uniform application", that "the diagnostic criteria were standardized at international level" and that "we can now diagnose mental disorders with the same certainty and precision as most common physical disorders" (Agency 2005c, 2005e).

Thus, it is for reasons of logical articulation of categories and a required compliance with the initial institutional order that the DSM (ICD being, in fact, never actually used, mainly because most scientific publications about depression use the DSM criterions) becomes the border guard on the passage from a common "depressive ill-being" to an internationally standardized "depressive pathology", conceptualized with a logic similar to that used for "common physical disorders". This is reflected in the working documents (original format) in which DSM criterions are used as the dividing line between normal and pathological as follows:

| Sub-goals | METHODS |
|---|---|
| **1.1** Enable (self) identification of depressed people in need of care | Definition of depressive disorders according to the DSM-IV symptoms, psychological distress, disability. |
| | Questionnaire (CIDIsf=DSM-IV). |
| | Testimonials |
| **3.1** Enable (self) identification of individuals with non-pathological depressive ill-being | Presentation of depressive ill-being: |
| | Differences between normal emotions and major depressive disorder (DSM-IV, ICD-10). |
| | Different types of depressive ill-being. |
| | Questionnaire (CIDIsf=DSM-IV). |
| | Testimonies. |

## Psychoanalytic Clinical Approach against Public Health Psychiatric Epidemiology

This general orientation of the project initially raises few objections within the experts group, as well as the first draft of the final booklet written in this general inspiration, as can be seen in an email from the head of communication service of the Agency who wrote: "We have sent the booklet to various experts, so far there have been mostly positive and constructive comments about the booklet". But things deteriorate with the comments made[23] by the representative of the French Federation of Psychiatry (FFP), on which we will focus now, since they are particularly representative of the violent conflict between the logic of public health mental health brought by government agencies and the logic supported by a still dominant part of French psychiatry that reasons from a psychoanalytic clinical point of view (Jeammet 1996; Effenterre et al. 2012; Gansel 2014; Lézé 2010), and of the present status of this conflict.

These comments are announced by the head of communication service of the Agency in a letter to a psychiatrist member of the experts group whom she seeks to align with the Agency against the criticisms of the FFP:

> However we received this morning some extremely aggressive comments from the FPP (see attached). [The Director of the Agency] and [the Director of Scientific Affairs] will be present at the beginning of February 9 meeting to answer the FFP but we know it will be very useful for us if psychiatrists, other than the representative of the FFP, may be present to counteract their speech (mail 30/01/2007).[24]

The head of scientific affairs says in response:

---

[23] Received 29 janvier 2007.

[24] All the mails used in this chapter were originally written in french, and translated in english by the author of this chapter.

> How to find an agreement with some psychiatrists who contest the very notion of diagnosis of depression from a list of criteria (or symptoms) (DSM, CIDI). It seems to me that we are constrained in such a document to have a public health and epidemiology of mental health approach and cannot enter into a diagnostic approach such as experienced by clinical specialists. How to get out of this problem? Moreover, we feel that we will be presented the usual equations: DSM-IV = anti-psychoanalytic attitude = reducing to symptoms = influence of Big Pharma (mail 30/01/2007).

As a matter of fact, these "equations" will take place in the comments of the FFP associated with different elements of the text of the booklet.

## Extension of the Depressive Domain

The FFP criticisms written in the document joined to the mail sent by the head of communication service of the Agency first bear on the indefinite extension of the depression diagnosis that would result from adopting the DSM-IV criteria used in the booklet to define depression.

Thus, for the minimum duration of two weeks of symptoms, the experts representing the FFP affix the following comment to the draft of the booklet: "Two weeks, even if this is the definition, it is a promotion of depression".

Regarding the affirmation of the booklet that "the state experienced during depression is characterized by [...] an extraordinary sadness, not a continuum with normal sadness": "It is an open door to everything despite the shade".

On a table that presents two pages of the symptoms of depression, "this is a 'catalogue à la Prévert', I do not know who would not be depressed".

Regarding the precision that "postpartum depressive episode (after delivery) should not be confused with the 'baby blues,' that is a transitory depressive state": "it does not mean anything and it opens the door to all drift, it is absolutely not suitable for the term baby blues".

Regarding the self-assessment questionnaire of depressive symptoms (CIDI directly issued from WHO (OMS)), that is still associated to the warning: "This questionnaire is designed to help you identify the symptoms of depression. It is by no means a diagnosis. A diagnosis of depression is a complex procedure, which requires taking into account all of your symptoms, your situation, your background, your personality...": "Is this a quiz to promote depression? I think we are going to prescribe a lot of drugs after the publication of this document, is the pharmaceutical industry part of sponsors? We should ask them a financial support".

Regarding the exclusion criteria of the diagnosis of Major Depressive Episode in a situation of grief formulated as "in the weeks following the loss of a loved one, it is common to experience depressive symptoms that are part of the normal grieving process. It is only if these symptoms persist over a long period (over 2 months) or if they have excessive impact on the person that it is necessary to treat": "this is where the problem lies, depression reduced to symptoms is associated to the fact that symptoms define depression and causes an infinite extension of the term depression, this is particularly inappropriate".

Regarding the question "During the last two weeks have you felt (e) sad, depressed (e), hopeless (almost) all day, (almost) every day?": "the game is over, the presupposition is here, a symbolic equation between a list of symptoms and depression, between the word depression used by lay people and depression".

## A Structural Conflict

The rudeness of the style used is absolutely not unusual in the French world of psychiatry and mental health. The style is even rather polite when compared to the comments made on the occasion of the release of the campaign in the editorial of No. 7 "Nouvel Ane", a journal of the Ecole de la Cause Freudienne (ECF),[25] written by a psychiatrist-psychoanalyst:

> [untranslatable play of words based on the acronym of the Agency] "Pestilence"? See the dictionary: "stench, putrid miasma, infection". The Agency has launched a massive nationwide campaign of disinformation on depression in adults, with TV spots, radio spots, a guide distributed to one million copies, brochures; media add: interviews, testimonies, photos. Surveys? There are few or not at all. This unprecedented hype is intended to impose seven theses: (1) that depression exists and (2) that it is a disease, and (3) that it is gaining ground in society to the point of becoming a public health problem, and that (4) development of medical care is therefore urgently needed, (5) it can be treated with medication and conditioning; (6) that depression has no existential dimension; (7) that psychoanalysis is of no use. Huge financial means from the State budget, not without the contribution, at least indirectly, of pharmaceutical industries, have been serving the unilateral promotion of these seven theses, all highly questionable.

Beyond the excesses of words that seem to suggest that something fundamental is being attacked, the text sheds light on seven critical points that correspond to the rhetorical structure initiated by the NIHM (see above). These seven points render the campaign of the Agency unacceptable for the ECF as well as for the FFP. These points are subsumed by the FFP under the question "structure or symptoms". Thus, about the "excessive consequences" of depressive symptoms that would justify the use of medical care in mourning, FFP wrote "excessive? What is it? You suffer too much from the loss of your child? This is again the problem of using a catalog of symptoms to define a disease (and not the underlying structure)". In other places, "They are all lining up to get into services and have a consultation yet, in contrast if you take the diagnosis by structure and not by symptoms it is clear that psychotic depressions and melancholies do not ask help"; "*psychiatrists* appear only in the second line, for sure if it is for the kind of depression detected by the test it is preferable (because everybody is concerned, including those who are hysterical, hypochondriacal, obsessive, psychasthenic, and others), but for depressive persons as *we* diagnose them, psychiatrists should be first for evaluation and it is not a question of severity, but of structure".

---

[25] http://www.causefreudienne.net/

"Structure" has long played a key role in the French intellectual debates in sociology and psychology, and even more so in psychopathology due in particular to the fact that the theories of Jacques Lacan, one of the most influent psychoanalysts in France, who relied heavily on this conceptualization of human beings (Corvez 1968; Kurzweil 1980). Together with the structure, it is the question of the meaning of symptoms that is raised by the FFP, depression being seen in this approach as a symptom integrated and having a meaning *inside* a psychic structure and not as a disease that *has* symptoms. Thus, a sentence in the booklet stating that "depression can manifest itself through excessive behaviors: alcohol, scarifications (cuts on purpose), states of agitation, verbal violence…" is deprecated by the French Federation of Psychiatry in their comments of the draft booklet in the following terms: "Society of soft-drinks, coca-cola, hamburger and in no case Camembert.[26] Alcohol use etc… are not excessive behaviors and their pathological character is not determined by whether they are excessive or not but by the meaning they have". In addition to the criticism addressed incidentally to the American culture from which the DSM comes, it is the very possibility of isolating the symptoms from the meaning they have for the patient that is questioned here. As a logical consequence, all the neurobiological explanations of depression (explanations by *causes* rather than by *reasons*) are violently disqualified by FFP on behalf of French psychiatry: "very bad, Reader's Digest of unassimilated false science at all levels [] it is everything and nothing, meaningless. Explanation without interest, the alibi for the scientist to say that this is a real illness, 'to exonerate' as it is fashionable to say". Logically, psychopharmacological recommendations, based on the neurobiological theories of depression, are also disqualified by this criticism. About the phrase "the duration of treatment of a depressive episode is therefore usually between 6 months and 1 year": "Wow, the pharmaceutical industry managed to convince everyone and now the machine will operate".

This conception of depression means that the position defended by the booklet, which is to send "people with major depressive disorder" – and not "depressed persons" – first to the general practitioner is unacceptable for the FFP, as well as the idea that psychiatric consultation might not be at once and always psychotherapeutic: "We do not agree on the implicit message of the booklet that psychiatrists are only second line". About the phrase: "the psychiatrist may also recommend to undergo psychotherapy": "Seeing a psychiatrist *is* having a psychotherapeutic relationship, it is not separated from his act even if he gives drugs". The idea that psychiatrists are "inherently" psychotherapists, and even the only possible psychotherapists amongst all medical or mental health professions, is a position that has been defended for decades by French psychiatrists (see for example [Hanon 2001] for more details).

---

[26] "Camenbert" is a French cheese made from unpasteurized cow milk that is quite strong in taste and smell. It is taken here as representative of a (supposed) French culture that would like and accept strong real things (psychoanalytical psychopathology) as opposed to a (supposed) American culture that would produce only pasteurized safe, fake, and tasteless things (DSM psychopathology).

# From Casus Belli...

For FFP holding this position is indeed a casus belli. They write in their comments "psychotherapy is an act that is inseparable from the act of the psychiatrist, it is not after, and this formulation is a condition of our agreement to the text, otherwise we will not sign [the agreement for publishing the booklet]" – thus relaying the dominant position defended for decades by French psychiatry that any psychiatrist is "in essence" a psychotherapist, a position that indeed does not really correspond to the quite incomplete training in psychotherapy that French psychiatrists have today (Effenterre et al. 2012, 2013). They write: "we ask that the term psychodynamic psychotherapy appears and be referenced as THE psychotherapy that occurs concomitantly with the psychiatric consultation". As a matter of fact, the way FFP conceptualizes psychotherapy *is* psychodynamic. About a paragraph in the booklet that reads as follows:

> Specific psychological mechanisms are also involved in depression: chronic feelings of loss, psychic conflicts, negative beliefs, low self-esteem (e.g. I can not do anything right, I'm no good ...). Some may find their origin in childhood, others may be linked to actual situations. The quality of early attachment relationships, significant experiences during childhood that may have been accompanied by a feeling of loss, loneliness, helplessness, guilt or shame, the consequences of traumatic situations or mourning (not only a person, but an ideal, or self-image), cognitive, emotional, and relational styles, specific modes of psychological defenses can play a role. */ The negative beliefs, or an excessive focus on the most pessimistic outlook, may also apply to the world around the person and his future. Certain events of everyday life, analyzed in their most negative angle automatically trigger in a depressed person a style of depressive thoughts without it being possible to use its other positive experiences. It is by acting on these psychic functioning problems that psychotherapy has an effect on depression. */

the associated comment is:

> If you insist on this very poorly written chapter, I propose the following paragraph: There are actually numerous mechanisms involved in the genesis of depression to be identified by a professional, specifically for each person. However, whatever the mechanisms involved, the depression is always a crisis characterized by a temporary or permanent inability to develop an acceptable compromise between the dynamic tension existing between the psyche and the reality on the one hand, the different forces at work in the psyche of the other.[27]

These elements – singularity of the mechanisms involved, reference to a professional having the skills to detect and understand these singular mechanisms, conflict between reality and psyche on the one hand and between the internal psychological dynamics on the other – are ones in which we recognize the fundamental Freudian approach of the psyche and its problems. They are completely antithetical to the logic driven by the DSM-IV and Evidence-Based Mental Medicine (EBMM), that results in: standardized nosographies, strictly symptomatic approaches without reference to the "unobservable" psychopathological underlying dynamics, standard-

---

[27] About the section between /* and */ that is from cognitive-behavioral inspiration, the added comment is « non sense ».

ized diagnostic procedures that require ideally almost no other expertise than the application of decision trees based on algorithms (First et al. 2002), and statistical evaluation of the effectiveness of standardized treatments as measured by standardized quantitative indicators using "uniform" groups, at least from the point of view of the nosography used (Briffault and Martin 2011).

We can see two approaches in this ideological conflict that involve radically different anthropological and epistemological positions (Briffault 2008; Castel 2006, 2010; Ehrenberg 2004c; Descombes 1995, 1996). Yet, far from generating a reflexive collective feedback on the content of the booklet and the categories used, the conflict between the two approaches is engaged and continues in a balance of power. FFP is the first to engage this positioning by accompanying the consignment of its comments by the following requirements, all of them trying to reinforce the leadership of the psychiatrist and of psychodynamic psychotherapy in the French mental health field:

Four of my remarks are essential for FFP:

1. The removal of some chapters.
2. The place of the psychiatrist.
3. The place of psychotherapy as inseparable from the psychiatric consultation.
4. The place of psychodynamic psychotherapy.

Without these elements I do not see how the FFP could sign the document but I'm sure these comments will be taken into consideration.


## ...to statu quo ante bellum

Receipt of the Agency is unfriendly, as illustrated by the message of the head of the communication service: "The comments of the FFP are saddening and they reveal an undisguised evil spirit. I wonder if we should not send a written response signed by the Director of the Agency". In fact, it is an appeal to authority that will be chosen to solve the problem. During the meeting of the experts group on February, 9 2007, not only the director of the Agency, but also the assistant director of DGS (*Direction Générale de la Santé*[28]), solicited for his support, will come at the beginning of the meeting to say again that:

Summary and priority messages of this book were presented and validated by the expert group (now reunited) in April 2006.

and that

The purpose of today's meeting is to validate the booklet. Its presentation will then be reworked by an editor to homogenize the writing style.

---

[28] An equivalent of the Surgeon General in the USA.

No place is given for major changes in the booklet, and even less for its main orientations. It is also clear in the notes written for the oral presentation in presence of the experts that:

> We received a number of very constructive comments that can for most of them be very easily integrated. On the other hand, some remarks (see if we mention FFP) cannot be integrated because they question the very logic of the document (explain why in 3 lines).

The so-called "three lines" consist in a reaffirmation of "the evidence-based orientation of the booklet, which requires going further than single expert opinions, to be based on data published in the international scientific literature". This orientation implies, in fact, the use of DSM, since so-called "evidence-based" studies all use this nosological standard to characterize depression. The Director of the Agency and assistant Director of the DGS then join together during the opening of the meeting to reaffirm that the use of DSM is not negotiable, and that the general direction of the booklet is not negotiable either, without directly addressing any of the comments made by the FFP, avoiding thus an overt conflict.

In truth, none of the "imperative" requirements of FFP will be satisfied. The term "psychodynamic" will not appear in the book, nor the term "psychoanalysis" or any other "brand name" of psychotherapy. No section will be removed, and the size of the booklet will not be diminished. The term "disease" to describe depression will be used 68 times in the 88-pages booklet. CIDI questionnaire will not be deleted even if the count of symptoms will not be mentioned – it will be replaced by the phrase "if you have observed several of these symptoms, this is a warning signal that should encourage you to talk with a doctor". Neither the place and role of the psychiatrists will be changed: they remain in second line after GPs for diagnosing and treating depression, have a specific role in prescribing psychotherapy, but are on par with clinical psychologists for their implementation.

## Vae Victis

The brief analysis that we have proposed illustrates the central, inescapable, and uncontestable place occupied by the DSM in the first French campaign about depression aimed at the general public, similar in this respect to other previous campaigns in other countries. This central role does not emerge from the interactions between experts to address the problem of what information is relevant to the general public about depression; it is raised at the outset and is a direct result of the way in which problems are initially formulated in institutional demand, including legislation that is binding on state agencies that implement this type of campaign. However, regardless of the mandatory nature of this axiomatic initially external to the Agency, it is integrated without difficulty, the ethos of public health being perfectly isomorphic to the logic carried by the DSM and the Evidence-Based Mental Medicine approach. The epidemiological and public health approach is presented as an obligation within the Agency: "we are constrained in such a document to have a public health and epidemiology of mental health approach and cannot enter into a diagnostic approach such as experienced by clinical specialists" (cited above). But if such an "obligation" exists, it is by no means seen as a constraint, but rather as an obligation of scientific rigor, and therefore, in the scheme of reasoning employed, as a moral obligation, to bring to the public the "best available scientific data". The science mentioned is necessarily based on epidemiology and quantitative psycho-metrics: "there is and there can be only one science. By definition there is only one scientific approach, you apply the same rules everywhere regardless of the object of study, be it parenting, tobacco, alcohol or mental health, the scientific rules are pre-determined... There is only one approach, one method, one protocol, the rest is meaningless verbiage by people who want to reconstruct reality ... What counts is an effective scientific approach and we now know where to find it [] I am always referring to data from the scientific literature to define [the concepts we use]... I always put myself behind an official definition" (remarks made by a member of the Agency coordinating the expert group).

Yet, to think that way is to go against the evidence, mentioned by sociologist Alain Ehrenberg, that "methods must be adapted to the object being observed and on which we try to have an effect" (Ehrenberg 2006b). To assume only one scientific approach is to pretend that the analytical methods of experimental science are the only one relevant in the analysis of psychological problems, including depression. This is a highly questionable postulate (Gorostiza and Manes 2011) which is, how-ever, never criticized if the fields of public health institutions, not only for the socio-logical reasons of necessary integration of agencies in the chain of public policy decision already mentioned, but also and especially because "they miss the [episte-mological and sociological] conceptual tools [needed]" (Ehrenberg 2007) to under-stand the complex interwoven nature of individual minds, meaning, social institutions, and mental disorders (Bolton and Hill 2004). The public health system that imposes its medical approach on mental health has neither the categories of thought, nor the reasoning methods or methodological tools to think of depression other than, according to DSM, as a meaningless disease that is ultimately com-pletely natural and without reasons or context. Indeed, the evidence-based medical paradigm in which "public health depression" is framed is seriously defended by an "immune system" that tolerates within that system only elements with an acceptable axiomatic. As said by an official of the Agency to a newcomer trainee in sociology as a welcome speech: "It's simple, Alex, it will be necessary that you choose your side, either you are engaged in the constructive logic of public health, as is done here, or you are engaged in a destructive logic, that of sociology that attempts to derail all actions. Anyway, these people have no actual solutions to offer to prob-lems related to poor mental health".

However, the conceptualization of depression generated by this paradigm "is not the result of an empirical scientific discovery (like the germs that cause infectious diseases). It is the effect of an heavily theory-laden rewriting of the ordinary moral content [that constitutes depression] in new neurobiology-compatible terms" (Castel 2010). And the new psychopathological knowledge that is deduced from this rewrit-ing "gives a much sharper hardness to the medically assisted strategies of normalization of intimate life, that is afterwards denounced by sociologists and psychoanalysts" (ibid.) – denunciations whose failure we have seen when examining the poor destiny of the FFP criticisms, and their complete failure to challenge the axiomatic DSM foundations of the whole making of the depression booklet and campaign.

If there is no denying that the condescending arrogance expressed by the tone of the criticism helps to reduce their chances of success, this is not the real problem. This contemptuous attitude only comes to diminish what is already almost zero. In fact, when we make "psychiatry a branch of natural science, this knowledge gives stakeholders (patients and caregivers) the insurance they lacked: that of acting in the name of the truth of the laws of nature, far from any "cosmetic" moral issue – when this moral reference is not simply held as an harmful filter preventing any objective understanding of depression" (ibid.).

The analysis presented above illustrates the difficulties encountered by the position of the "socialized and speaking" human being (Ehrenberg 2004a, c) – at least as it is defended by those French psychiatric institutions who endorse it – to retain an efficient position in the overwhelming public health approach extended to mental health: " the existence of a nosographic standard entails a high level of coherence at all levels of the stakeholders involved in depression and its treatment, which determines an extremely coherent and highly interdependent system. The normative power thus generated leads to a strong inertia to change. From the definition of the scales measuring the way people think, live and act their 'depression', through the definition of treatments, clinical trials, recommendations for good practice, training of practitioners, national information campaigns, the media, the categories of the common social grammar … is a complete 'social construct' that is 'held together' by the DSM and the 'depression' to which it gives an existence" (Briffault and Martin 2011; Briffault 2013): "the object, initially the product of a convention becomes real after having been transmitted off the shelf and reused by others" (Desrosieres 2002). The Major Depressive Disorder of the DSM, initially the product of a convention, becomes real in its use by the public (mental) health system. And it has to, if stakeholders are to avoid unmanageable epistemological, sociological, and moral choices, and conflicts that would prevent any attempt to produce a common, coherent, single voice public health campaign. We need a common frame and a common language to be able to co-operate. This is the reason why DSM is used as a kind of "Planck's wall", the ultimate possible point of view on the reality of mental disorders, and thus on mental health.

Finally, the major difficulties encountered by the French psychiatrists to have an accepted voice during the making of this campaign might suggest that the "French exception" in psychiatry, made of psychoanalytically informed systematic opposition to the extension of the field of public health and standardized medical nosology to the field of the psyche, begins to seriously fizzle. Indeed, from the point of view of public health actors, there is no doubt that this is already the case, as seen in the opinion of a high level member of the Agency: "These people are paranoid. But as in any paranoia, there's a little truth. The problem is that times are changing, and they feel it as an attack against them, while it is much worse: we almost do not listen to them anymore".

# References

Abbott, A. (1988). *The system of professions: An essay on the division of expert labor*. Chicago: University of Chicago Press.

Agency. (2005a). *Cahier des charges remis aux agences de communication*.

Agency. (2005b). *Compte-rendu de réunion Groupe de travail sur la campagne d'information dépression (INPES) 20 juin 2005*

Agency. (2005c). *Conception et réalisation d'un programme d'information sur les troubles dépressifs : Programme fonctionnel*.

Agency. (2005d). *Programme d'information sur les troubles dépressifs et leur prise en charge*.

Agency. (2005e). *Troubles dépressifs : définition et prise en charge – Synthèse des recommandations françaises*.

Agency. (2007). *la dépression : en savoir plus pour en sortir*.

Althaus, D., & Hegerl, U. (2003). Concept and results of an awareness campaign: The "Nuremberg Alliance against Depression". *MMW Fortschritte der Medizin, 145*, 42–44.

Baldwin, D., Kempe, D., & Priest, R. (1996). The Defeat Depression Campaign: Interim results and future directions. *International Journal of Methods in Psychiatric Research, 6*, S21–S26.

Ballenger, J. C., Davidson, J. R., Lecrubier, Y., Nutt, D. J., Kirmayer, L. J., Lepine, J. P., Lin, K. M., Tajima, O., & Ono, Y. (2001). Consensus statement on transcultural issues in depression and anxiety from the International Consensus Group on Depression and Anxiety. *The Journal of Clinical Psychiatry, 62*(Suppl 13), 47–55.

Beck, F., Guignard, R., Du Roscoat, E., & Briffault, X. (2009a). Attitudes et opinions vis-à-vis de la dépression. In INPES (Ed.), *La dépression en France : enquête ANADEP 2005*. Saint-Denis: INPES.

Beck, F., Sapinho, D., Chan Chee, C., Briffault, X., & Lamboy, B. (2009b). Méthodologie de l'enquête ANADEP. In INPES (Ed.), *La dépression en France : enquête ANADEP 2005*. Saint-Denis: INPES.

Benbow, A. (2007). Mental illness, stigma, and the media. *The Journal of Clinical Psychiatry, 68*(Suppl 2), 31–35.

Bolton, D., & Hill, J. (2004). *Mind, meaning and mental disorder: The nature of causal explanation in psychology and psychiatry*. Oxford: OUP.

Briffault, X. (2008). Liberté, sécurité, évaluation : à propos de quelques organisateurs des polémiques autour de l'évaluation des psychothérapies. In C. Françoise (Ed.), *Psychothérapie et Société*. Paris: Armand Colin.

Briffault, X. (2009). Conflits anthropologiques et stratégies de lutte autour de l'évaluation des psychothérapies. *Nouvelle Revue de Psychosociologie, 8*, 105–118.

Briffault, X. (2013). Sur la classification et sa signification en santé (mentale) publique. *Psychiatrie Française, 43*(4), 73–82.

Briffault, X., & Beck, F. (2009). Perspectives pour les études et recherches en épidémiologie de la santé mentale en France. In INPES (Ed.), *La dépression en France : enquête ANADEP, 2005*. Saint-Denis: INPES.

Briffault, X., & Martin, O. (2011). Déprimer par les nombres. *Sociologie et Societes, 43*, 67–89.

Briffault, X., Caria, A., Finkelstein, C., Hérique, A., Nuss, P., Terra, P., & Wooley, S. (2007). *La dépression, en savoir plus pour en sortir*. Saint-Denis: INPES.

Briffault, X., Morvan, Y., Guilbert, P., & Beck, F. (2008). Évaluation de la dépression dans une enquête en population générale. *Bulletin Epidémiologique Hebdomadaire, 48*, 35–36.

Briffault, X., Morvan, Y., & Roscoat, E. (2010a). Les campagnes nationales d'information sur la dépression : une anthropologie bio-(psycho)-sociale ? *Encephale, 36*(Suppl 2), D124–D132.

Briffault, X., Morvan, Y., Rouillon, F., Dardennes, R., & Lamboy, B. (2010b). [Factors associated with treatment adequacy of major depressive episodes in France]. *Encephale, 36*(Suppl 2), D59–D72.

Briffault, X., Morvan, Y., Rouillon, F., Dardennes, R., & Lamboy, B. (2010c). [Use of services and treatment adequacy of major depressive episodes in France]. *Encephale, 36*(Suppl 2), D48–D58.

Castel, P.-H. (2006). *A quoi résiste la psychanalyse ?* Paris: Presses Universitaires de France – PUF.

Castel, P.-H. (2010). *L'Esprit malade. Cerveaux, folies, individus.* Les Editions d'Ithaque. Paris.

CCNE. (2006). *Problèmes éthiques posés par les démarches de prédiciton fondées sur la détection de troubles précoces du comportement chez l'enfant.* Paris.

Corvez, M. (1968). Le structuralisme de Jacques Lacan. *Revue Philosophique de Louvain, 66,* 282–308.

Crisp, A. H., Gelder, M. G., Rix, S., Meltzer, H. I., & Rowlands, O. J. (2000). Stigmatisation of people with mental illnesses. *The British Journal of Psychiatry, 177,* 4–7.

Crisp, A., Gelder, M., Goddard, E., & Meltzer, H. (2005). Stigmatization of people with mental illnesses: A follow-up study within the Changing Minds campaign of the Royal College of Psychiatrists. *World Psychiatry, 4,* 106–113.

Descombes, V. (1995). *La denrée mentale.* Paris: Editions de Minuit.

Descombes, V. (1996). *Les institutions du sens.* Paris: Editions de Minuit.

Desrosieres, A. (2002). *The politics of large numbers: A history of statistical reasoning.* Cambridge, MA: Harvard University Press.

Dumesnil, M. S., & Verger, M. D. (2009). Public awareness campaigns about depression and suicide: A review. *Psychiatric Services, 60,* 1203–1213.

Effenterre, A. V., Azoulay, M., Briffault, X., & Champion, F. (2012). Psychiatres… et psychothérapeutes ? Conceptions et pratiques des internes en psychiatrie. *L'Information Psychiatrique, 88,* 305–313.

Effenterre, A. V., Azoulay, M., Champion, F., & Briffault, X. (2013). La formation aux psychothérapies des internes de psychiatrie en France : résultats d'une enquête nationale. *L'Encéphale, 39,* 155–164.

Ehrenberg, A. (2004a). Le sujet cérébral. *Esprit, 309*(11), 130–155.

Ehrenberg, A. (2004b). Les changements de la relation normal-pathologique. A propos de la souffrance psychique et de la santé mentale. *Esprit, 304,* 133–156.

Ehrenberg, A. (2004c). Les guerres du sujet. *Esprit, 309*(11), 74–84.

Ehrenberg, A. (2006a). La dépression, un succès médical et social *Panorama du Médecin, 5010,* 42–44.

Ehrenberg, A. (2006b). Malaise dans l'évaluation de la santé mentale. *Esprit, 5,* 89–102.

Ehrenberg, A. (2007). Épistémologie, sociologie, santé publique: tentative de clarification. *Neuropsychiatrie de l'enfance et de l'adolescence, 55*(8), 450–455.

Ellis, P. M. & Smith, D. A. (2002). Treating depression: The beyondblue guidelines for treating depression in primary care. "Not so much what you do but that you keep doing it". *Med J Aust,* 176(Suppl), S77–S83.

First, M. B., Frances, A., & Pincus, H. A. (2002). *DSM-IV-TR handbook of differential diagnosis.* Washington, DC: American Psychiatric Press.

Française, R. LOI no 2004-806 du 9 août 2004 relative à la politique de santé publique.

Gansel, Y. (2014). La bipolarité épistémologique de la psychiatrie française. *L'Évolution Psychiatrique.*

Gorostiza, P. R., & Manes, J. A. (2011). Misunderstanding psychopathology as medical semiology: An epistemological enquiry. *Psychopathology, 44,* 205–215.

Greenfield, S. F., Reizes, J. M., Magruder, K. M., Muenz, L. R., Kopans, B., & Jacobs, D. G. (1997). Effectiveness of community-based screening for depression. *The American Journal of Psychiatry, 154,* 1391–1397.

Greenfield, S. F., Reizes, J. M., Muenz, L. R., Kopans, B., Kozloff, R. C., & Jacobs, D. G. (2000). Treatment for depression following the 1996 National Depression Screening Day. *The American Journal of Psychiatry, 157,* 1867–1869.

Hanon, C. (2001). *La formation des internes en psychiatrie.* MD thesis, Université Paris 6.

Hegerl, U., Althaus, D., Schmidtke, A., & Niklewski, G. (2006). The alliance against depression: 2-year evaluation of a community-based intervention to reduce suicidality. *Psychological Medicine, 36,* 1225–1233.

Hegerl, U., Wittmann, M., Arensman, E., Van Audenhove, C., Bouleau, J. H., Van Der Feltz-Cornelis, C., Gusmao, R., Kopp, M., Lohr, C., Maxwell, M., Meise, U., Mirjanic, M., Oskarsson, H., Sola, V. P., Pull, C., Pycha, R., Ricka, R., Tuulari, J., Varnik, A., & Pfeiffer-Gerschel, T. (2007). The 'European Alliance Against Depression (EAAD)': A multifaceted, community-based action programme against depression and suicidality. *The World Journal of Biological Psychiatry, 9,* 1–8.

Highet, N. J., Luscombe, G. M., Davenport, T. A., Burns, J. M., & Hickie, I. B. (2006). Positive relationships between public awareness activity and recognition of the impacts of depression in Australia. *The Australian and New Zealand Journal of Psychiatry, 40,* 55–58.

Horwitz, A. V., & Wakefield, J. C. (2007). *The loss of sadness: How psychiatry transformed normal sorrow into depressive disorder.* Oxford: Oxford University Press.

INSERM. (2004). *Psychothérapies : trois approches évaluées.*

INSERM. (2005). *Trouble des conduites chez l'enfant et l'adolescent.*

Jeammet, P. (1996). Psychanalyse et psychiatrie : des relations toujours actuelles. *Revue Française de Psychanalyse, 60,* 351.

Jorm, A. F. (2006). National surveys of mental disorders: Are they researching scientific facts or constructing useful myths? *The Australian and New Zealand Journal of Psychiatry, 40,* 830–834.

Jorm, A. F., Christensen, H., & Griffiths, K. M. (2005). The impact of beyondblue: The national depression initiative on the Australian public's recognition of depression and beliefs about treatments. *The Australian and New Zealand Journal of Psychiatry, 39,* 248–254.

Jorm, A. F., Christensen, H., & Griffiths, K. M. (2006). Changes in depression awareness and attitudes in Australia: The impact of beyondblue: The national depression initiative. *The Australian and New Zealand Journal of Psychiatry, 40,* 42–46.

Kendell, R., & Jablensky, A. (2003). Distinguishing between the validity and utility of psychiatric diagnoses. *The American Journal of Psychiatry, 160,* 4–12.

Kirk, S. A., & Kutchins, H. (1992). *The selling of DSM: The rhetoric of science in psychiatry.* New York: Aldine de Gruyter.

Kravitz, R. L., EPSTEIN, R. M., Bell, R. A., Rochlen, A. B., Duberstein, P., Riby, C. H., Caccamo, A. F., Slee, C. K., Cipri, C. S., & Paterniti, D. A. (2013). An academic-marketing collaborative to promote depression care: A tale of two cultures. *Patient Education and Counseling, 90,* 411–419.

Kurzweil, E. (1980). *The age of structuralism: Lévi-Strauss to Foucault.* New York: Columbia University Press.

Lanfredi, M., Rossi, G., Rossi, R., Van Bortel, T., Thornicroft, G., Quinn, N., Zoppei, S., & Lasalvia, A. (2013). Depression prevention and mental health promotion interventions: Is stigma taken into account? An overview of the Italian initiatives. *Epidemiology and Psychiatric Sciences, 22,* 363–374.

Lézé, S. (2010). *L'autorité des psychanalystes.* Paris: Presses Universitaires de France – PUF.

Magruder, K. M., Norquist, G. S., Feil, M. B., Kopans, B., & Jacobs, D. (1995). Who comes to a voluntary depression screening program? *The American Journal of Psychiatry, 152,* 1615–1622.

Mccollam, A., Maxwell, M., Huby, G., Woodhouse, A., Maclean, J., Themessl-Huber, M. & Morrison, J. (2006). *A report of the three year programme to enhance services in primary care for people with mild to moderate depression.*

Moncrieff, J., & Moncrieff, J. (1999). The Defeat Depression Campaign and trends in sickness and invalidity benefits for depressive illness. *Journal of Mental Health, 8,* 195–202.

OMS. (1986). *Charte d'Ottawa.*

OMS. (1998). *World Health Assembly resolution WHA51.12 – Health promotion.*

OMS. (2001). *Rapport sur la santé dans le monde 2001. Santé mentale : nouvelle conception, nouveaux espoirs.*

OMS. (2005). *Déclaration sur la santé mentale pour l'Europe : Relever les défis, trouver des solutions.*

Parslow, R. A., & Jorm, A. F. (2002). Improving Australians' depression literacy. *The Medical Journal of Australia, 177*(Suppl), S117–S121.

Paton, J., Jenkins, R., & Scott, J. (2001). Collective approaches for the control of depression in England. *Social Psychiatry and Psychiatric Epidemiology, 36*, 423–428.

Paykel, E. S., Tylee, A., Wright, A., Priest, R. G., Rix, S., & Hart, D. (1997). The Defeat Depression Campaign: Psychiatry in the public arena. *The American Journal of Psychiatry, 154*, 59–65.

Paykel, E. S., Hart, D., & Priest, R. G. (1998). Changes in public attitudes to depression during the Defeat Depression Campaign. *The British Journal of Psychiatry, 173*, 519–522.

Priest, R. G., Vize, C., Roberts, A., Roberts, M., & Tylee, A. (1996). Lay people's attitudes to treatment of depression: Results of opinion poll for Defeat Depression Campaign just before its launch. *BMJ, 313*, 858–859.

Quinn, N., Knifton, L., Goldie, I., Van Bortel, T., Dowds, J., Lasalvia, A., Scheerder, G., Boumans, J., Svab, V., Lanfredi, M., Wahlbeck, K., & Thornicroft, G. (2013). Nature and impact of European anti-stigma depression programmes. *Health Promotion International, 29*, 403–413.

Regier, D. A., Hirschfeld, R. M., Goodwin, F. K., Burke, J. D., Jr., Lazar, J. B., & Judd, L. L. (1988). The NIMH depression awareness, recognition, and treatment program: Structure, aims, and scientific basis. *The American Journal of Psychiatry, 145*, 1351–1357.

Rix, S., Paykel, E. S., Lelliott, P., Tylee, A., Freeling, P., Gask, L., & Hart, D. (1999). Impact of a national campaign on GP education: An evaluation of the Defeat Depression Campaign. *The British Journal of General Practice, 49*, 99–102.

Rochlen, A. B., Whilde, M. R., & Hoyer, W. D. (2005). The real men. Real depression campaign: Overview, theoretical implications, and research considerations. *Psychology of Men & Masculinity, 6*, 186–194.

Rochlen, A. B., Mckelley, R. A., & Pituch, K. A. (2006). A preliminary examination of the 'Real Men Real Depression' campaign. *Psychology of Men & Masculinity, 7*, 1–13.

Santé, M. D. L. (2004). *Plan Psychiatrie et Santé mentale 2005–2008.*

Thurin, J. M., & Briffault, X. (2006). Distinction, limits and complementarity between efficacy and effectiveness studies: New perspectives for psychotherapy research. *Encephale, 32*, 402–412.

# Extrapolation from Animal Model of Depressive Disorders: What's Lost in Translation?

Maël Lemoine

**Abstract** Animal models of depression are problematic and results drawn from them is moderately convincing. The main problem, it is often argued, is that it is impossible to model a mental disorder, i.e. specifically human, in animals like rodents: it is a matter of resemblance of symptoms. Yet in this field it is generally assumed that animal models of depression are more or less 'valid' according to three criteria: predictive, construct, and face validity, with only the latter concerned with the resemblance of symptoms. It is argued here that the problem is actually not with resemblance to the clinical features or to the factors of depression: it is not their being *mental* parameters. It lies, rather, in the fuzziness of the definition of a human entity and in the difficulty of linking together supposedly involved biological mechanisms into a consistent picture of the underlying process of the disease. It is therefore not that we cannot model what we know to be depression, it is rather that we do not know *what* to model.

## Introduction: Translational Research and Extrapolation in Psychiatry

Philosophers tend to import their own problems into foreign domains, not always for the sake of the greater good. An alternative strategy in the philosophy of science consists in trying to illuminate problems as scientists encounter them. Modeling mechanisms of diseases in organisms belongs to what is called 'translational research'. As a matter of fact, in contemporary medicine, 'translational research' is summarized through the rhetorical motto 'from the bench to the bedside'. As defined more specifically by the Translational Research Working Group regarding cancer research,

> Translational research transforms scientific discoveries arising from laboratory, clinical, or population studies into clinical applications to reduce cancer incidence, morbidity, and mortality. (Translational Research Working Group 2007, 99)[1]

---

[1] Other definitions have been proposed (see McArthur and Borsini 2008, xix).

M. Lemoine (✉)
University of Tours, INSERM U930, IHPST, Paris, France
e-mail: lemoine@univ-tours.fr

© Springer Science+Business Media Dordrecht 2016
J.C. Wakefield, S. Demazeux (eds.), *Sadness or Depression?*
History, Philosophy and Theory of the Life Sciences 15,
DOI 10.1007/978-94-017-7423-9_11

Yet this simple definition contains multiple meanings. In an editorial for the first issue of *Science Translational Medicine*, Elias A. Zerhouni, a former director of the National Institutes of Health and formerly a strong advocate of this approach, states that the term 'translational' can be understood in at least three senses: the rendering in clinical terms of what is *understood* at the basic level; the therapeutic *application* of basic biological knowledge; and the *extrapolation* made possible by the "profound unity of biology" resulting from "shared evolutionary pathways" (Zerhouni 2009). Indeed, application does not automatically follow understanding. This seems to be all the more true in psychiatry, where translational research has recently become a motto (the first issue of *Translational Psychiatry*, a publication by Nature Publishing Group was released in April 2011). Many potential treatments have resulted in disappointment and many exciting *in vivo* and *in vitro* models have failed to tackle the issue of human mental disorders.

As regards *in vivo* or animal models, experimental as well as more theoretical issues have been raised. As a matter of fact, concerns about the rationale of extrapolation from animal models have been both objected to and dismissed by philosophers (LaFollette and Shanks 1995; Schaffner 1998a, b, 2000; Ankeny 2001; Weber 2005), so the question may need further consideration in the specific case of animal models *of mental disorders*. More specifically still, scientists spontaneously distinguish disorders that seem to hit potentially anyone, such as anxiety and depressive disorders, and those disorders that seem to threaten only a clinical subpopulation, such as autistic disorders and schizophrenia; the latter seem to be even harder to model in animals than the former. The main reason seems to be the impossibility of modeling mental features that we find hard to understand 'intimately' in humans, a problem scientists apparently consider to be less stringent in the case of mood and anxiety disorders, where cognitive traits look less mysterious and behavioral traits far more recognizable.

Is modeling depression along with its mental processes, factors, and symptoms in animals truly unproblematic? My contention in this chapter is that the main problem scientists encounter in the field of mental health is not the fact that depression is difficult to model because its symptoms are 'mental', that is, personal, experienced, and contextual (1); rather, it is the fact that human depression is a fuzzy target of modeling, and that "piecemeal theorizing" (Murphy 2006) is required, which is a challenge to causal reasoning in medicine in general (2).

## Translation and Extrapolation about Depression: The Mind-Body Problem?

If rodents cannot conceive of guilt, worthlessness, despondency and dejection, or if they cannot worry about what the future may bring and 'consider' suicide, is there any causal pathway left for them to develop genuine depression? Broadly speaking, there are two series of objections here:

1. the target condition, i.e. *mental* disorders, cannot exist in animals (*dissimilarity of animal models to their human target*);
2. the causal network relevant to this condition, including *mental factors*, is not relevant for animals (*impossibility of bypassing mental causality*).

In this section, I consider the way translational psychiatry deals with both problems and conclude that problems raised by modeling mental disorders in animals are not relevant to the mind-body problem.

## How Translational Psychiatry Deals with the Problem of Similarity to Depressive Symptoms in Animal Models

### Feature-to-Feature Resemblance

In this section, I attempt to give a brief presentation of a field largely unknown to philosophers of psychiatry. When submitted to environmental factors similar to some of those precipitating depression in humans, like moderate chronic stress, animal models are expected to produce some behavioral symptoms and biological changes similar to those found in humans. In an experimental test of a pharmacological treatment, the animal should not only resemble the human, but the whole experimental situation should resemble the whole human situation too. This 'situation' is generally construed in the following way:

1. A disease entity instantiates in a human population marked by a genetic vulnerability through the occurrence of a pathogenic sequence of events enticing a neurobiological dysfunction.
2. This dysfunction can be assessed on the basis of clinical symptoms and biological markers thanks to diagnostic tests.
3. Any possible chemical treatment is a molecule with a pharmacological target called the endpoint.

The relevant features of resemblance in this situation are reduced to abstracted and idealized parameters (see Table 1).

Each parameter in itself is a matter of concern:

- *Disease entities* do not necessarily cross the boundaries of species.
- *Animal species* display specific natural and artificial properties with known and unknown advantages and drawbacks for modeling a specific disease.
- *Animal strands* are known for specific genetic vulnerabilities, some being an exaggeration of what can be encountered "in the wild", that is in a natural human population.
- *Pathogenic sequences of events* in humans have only partial correspondents in mice.
- Too many *neurobiological mechanisms* are potentially dysfunctional in depression.

**Table 1** Animal models of depression: Parameters of feature-to-feature resemblance

| Parameters (human condition) | Corresponding parameters (animal experiment) |
| --- | --- |
| Human depressive disorder | Animal equivalent of the depressive disorder |
| Genetic and environmental vulnerability factors | Animal species and strand |
| Depressogenic sequence of events | Stress protocol |
| Dysfunctional neurobiological mechanism | Dysfunctional neurobiological mechanism |
| Clinical symptoms | Behavioral and cognitive changes |
| Biomarkers | Biomarkers |
| Diagnostic tests | Biological, behavioral and cognitive tests |
| Endpoint | Endpoint |
| Treatment (molecule, vehicle and posology) | Treatment (molecule, vehicle and posology) |

- Some *clinical symptoms* of human depression have reasonably convincing equivalents in mice like psychomotor agitation or retardation, insomnia, weight loss, and even anhedonia, while others do not, such as feeling of guilt or worthlessness, irritability, or suicidal ideation.
- *Biomarkers*, that is, evaluated indicators of the intrinsic causes of an illness, its clinical course, and its modification by treatment (Frank and Hargreaves 2003), not pathognomonic or cutting-off signs, cannot generally be measured *in situ*, but only indirectly, and a thorough knowledge of the specifics of human and animal physiology is required to translate.
- Usual *clinical tests* differ in humans (questionnaires) and in animals (measurement and observation of activity).
- *Endpoint* of a candidate treatment, i.e. is the locus of action (receptor, behavior), is ideally the same in both humans and mice, but species may have different potential acceptors of the molecule leading to different potential side effects.
- A potential *treatment* itself has to be adapted in many ways, because of differences in required dosage (Lin 1998), or transposition of places to be stimulated in the case of transmagnetic stimulation (TMS).

Two concluding remarks are noteworthy. The first is that there are many more features to compare between species than it seems at first sight. Some are deeply problematic, others, not at all. The second remark is that scientists generally do not focus on the possibility of modeling, but rather on the strategic choices to make in order to design the best model possible. There are obviously good choices and bad choices, given what biologists generally assume about the inner working or main symptoms of depression. Nevertheless, all this indeed does not prove skepticism wrong about the potential results of animal research on depression. My main claim in this chapter is the reverse, i.e. that skepticism about resemblance of animal models to psychiatric conditions, if justified, does not entail that no significant result can come from this field.

## Face Validity, Predictive Validity, and Construct Validity

It is crucial to understand that translational research does not assess an animal model by *similarity* to the target, but by the *validity* of the inference. The similarity of the animal model to its human counterpart is neither a sufficient nor even a necessary condition of the validity of the extrapolation of a result based on animal experiments to a human population.

Many conditions of validity have been proposed and considered, for instance, in the field of the study of mood disorders, where this reflection happens to be most developed in translational psychiatry (Van der Staay 2006; van der Staay et al. 2009; Belzung and Lemoine 2011). Paul Willner proposed the most often cited conception of validity in this field (Willner 1984, 1994; Willner and Mitchell 2002); he distinguishes:

- *Face validity*: "the extent of similarity between the model and the disorder (…) on as wide as possible a range of symptoms and signs" (Willner and Mitchell 2002);
- *Predictive validity*: "similar response to treatment" (Willner 1984);
- *Construct validity*: specific similarity of the animal experiment to the theoretical entity referred to as the disease and supposed to explain its symptoms, and to this theoretical entity only.

These three aspects of validity are not only different, but also independent of one another, so that when one is fulfilled, the others are not necessarily satisfied.

Face validity is what is commonly understood by the 'resemblance' of the animal model to its human target, especially in critical assessments of translational psychiatry. Yet face validity is not considered as equally important as construct and predictive validity. About the relations between construct validity and face validity, for instance, Willner says:

> Face validity only requires the demonstration of similarity between the model and symptoms of the disorder being modelled. *Construct validity does not require superficial similarity which may, indeed, be absent.* It does, however, require the demonstration of homology – the same theoretical constructs must be applicable in the two cases – and an empirically supported rationale for believing that the construct in question is fundamental to the disorder, rather than an epiphenomenon. (Willner 1986, 684, my emphasis)

For instance, when examining two standard protocols, the Tail Suspension Test (TST) and the Unpredictable Chronic Mild Stress (UCMS), Willner notes that while the first has poor face validity and construct validity but strong predictive validity, the second has fair face validity and less convincing construct validity (depending on one's hypothesis on the relation between stress and depression). A mouse that stops moving when suspended by its tail bears little resemblance to either the observable features or any received explanatory model of depression. Yet it is strongly predictive of the action of a drug in depression, and this is considered sufficient to assess whether a treatment should be tested on humans. A mouse submitted for a protracted time to mild stressors such as nocturnal light, humidified soil, predator sounds, etc., shows signs very much alike to some of those depressed human subjects display, but it can be, and actually is, discussed on a theoretical level whether what stress entails is indeed an equivalent of depression.

It might be objected that predictive and construct validity also are specific forms of resemblance. As a matter of fact, predictive validity is more readily interpreted as a correlation of results of experiments than as a degree of resemblance between, say, effects of a treatment on mice and on humans. It says, roughly, that when the experiment is successful on mice, it will also be on humans. As to construct validity, it is not exactly the *similarity* of a model to its target, but rather the *conformation* of both the model and its target to a *theoretical* construct. Both what is observed in the model and in its target must be explained by the same underlying theoretical disease entity, all other theoretical disease entities excluded. It therefore depends on the nature of the theoretical construct, that is, whether animal modeling of depression is possible or not: as a highly sophisticated mental process, depression is hardly what rodents undergo. Nevertheless, the problem is that there is no consensual theoretical model of what depression consists of in translational research. Experimenting on animal models does not beg the question, but indeed excludes possible explanations – like highly elaborated psychodynamic models. This should not be considered a reductive claim, but a biological bet. What scientists really expect is not to make a point, but depends on the results of the experiments: it is a strategy, good or bad, not dogma. Of course, some scientists may try to make reductionist points. Yet objecting that experimenting on animal models cannot achieve any knowledge of the allegedly corresponding human condition is indeed both dogmatic and bad strategy.

Some may ask: what if the success of antidepressant medication was precisely defined through the very hypothesis that animal models implement? For instance, if 'depression' was defined as a 'low level of serotonin in the brain', then surely a certain animal model with a low level of serotonin in the brain could provide a wonderfully predictive model... at a small price. This objection of circularity is to be carefully considered. So far, the efficiency of antidepressant medication has not been assessed through biological markers, but rather as a result of scales, like the MADRS or the HAMD described above, that are not semantically, but empirically connected (or not) with drug intake.

For all these reasons, the resemblance of the animal model to its human target is but one series of problems among the more general question of the validity of the extrapolation, probably the less important, because what matters most is both the power of prediction and the theoretical interpretability of the model.

## How Psychiatry Deals with the Problem of Heterogeneous Factors

An additional problem comes from modeling causal factors of depression. This section presents how it is addressed.

## Multifactorial Determinants of Psychiatric Disorders vs. Animal Research

By famously urging the use of multifactorial models in psychiatry as well as in somatic medicine, Engel (1977) clearly opposed two attitudes he labeled reductionism and exclusionism. Whereas 'reductionism' was the view that biomolecular models should suffice to account for diseases both somatic and mental, 'exclusionism' was the view that conditions not amenable to biomolecular models were simply not diseases, which to some is the case for mental disorders (Szasz 1960). He proposed instead that the interaction of all factors, biological, psychological, and social, be studied in a system-theoretic approach. Since then, epidemiological studies of depression have repeatedly shown the importance of sociological and economical factors in its pathogenesis.

It requires a body and a nervous system to produce a sadness reaction, but it does not necessarily require stressful or demoralizing environmental conditions to deplete serotonin, stop hippocampal neurogenesis, or produce chronically high levels of cortisol. Psychological and social factors obviously supervene on some biological factors, whereas other biological factors do not make any psychological or social sense. Systemic approaches should therefore take great care to avoid considering the same factor twice, that is, as a biological as well as a sociological or a psychological factor. That is obviously not easily operationalized.

On the other hand, it is not necessary for someone working on animal models of depression to deny or even neglect the causal power of meaningfulness on an intelligent system (Bolton and Hill 2004). It is natural, on the contrary, to assume that if they exist at all in animals, mental causal factors, i.e. meanings, are already taken into account in their biological form and should not be 'added' somehow. In any case, cognitive bias, personality types, early-life events such as maternal care deprivation, neuroticism, and so on, all have proposed animal equivalents.

The problem is therefore not that some causal factors are not taken into account, but rather that in animals, the underlying biological phenomena of meanings might be absent or might underlie something else, so that in the best of cases, only an incomplete part of the biological mechanisms of depression can be studied. I assume that most scientists in the field would acknowledge that. I also assume that here again, what they are doing is a methodological bet rather than an ontological claim: it is possible to study some essential aspects of depression in a system that does not display other essential aspects of this mental disorder.

## Knowledge Approach vs. Treatment Approach

This methodological bet is an essential thing to understand. Let us take the example of drug discovery research. The point in modeling is not to create a homolog on which testing drugs is acceptable. It is not *knowledge-based* in the sense that scientists would think:

- If we knew how mental disorders worked, we could devise efficient treatments;
- We must experiment to know how they work;

- We cannot safely experiment directly on humans, we must therefore experiment on animals;
- What are the best animals to experiment on in order to know how the human disease works?
- Once we have good models, test of treatments on them will be trustworthy.

This line of thought can be encountered as a rhetorical justification of the method. However, as a matter of fact, the actual reasoning is rather *treatment-based*, and consists in the following:

- We know that some chemical agents have dramatic effects on mental disorders;
- These agents have effects on animals too;
- Which effects, on which animals, will guide us toward selecting the right chemical agents, i.e. with efficient and specific action, to test on humans?
- In order to restrain the possibilities of further agent candidates, we want to know how the right treatments work both on animals and on humans, i.e. what the targets could be.

The crucial point is that the analogy of causal effects is not assessed as a result of a previously existing theory, but rather that whatever the theory, any effective treatment on humans will have effects on some animals too; the question remains, though, which molecules affect which animals. Theories are not a starting point, but only a heuristic tool to restrain the domain of testable molecules.

### Relevant Differences: A Philosophical Account of How the Problem of Heterogeneous Factors Is Successfully Dealt With

A final concern is the possibility of modeling when significant factors differ – such as guilt, despair, and feelings of worthlessness. Modeling mental disorders such as depression is but a case of what philosopher Daniel Steel addresses as "the problem of extrapolation in heterogeneous populations" (Steel 2008). This refers to the possibility of inferring from one experiment on a test population to properties of a target population, when both populations differ in causal aspects *relevant* to the inferred properties. What is needed, according to Steel, is knowledge that relevant dissimilarities at corresponding stages of the mechanism of interest in the model and target have no significant effect on the point of comparison, 'significant' meaning affecting the extrapolation. He calls this approach "comparative process tracing" (Steel 2008, 89).

A facilitating condition is that it is possible to abstract some relevant factors, namely, upstream factors (resulting in the same starting point of the mechanism of interest), and downstream factors (intervening after the last stage of the mechanism of interest). The former can be abstracted away provided that there is no bypassing mechanism linking the upstream factor to a given stage in the mechanism of interest (Steel 2008, 90). The latter can also be abstracted away, provided that there is no feedback loop. Mental factors in depression are considered upstream factors, whereas mental reactions such as rumination are considered downstream factors. What is at stake is the mechanism that takes place in-between.[2]

Moreover, what is sought for is not a deterministic, but rather a probabilistic claim. The existence of any mechanism from X (cause) to Y (effect) in any individual in the animal population increases the probability of Y in the animal population when X is the case (Steel 2008, 109). At least, this is true if and only if there is at least one undisrupted mechanism from the cause to the effect, which in turn has the experimental consequence that any intervention on the cause makes a difference to the probability of the effect (*sublata causa, tollitur effectus*). This makes the case of mental phenomena a particularly difficult experimental problem. The reason is that they are very sensitive, or causally central, that is, possibly influenced by many more causal factors than most physical phenomena. Anything, from deprivation of a particular kind of food (say, chocolate) to living in a particular place, having undergone such or such experience in the past or having to in the future, can affect the mood in the most radical way. But this does not make it specific in nature, and it does not preclude a carefully designed animal model that can teach us something about causal mechanisms in depression.

All in all, in the case of the study of depression in animal models, the treatment approach I described above entails the preliminary assumption that what is directly at stake are the molecular interactions within the brain, and only indirectly the mental or social factors that supervene on them. This, however, does not completely abstract away mental factors, for it does not abstract away the molecular causal effects that underlie these factors in the brain. The problem is therefore, to identify

– the modular neuronal mechanism where some dysfunction is implied in the mental disorder in human subjects as well as in animal models;
– the modular neuronal mechanism realizing this particular kind of cognitive process that presumably does not take place in rodents (say, despondency after losing a job, despair at the perspective of the void of a life to come without a loved one, and so on);
– the causal interactions between both modules.

That done, animal modeling applies to the case of mental disorders without any specificity, provided that what is looked for is a picture of crucial parts of the mechanism, not the entirety of the mechanism, and that the approach is treatment-driven rather than knowledge-driven.

The conclusion is that modeling depression in animals does not raise specific problems because it is a mental disorder. The reasons why are: *(1)* most relevant features can be reasonably considered similar in both animals and humans; *(2)* face validity (i.e. resemblance) is but a minor point in extrapolation; *(3)* mental factors

---

[2] Steel also refers to another facilitating condition, namely, that the inference is about negative or positive causal relevance only, not on the effect size. Thereby, a certain degree of dissimilarity in corresponding stages of the mechanism does not affect the soundness of the extrapolation. This obviously applies to the problem of metabolism referred to above in the case of modeling depression.

can be considered as supervening on neurobiological mechanisms; *(4)* the approach is generally treatment-based, that is, does not presuppose a known mechanism to be similar, but rather, an interesting effect to occur in animals too; and *(5)* relevant factors can be abstracted away consistently even in the case of mental disorders. However, this does not mean that mental disorders in general, and depression in particular, do not pose specific problems to animal modeling. The problem with animal models of depression is therefore not an instance of the mind-body problem. What is it, if any?

## Something Is Modeled in Translational Psychiatry: What, Exactly?

The problem of inferring causal relations from animal models of depression to human targets is not the similarity of the model, but the indeterminacies of the target. Depressed human subjects are a fuzzy target. The definition of depression as a syndrome contributes to this fuzziness, and that must have consequences on the relevance of likely animal models: should they display all the symptoms animal models can, or a significant subset of them? So does the fact that the various mechanisms known to be possibly involved in depression do not fall neatly in place. In this situation, the scope of the extrapolation cannot be precisely determined.

### Fuzziness

The target population is fuzzily determined, first, through the uncertainty of the disease entity due to its polythetic semiology, second, through the width of the spectrum of mood disorders, and third, through the dimensionality of the criteria of depressive disorders. Consequently, the poor results of factor analysis and principal component analysis have repercussions on the evidential power of animal models of such conditions.

In the *Diagnostic and Statistical Manual of Mental Disorders* (DSM), a major depressive episode (MDE) is defined through alternative combinations of symptoms. This kind of diagnostic definition, called *polythetic*, leads to much heterogeneity in the population of people suffering from a MDE. Ostergaard et al. (2011) calculated that for 5 items out of 9, the first or the second being necessary, the possibilities number up to 227. Moreover, considering that three criteria contain alternate but incompatible subcases (*either* weight gain *or* weight loss, etc.), the number of possible forms of MDE could amount to 1497. The result is that many configurations of symptoms have not even one symptom in common, and many more share only nonspecific symptoms (such as insomnia and weight loss). The problem is that no common underlying dysfunctional system has yet been discovered from which such heterogeneous patterns could be causally derived, and thereby the unity of the syndrome, justified. What is, then, the possible configuration, or the core symptom, that animal models should display? Anhedonia and 'helplessness' behaviors are most often proposed; this is a strong theoretical claim, which clinicians may question.

MDEs occur within the course of many mental disorders, including major depressive disorder (MDD) but also bipolar disorders or schizophrenia. It is a question whether the nature of the MDE is the same under the surface of symptoms in these different cases. Moreover, major depressive disorder is different from but next to disruptive mood dysregulation disorder, chronic depressive disorder (formerly known as dysthymia), premenstrual dysphoric disorder, the controversial and abandoned 'mixed anxiety/depression', substance-induced depressive disorder, depressive disorder associated with a known general medical condition, and a few other specified depressive disorder and unspecified depressive disorder. It is not so clear whether there are biological differences underlying these distinctions and above all how, if biological, these differences could be modeled in animals. Moreover, one can wonder whether what is induced or observed in animals is specific to MDE. The Novelty Suppressed Feeding test (i.e., testing whether a rodent will or will not eat in an unknown environment), for instance, is sometimes considered as a test of anxiety, and sometimes as a test of depression.[3] This uncertainty unintentionally reflects many hesitations in the clinic about the distinction to be made between these two disorders. The upshot is that whereas animals are supposed to model one mental disorder, this specificity is highly questionable and there is a genuine problem in knowing what, exactly, is modeled in a 'depressed' mouse.

Two further problems are worth mentioning. The first is the dimensionality of criteria. Most features of depression can, and maybe should, be assessed quantitatively: disturbed sleep and weight change, for example; but things such as loss of interest and feelings of worthlessness can be quantified as moderate, mild or severe (see the Beck Depression Inventory (BDI), the Hamilton Rating Scale for Depression (HDRS/HAMD) and the Montgomery-Åsberg Depression Rating Scale (MADRS)). It is often noted that the main outcome of such continuity is fuzzy boundaries between normal and pathological sadness and pessimism. This, too, is a difficulty for modeling: should only severe cases be modeled? However, these scales are generally used as a measure of severity rather than presence of a MDE.

Second, there is the problem of the poor results of factor and cluster analyses. For instance, the key result of Paykel's study in the 1970s was that the main distinction was between old subjects with severe depression and young subjects with mild depression, the former subdividing between psychotic and anxious types, the latter, between hostile types and those with personality disorders (Paykel 1971). A classical factor analysis of depression found three profiles, "anxious-tense depression", "hostile depression" and "retarded depression" (Overall et al. 1966); yet another found that the main factors were the neurotic-psychotic axis and the depressive vs. paranoid factor (Kay et al. 1969). As philosopher Rachel Cooper rightly emphasized, the problem with all studies of this kind is theoretical and comes either with

---

[3] As neurobiologist Catherine Belzung explained to me (personal communication).

the choice or with the interpretation of variables and results (clusters or profile) (Cooper 2010). In other terms, the problem is the elaboration of the relevant construct. Animal models should conform to that construct, but a prior decision is to be made: should psychiatrists include observable variables that have clear equivalents in mice? The second question is: can the result of a cluster or factor analysis in humans be back-translated into mice?

## Mosaicism and Chimerism of Models

Despite the treatment approach I emphasized in the first section, some knowledge of the whole biological picture is necessary to model the disease. We have some indeed, but it is very patchy: areas of known mechanisms upon which used treatments act are surrounded by largely unknown causal chains. This situation leads to what philosopher Dominic Murphy calls, in *Psychiatry in the Scientific Image*, "piecemeal theorizing", that is, the fact that psychiatry about mental disorders in general employs "generalizations or causal models of limited scope at different levels" rather than "one big elegant theory" (Murphy 2006, 240–1). In the more specific case of one given mental disorder in turn, Murphy distinguishes global models, designed to explain all symptoms by one general dysfunction, and modular models, designed to explain all symptoms by a series of part-dysfunction, each explaining one symptom or one part of the symptoms.

The requirements of animal experiments are partly responsible for the prevalence of piecemeal theorizing and modular models in biological approaches to depression. One has to choose *one* putative mechanism to model it. In translational psychiatry, scientists therefore consider their animal models to instantiate *one* component mechanism of the disease (hopefully *the key* mechanism). But they do not exactly know where, in the global plan of the disease, this mechanism stands – that is, what are its causal relations with the rest. It may be central or peripheral, it may precede, follow, or add up to other mechanisms in the course of the mental disorder.

The main biological hypothesis on depression until recently, the monoamine hypothesis, is an illustration of piecemeal theorizing. The serendipitous discovery of seemingly effective treatments of depression, tricyclic antidepressant (imipramine), and monoamine oxidase inhibitors (iproniazid), led to research on their target, mainly, the serotonergic system (Maxwell and Echhardt 1990; McArthur and Borsini 2008). Further exploration of this biological mechanism in animal models led in turn to better animal models on the one hand, and better molecules on the other hand (mostly, with less side effects): chiefly, fluoxetine. Many have thought that an imbalance in the serotonergic system, grossly in the form of a depletion of synaptic serotonin, expressed the main mechanism of depression (Hirschfeld 2000). Yet this position hides a paradox, that of the delay of action of mood regulators: how can depression consist mainly in a serotonin deficit if normal levels are restored almost immediately under medication, but improvement occurs only 3 weeks after the treatment begins? This question has more recently lead scientists to question the centrality of serotonergic system in depression, and look for complementary, alternative, or competing hypotheses. Among others, a possible disruption in hippocampal neurogenesis, which has in turn been linked to a mechanism known to be crucial in anxiety disorders, the so-called hippothalamo-pituitary-adrenergic axis of stress, and so on to a dozen other mechanisms possibly involved in depression (Licino and Wong 2005).

This situation, i.e. many different animal models of various mechanisms of mostly unknown importance and causal relations with one another, though referring to the same mental disorder, I propose to call *mosaicism* of animal models. I distinguish it from *chimerism* of animal models, i.e. the fact that several different animals are usually required for the instantiation of one hypothesis, each instantiating one part of the component mechanism of the disease, none instantiating the whole mechanism. In other terms, there is not one animal model similar to the mental disorder according to hypothesis $X$ on its inner mechanisms, but rather several animal models implementing parts of the whole mechanism supposed to take place in the disease in humans. For instance, the hypothesis that the s/s polymorphism of the serotonin transporter gene is a vulnerability factor to depression, and requires that a whole chain of events from this polymorphism to symptoms of depression be established. As a matter of fact, it has been, but not the whole chain into a single model – it required at least three different rodent models.

Both mosaicism and chimerism of animal models are consequences of modeling in the dark about the ins and outs of mental disorders. The main outcome of that necessity to model piecemeal is on the scope of the extrapolation. First, one does not know the strategic place of the part of the human disease modeled in the animal and, second, one does not extrapolate from one type of animal to the human target population on the basis of a one-to-one resemblance, but from several types of animals to the human target population on the basis of a many-to-one resemblance.

# Conclusion

What is lost in the translation of animal models to human targets? It was not a well-formed meaning, but rather the conviction that there was one in the first place. The question is not the impossibility of translating mental properties and mental factors into 'animal language'. The real problem with animal models of depression is depression itself. First, the human population to be modeled is not itself strictly determined, and second, animal models cannot be thought of as experiments about mechanisms precisely placed and fitting nicely into the sound template of a biological theory of this mental disorder, for there is no such theory. They indicate fixed directions and sound natural facts about those mechanisms, but we do not know which directions and which facts.

In the face of this problem, there have been theoretical attempts at gathering all we know about the biology of depression (Kendler et al. 2002, 2006; Willner et al.

2012). The problem is always about searching either for consistent, if alternative, underpinning mechanisms of a same clinical condition, or for a relevant definition of the clinical presentation of the same biological dysfunction. Should we redefine depression after what we think we know of its underlying biology or should we search for a biological rationale of what we think we observe of its clinical presentation? Translational psychiatry of depression is at the heart of this problem. It tends to use concepts, such as that of 'endophenotypes', to resolve the question. As opposed to exophenotypes, that is, clinical presentations of depression affected by many environmental and developmental factors, endophenotypes are hypothetical underlying presentations of genetic factors of depression. In the present field, they consist in behavioral patterns affected by genetics only, that is, hereditary, possibly hidden or disguised by cultural or biographical events (John and Lewis 1966; McArthur and Borsini 2008). Their function is obviously to deconstruct the clinically defined syndromes into (yet) undetermined alternative phenotypes, of which traditional clinical entities might have been an approximate picture. As endophenotypes would not necessarily be species-bound, and could be defined after whatever genetic determinants of depression can be discovered, they would totally redefine the human condition that depression is into a biological, trans-species condition. If the unity and reality of the condition were specifically human and relied on meanings, then this attempt would be doomed to failure.

This ultimate consequence of animal modeling – to rewrite the very notion of what depression is about – is neither to be fought nor favored by philosophers. As a matter of fact, scientific progress is about the naturalization of prescientific notions such as movement, heat, reproduction, species, but also diabetes, epilepsy, and, possibly, schizophrenia and depression. Some of these attempts at naturalization seem to be bound to fail, some, to succeed: how could a philosopher know which ones can successfully be naturalized before they are? For a successful naturalization, i.e., roughly, an explication of a profane notion through the terms of natural sciences, is not about the faithfulness of the scientific concept to the prescientific concept (Murphy 2006; Lemoine 2014). It is about capturing, in a consistent picture, how nature works.

**Acknowledgments** Professors C. Belzung, neurobiologist, and V. Camus, psychiatrist, have read and discussed the paper. Thanks to them for having always been an invaluable help since the beginning of my philosophical work in their team.

# References

Ankeny, R. A. (2001). Model organisms as models: Understanding the "Lingua Franca" of the human genome project. *Proceedings of the Philosophy of Science Association 2001, 68,* S251–S261.

Belzung, C., & Lemoine, M. (2011). Criteria of validity for animal models of psychiatric disorders: Focus on anxiety disorders and depression. *Biology of Mood and Anxiety Disorders, 1,* 9. doi:10.1186/2045-5380-1-9.

Bolton, D., & Hill, J. (2004). *Mind, meaning and mental disorder: The nature of causal explanation in psychology and psychiatry* (2nd ed.). Oxford: Oxford University Press.

Cooper, R. (2010). *Classifying madness: A philosophical examination of the diagnostic and statistical manual of mental disorders* (1st ed.). Softcover of orig. ed. 2005. New York: Springer.

Engel, G. (1977). The need for a new medical model: A challenge for biomedicine. *Science, 196*, 129–136.

Frank, R., & Hargreaves, R. (2003). Clinical biomarkers in drug discovery and development. *Nature Reviews Drug Discovery, 2*, 566–580. doi:10.1038/nrd1130.

Hirschfeld, R. M. A. (2000). History and evolution of the monoamine hypothesis of depression. *The Journal of Clinic Psychiatry, 61*(supp. 6), 4–6.

John, B., & Lewis, K. R. (1966). Chromosome variability and geographic distribution in insects. *Science, 152*, 711–721. doi:10.1126/science.152.3723.711.

Kay, D. W., Garside, R. F., Beamish, P., & Roy, J. R. (1969). Endogenous and neurotic syndromes of depression: A factor analytic study of 104 cases. Clinical features. *The British Journal of Psychiatry, 115*, 377–388.

Kendler, K. S., Gardner, C. O., & Prescott, C. A. (2002). Toward a comprehensive developmental model for major depression in women. *The American Journal of Psychiatry, 159*, 1133–1145.

Kendler, K. S., Gardner, C. O., & Prescott, C. A. (2006). Toward a comprehensive developmental model for major depression in men. *The American Journal of Psychiatry, 163*, 115–124. doi:10.1176/appi.ajp.163.1.115.

LaFollette, H., & Shanks, N. (1995). Two models of models in biomedical research. *Philosophical Quarterly, 45*, 141–160.

Lemoine, M. (2014). The naturalization of the concept of disease. In G. Lambert, M. Silberstein, & P. Huneman (Eds.), *Classification, disease and evidence. New essays in the philosophy of medicine* (pp. 19–41). Amsterdam: Springer.

Licino, J., & Wong, M. L. (Eds.). (2005). *Biology of depression. From novel insights to therapeutic strategies*. Weinheim: Wiley.

Lin, J. H. (1998). Applications and limitations of interspecies scaling and in vitro extrapolation in pharmacokinetics. *Drug Metabolism and Disposition, 26*, 1202–1212.

Maxwell, R. A., & Echhardt, S. B. (1990). *Drug discovery: A casebook and analysis*. Clifton: Humana Press Inc.

McArthur, R. A., & Borsini, F. (2008). *Animal and translational models for CNS drug discovery: Psychiatric disorders*. Burlington: Academic.

Murphy, D. (2006). *Psychiatry in the scientific image*. Cambridge, MA: MIT Press.

Ostergaard, S. D., Jensen, S. O. W., & Bech, P. (2011). The heterogeneity of the depressive syndrome: When numbers get serious. *Acta Psychiatrica Scandinavica, 124*(6), 495–496 doi:10.1111/j.1600-0447.2011.01744.x.

Overall, J. E., Hollister, L. E., Johnson, M., & Pennington, V. (1966). Nosology of depression and differential response to drugs. *JAMA, 195*, 946–948.

Paykel, E. S. (1971). Classification of depressed patients: A cluster analysis derived grouping. *The British Journal of Psychiatry, 118*, 275–288.

Schaffner, K. F. (1998a). Genes, behavior, and developmental emergentism: One process, indivisible? *Philosophy of Science, 65*, 209–252.

Schaffner, K. F. (1998b). Model organisms and behavioral genetics: A rejoinder. *Philosophy of Science, 65*, 276–288.

Schaffner, K. F. (2000). Behavior at the organismal and molecular levels: The case of C. Elegans. *Philosophy of Science, 67*, 288.

Steel, D. (2008). *Across the boundaries: Extrapolation in biology and social science*. Oxford: Oxford University Press.

Szasz, T. S. (1960). The myth of mental illness. *American Psychologist, 15*, 113–118. doi:10.1037/h0046535.

Translational Research Working Group. (2007). *Transformation translation – Harnessing discovery for patient and public benefit*. Washington, DC: National Cancer Institution/National Institutes of Health/U.S. Department of health and human services.

Van der Staay, F. J. (2006). Animal models of behavioral dysfunctions: Basic concepts and classifications, and an evaluation strategy. *Brain Research Reviews, 52*, 131–159. doi:10.1016/j.brainresrev.2006.01.006.

Van der Staay, F. J., Arndt, S. S., & Nordquist, R. E. (2009). Evaluation of animal models of neurobehavioral disorders. *Behavioral and Brain Function, 5*, 11. doi:10.1186/1744-9081-5-11.

Weber, M. (2005). *Philosophy of experimental biology*. Cambridge: Cambridge University Press.

Willner, P. (1984). The validity of animal models of depression. *Psychopharmacology, 83*, 1–16.

Willner, P. (1986). Validation criteria for animal models of human mental disorders: Learned helplessness as a paradigm case. *Progress Neuro-Psychopharmacology and Biology Psychiatry, 10*, 677–690.

Willner, P. (1994). Animal models of depression. In J. den Boer & J. Ad Sitsen (Eds.), *Handbook of depression and anxiety. A biological approach* (pp. 291–316). New York/Basel/Hong Kong: Marcel Dekker.

Willner, P., & Mitchell, P. J. (2002). The validity of animal models of predisposition to depression. *Behavioural Pharmacology, 13*, 169–188.

Willner, P., Scheel-Krüger, J., & Belzung, C. (2012). The neurobiology of depression and antidepressant action. *Neuroscience and Biobehavioral Reviews*. doi:10.1016/j.neubiorev.2012.12.007.

Zerhouni, E. A. (2009). Space for the cures: Science launches a new journal dedicated to translational research in biomedicine. *Science Translational Medicine, 1*, 1ed1. doi:10.1126/scitranslmed.3000341.

# Psychiatry's Continuing Expansion of Depressive Disorder

Jerome C. Wakefield and Allan V. Horwitz

**Abstract** In our book, *The Loss of Sadness* (LoS), published in 2007, we argued that DSM symptom-based diagnostic criteria for depressive disorder confuse intense normal sadness with depressive disorder, thus potentially misdiagnosing large numbers of individuals with a psychiatric disorder when in fact they are responding to loss or stress with normal human emotions. We detailed the many negative effects of such misdiagnosis, from unnecessary treatment to meaningless research results to distorted mental health policy. In this chapter, we review the main developments since LoS's publication that bear on its thesis. For example, recent epidemiological surveys have confirmed that the majority of individuals experience DSM-defined depression at some point in life, antidepressant medication use continues to rise sharply, and depression is increasingly treated by general physicians rather than mental health professionals. Most importantly, the recently published fifth edition of the DSM (DSM-5) further expanded major depression by eliminating the "bereavement exclusion," a clause that acknowledged that mild depressive symptoms could be normal when they occurred shortly after the death of a loved one. The DSM-5's elimination of the bereavement exclusion, we find, was based on largely spurious arguments, while ample research evidence has confirmed the exclusion's validity. In addition, DSM-5 greatly expanded the overall domain of depressive disorders by adding several new diagnostic categories that are each open to overdiagnosing the intensely sad individual as being psychiatrically disordered. The trends we observed in LoS, we conclude, are confirmed by subsequent developments and are if anything accelerating.

In 1980, the American Psychiatric Association published the third edition of its official diagnostic manual, *The Diagnostic and Statistical Manual of Mental*

J.C. Wakefield (✉)
Silver School of Social Work and Department of Psychiatry,
New York University, New York, NY, USA
e-mail: jw111@nyu.edu

A.V. Horwitz
Department of Sociology, Rutgers University, New Brunswick, NJ, USA
e-mail: ahorwitz@sas.rutgers.edu

© Springer Science+Business Media Dordrecht 2016
J.C. Wakefield, S. Demazeux (eds.), *Sadness or Depression?*
History, Philosophy and Theory of the Life Sciences 15,
DOI 10.1007/978-94-017-7423-9_12

*Disorders* (DSM-III; American Psychiatric Association 1980) at a time when psychiatry was being severely criticized for the unreliability of its diagnoses. To address these complaints, rather than providing the traditional diagnostic labels with a sentence or two of vague description, DSM-III for the first time provided lists of symptoms by which to diagnose each psychiatric disorder, increasing the reliability and precision of diagnosis and allowing for more productive research. This turned out to be a watershed moment, providing American psychiatry with a scientific legitimacy that had previously eluded it. Subsequent editions of the DSM through to the current fifth edition, DSM-5 (American Psychiatric Association 2013), refined the criteria but did not alter DSM-III's basic approach. Moreover, through the widespread adoption of the DSM system by other countries, and through the DSM's powerful influence on the subsequent development of the World Health Organization's (WHO) International Classification of Disease (ICD-10; World Health Organization 1992), DSM-III reshaped psychiatric diagnosis worldwide. The ICD followed DSM-III's lead with symptom-based guidelines for psychiatric diagnosis – although it never attempted the precise necessary-and-sufficient algorithms included in DSM.

Among the disorders that DSM-III newly defined in this precise manner was major depressive disorder (MDD). MDD was defined in terms of symptoms such as sadness, loss of interest or pleasure in usual activities, insomnia, lessened appetite or weight loss, difficulty concentrating, a sense of worthlessness or guilt, suicidal thinking, and other such symptoms. To be diagnosed with MDD, one had to have symptoms from at least 5 out of 9 symptom groups for at least 2 weeks.

Once this symptom-based definition was in place and widely applied, MDD became the most important of the several hundred diagnostic categories in the manual. It was by far the most common condition diagnosed in outpatient practices (Olfson et al. 2002). Community surveys indicated that MDD was the single most prevalent mental illness in the population (Kessler et al. 2003). The World Health Organization, calculating the actual and prospective burden of disease imparted by MDD, found that MDD was the fourth leading cause of disability due to disease worldwide in 2002 (Ustun et al. 2004), and warned that MDD would become the second most disabling of any medical condition worldwide by 2030, save only for HIV/AIDS (Mathers and Loncar 2006). It appeared that we had entered an "Age of Depression" that replaced or perhaps supplemented the "Age of Anxiety" that dominated the Western world in the post-World War II era.

However, we do not view this new age of depression as the result of a genuine epidemic of depressive mental illnesses. In our book, *The Loss of Sadness: How Psychiatry Transformed Normal Sorrow into Depressive Disorder* (LoS; Horwitz and Wakefield 2007), we observed that intense normal sadness and depressive disorder are distinct conditions that can be manifested by very similar symptoms and thus can easily be confused, a point already recognized in antiquity. We thus argued that the seeming epidemic of major depression mainly stemmed from the DSM's symptom-based diagnostic criteria that conflated normal sadness and depressive disorder and mistakenly categorized both of these conditions as psychiatric disorders.

Contrary to antipsychiatric critics who see psychiatry primarily as social control masquerading as a medical field, we do acknowledge in LoS the obvious existence of genuine and serious mental disorders that should be the target of medical treatment efforts, including depressive disorders. Just as any biologically designed bodily process can fail to function properly and can yield a physical disorder, so any biologically shaped psychological process, such as sadness or grief, can fail to function properly and can yield a mental disorder (First and Wakefield 2013; Horwitz and Wakefield 2007; Wakefield 1992, 2006). The problem was not that depressive disorder does not exist, but that its domain was inflated by DSM's symptom-based criteria to encompass much normal human emotion.

LoS received wide publicity and positive reviews, and was named the best psychology book of the year by the Association of American Publishers. The question remained of what impact it would have on psychiatric diagnosis.

The time was right to reconsider psychiatry's approach to depression. LoS was published just as American psychiatrists, after almost a decade of quiet preparation, began more actively and publicly to prepare the new fifth edition of the DSM (DSM-5; American Psychiatric Association 2013). LoS provides what we believe is a compelling critique of the DSM-IV criteria for major depressive disorder (MDD) and a critical analysis of how psychiatry came to mistakenly categorize so many people who experience intense normal sadness as psychiatrically ill with MDD. Our hope was that LoS would stimulate changes in the way the forthcoming DSM-5 would define this diagnosis, hopefully causing the criteria to be amended to narrow the range of conditions classified as depressive disorders. Our critique, as we will explain below, did indeed influence the DSM-5 classification of MDD, although not in the way that we intended.

Proposals for changes to be made to the diagnostic criteria used to identify mental disorders in DSM-5 were made public by the DSM-5 Task Force and by the many DSM-5 work groups concerned with specific groups of disorders in 2010. The French edition of LoS (Horwitz and Wakefield 2010), translated by Francoise Parot, was published just at the time when the proposed revisions were starting to be hotly debated. That debate intensified over time and absorbed American psychiatry right up to the publication of DSM-5 in May 2013. This volume of reflections on depression is appearing a couple of years after DSM-5's publication. This chapter endeavors to bring the story of depression's fate in the DSM and society more generally up to date, filling in the main developments from the time of the publication of LoS to the publication of DSM-5. Many of the changes in the DSM-5 that we describe are likely to be reflected as well in the upcoming eleventh revision of the ICD, currently in preparation.

## Terminology

Terminology poses a challenge when discussing whether certain conditions classified by DSM-5 as depressive disorders are in fact normal sadness. The two domains of psychiatric disorder and normal suffering usually involve quite different terminology. The medical conditions are described by medical terms such as "diagnosis," "symptoms," and "depression," whereas normal sadness is generally described by terms such as "feelings," "grief," "suffering," and so on. However, when considering whether certain conditions are disorders or normal sadness, the discussion can become quite tortured if one flips back and forth between vocabularies. More importantly, one's choice of vocabulary in disputed cases can beg the very question under consideration by presupposing or at least suggesting the nature of the condition being described.

Consequently, as in LoS, for convenience we adopt here the standard terminological convention one finds in most writing on this topic, which is to use the medical vocabulary of "symptom," "diagnosis," and "depression" throughout as a uniform way to describe both disorders and non-disorders, including conditions whose status is under dispute. These medical terms are to be understood as purely descriptive and as neutral with regard to disorder versus normality, so that they do not imply the presence of a medical disorder. Thus, as used here, normal sadness has "symptoms" such as insomnia and lessened interest in one's usual activities, "depression" is sometimes a normal emotion (a usage that has become quite common), and a clinician can "diagnose" a condition as normal sadness. We also use the DSM's phrase "depressive episode" as well as the phrase "DSM depression" to denote any condition that satisfies the DSM's symptom and duration criteria for MDD (i.e., at least 5 symptoms for at least two weeks), but again neutrally with respect to whether such episodes are disorders or, contrary to DSM, are sometimes periods of intense normal sadness. We do not intend for this terminological convenience to in any way demean, implicitly medicalize, or simplify the all-too-human experience of grieving the loss of that which we love.

## The Ubiquity of Depression

One of the most revealing recent scientific developments for an understanding of the nature of DSM-defined MDD is the improved measurement of the prevalence of DSM-defined depressive episodes in the general population. In LoS, we documented a dramatic rise in the estimated lifetime prevalence (i.e., how many people have the condition at some point in their lives) of major depressive disorder in the United States. Just a few decades ago, psychiatrists were trained to believe that perhaps 2–3 % of the population would suffer from depressive disorder, which was considered a relatively rare but severe disorder (Klein and Thase 1997). Others considered the true prevalence to be in the vicinity of 1–2 %, if they believed that "endogenous" depression, a more severe form, was the only form legitimately diagnosed as a medical disorder (Parker 2007). These views corresponded to the more demanding approach to depression diagnosis taken throughout much of medical history (Horwitz & Wakefield 2007).

The most methodologically advanced studies of the national prevalence of DSM-defined MDD in the community that were available at the time of LoS's publication were cross-sectional studies that interviewed a sample of subjects during one period of time and asked them to recall whether they had ever experienced each of the depressive symptoms in the past, and if so, whether they had experienced them together during a common episode. These recollections were then transformed into diagnoses and used to calculate how many people have depressive disorders at any point over a lifetime.

Major DSM-based cross-sectional studies of nationally representative samples, some of which were reported in LoS, revealed increasingly large numbers of individuals who at some point satisfied the DSM diagnostic criteria for MDD. The initial DSM-based study, the Epidemiological Catchment Area Study (ECA), found a national lifetime MDD prevalence rate of 5.2 % (Robins and Regier 1991). Further studies with improved methodology trended much higher, including the National Comorbidity Survey (NCS) rate of 17 % for depressive episodes of all kinds (Kessler et al. 1994) and 15 % for MDD strictly defined (Kessler et al. 1996), the National Comorbidity Survey Replication (NCS-R) rate of 16 % (Kessler et al. 2003), and the National Epidemiologic Survey of Alcoholism and Related Conditions (NESARC) rate of 13 % (Hasin et al. 2005). Although the NCS's 17 % rate tends to get cited, perhaps the most authoritative estimate was Kessler et al.'s (2005) projection of lifetime risk from the NCS-R data, yielding an overall lifetime MDD risk up to age 75 years old of 23 %, about a quarter of the entire population. Similar lifetime rates were arrived at in many other countries at about the same time using similar cross-sectional methodology, including rates in Germany, the Netherlands, Norway, Italy and Hungary ranging from 15 to 18 % (Hasin et al. 2005).

The magnitude of these prevalence rates puzzled even some prominent epidemiologists, who acknowledged that normal reactions to stress might have been misclassified as depressive disorder (Narrow et al. 2002; Regier et al. 1998). Attempts to resolve the problem by limiting diagnosis to conditions in which there was distress or role impairment were not very successful in reducing prevalence (Wakefield and Spitzer 2002), perhaps because normal negative emotions such as sadness can be intense and are inherently distressing and often impairing of one's usual role performance. Consequently, these "clinical significance" criteria did not really distinguish disorder from normality (Spitzer and Wakefield 1999; Wakefield 2009; Wakefield and First 2013; Wakefield et al. 2010). Moreover, a troubling question went unexpressed at the time: if the DSM criteria do in fact confuse normal sadness with psychiatric disorder, then is it possible that even these high rates are too low and that with full information we would find even more people in the community that satisfy the DSM-defined MDD criteria?

In terms of full information, the question about all of these cross-sectional studies was the accuracy and completeness of memory; were respondents recalling all of the symptoms they had experienced years before the interview? In fact, memory is known to be notoriously unreliable about such feelings when recalled many years later (Kruijshaar et al. 2005). The only way to establish the true prevalence of DSM-defined MDD in the community would be to follow individuals longitudinally and periodically assess them while symptoms were still fresh in their minds.

At the time that LoS's manuscript was in preparation, two initial longitudinal studies that were methodologically limited but still quite informative had been recently published, but did not come to our attention in time to be reported in the book. First, Wells and Horwood (2004) reported on a representative sample of a cohort of youths born in the New Zealand city of Christchurch in 1977, who were given mental health assessments starting at age 15 (in 1992) that included questions about the depressive symptoms they had experienced the previous year. The youths were re-interviewed at ages 16, 18, and 21 years. In just the 7-year study period between the ages of 14 and 21 years old, 37 % of Wells and Horwood's (2004) sample satisfied DSM MDD criteria at one or more points, supporting the notion of radically higher prevalence rates than were reported in cross-sectional studies. Moreover, 54 % reported key depressive symptoms of depressed mood or loss of interest, so even those who did not qualify for MDD often would have qualified for minor or subthreshold depression or adjustment disorder with depressive features.

The second study not reported in LoS was a longitudinal study starting in 1978 but continuing through to 2007 (Parker 1979, 2007), in which Wilhelm and Parker followed a cohort of students who took a one-year post-graduate course in teacher education at a Sydney college, measuring a variety of depression-related variables every 5 years. When the study began, they asked participants whether they had experienced depression in the broad sense that includes normal mood variation, defining depression as any "significant lowering of mood, with or without feelings of guilt, hopelessness and helplessness, or a drop in one's self-esteem or self-regard" (Parker 1979, p. 128). Fully 95 % of the sample reported having such experiences, with 91 % reporting having had them in the past year, and with a mean number of episodes occurring in the past year of 6.3 episodes (Parker 1979, 2007). This nicely illustrates the ubiquity of normal depressive mood shifts. Regarding lifetime prevalence of MDD, based on the initial interview and three subsequent interviews, Wilhelm and Parker's sample had a lifetime MDD prevalence rate over a period of 15 years of 35 % (Wilhelm et al. 1996). If one includes in depressive disorder both major depression and DSM minor depression (the latter requiring 3–4 symptoms for 2 weeks), then 57 % of the sample had experienced a depressive disorder. When the sample was examined after 25 years, with the sample's average age having increased from 23 to 48 years old, the lifetime cumulative MDD prevalence rate was 42 % (Wilhelm et al. 2006).

Two more incisive studies with improved methodology that appeared subsequent to LoS's publication have come close to satisfactorily resolving the question of lifetime prevalence of DSM-defined MDD for a substantial age range, though not yet for the entire lifespan. Moffitt et al. (2007, 2010) longitudinally followed a representative cohort of individuals in Dunedin, New Zealand over the years from childhood to adulthood. The respondents were periodically interviewed only about symptoms they had experienced during the past year before the interview, maximizing accuracy of recall. The result was that, in contrast to the standard estimate of 17 % lifetime prevalence of MDD derived from cross-sectional studies, the Dunedin study yielded roughly a 17 % prevalence rate of MDD *in any one given year*. The cumulative Dunedin lifetime rate of MDD over the four one-year measurements at ages 18, 21, 26, and 32 (i.e., the percentage who satisfied DSM criteria for MDD at any one or more of the four one-year evaluation points) was 41.4 %. This lifetime rate does not include individuals who had depressive episodes only before age 18 or after age 32, or had them only during the other 10 years between the ages of 18 and 32 that were not sampled in the four one-year evaluations, so full lifetime prevalence would be considerably higher.

A second longitudinal study by Rohde et al. (2013) essentially replicated the main results of the Moffitt et al. study. Rohde et al. found a 51 % cumulative incidence of MDD in a U.S. cohort of Oregon children followed longitudinally from childhood to age 30, with interviews at roughly 6-year intervals covering the time since the previous interview rather than just the previous year. MDD prevalences just during the "emerging adult" (ages 18–23 years) and "adult" (ages 24–30 years) periods were 28 % and 26 %, respectively. Recalculating from Rohde et al.'s tables and counting only MDD in emerging adulthood and newly emerging cases in adulthood, Rohde et al.'s findings indicate a minimum incidence of DSM MDD between ages 18 and 30 of 44 % (an underestimate because cases in adulthood recurrent with episodes experienced before emerging adulthood are missed in this count). This result is comparable to Moffitt et al.'s (2010) finding for the same ages of 41 %.

However, neither the Moffitt et al. nor the Rohde et al. studies considered MDD first-onsets that occurred after the early thirties. We don't yet have longitudinal studies for the lifetime of community samples, so we don't know what the prevalence of DSM-defined MDD would be across the entire lifespan. The best that can be done at present is speculatively to extrapolate total prevalence, using cross-sectional studies to indicate roughly how many first onsets occur in older individuals.

For example, in the cross-sectional National Comorbidity Survey Replication (NCS-R), using careful life-history-review methodology, Kessler et al. (2005) found that 50 % of the cases reported first onset after the age of 32. Eaton et al. (1995) similarly found in the ECA that of those satisfying the DSM MDD criteria, "50 % meet the criteria before they are 35" (p. 969). Because the NCS-R and ECA are cross-sectional studies, the first onsets in later years are overestimated because some failed to recall earlier episodes. But even if we assume that the actual first-onset rate is half of what was reported, that would mean that about 25 % (instead of 50 %) of all DSM-defined MDD cases have first onset after the early 30s. That would mean that the prevalence from the Rohde et al. study represents 75 % of the overall rate, and the overall rate would then be 4/3 of the Rohde rate (because the additional 25 % is one-third of 75 %). Extrapolating from the Rohde et al. report, the projected (speculative) lifetime DSM-defined MDD prevalence would then rise to about the two-thirds of the entire population (i.e., $4/3 \times 51$ % $= 68$ %).

In sum, recent studies confirm that even the implausibly high prevalence estimates available at the time LoS was published were much too low. Depressive disorder, a condition considered relatively rare just a few decades ago, if defined via DSM symptom-based criteria, occurs in the majority of individuals. This is just what one might expect if disorder and normal sadness are being confused by the use of symptom-based criteria. These astonishingly high rates have led to fresh calls by leading scholars to rethink the diagnostic threshold between normal sadness and depressive disorder (Goldberg 2011; Maj 2011a, b; Parker 2011; Tyrer 2009), the very task we began in LoS.

# The Tidal Wave of Antidepressant Use

Since LoS's completion, the rates of antidepressant use have continued to skyrocket in the United States, with multiple studies showing a rise of about 400 % in just a decade from the early or mid 1990s to the early or mid 2000s (Mojtabai 2008; Pratt et al. 2011). Moreover, the rise is taking place fastest among the less severe depressions for which the evidence of benefit is weakest (Mojtabai 2008). Recent reports indicate that in the United States about one in every nine adults and, shockingly, about of a quarter of all adult women in their forties and fifties, are taking these drugs at any given time (Pratt et al. 2011).

The international data indicate a worldwide trend towards expanding use of antidepressant medication beyond any plausible application to genuine depressive disorders or related disorders. According to the Organization for Economic Cooperation and Development (OECD), countries such as Iceland, Australia, Canada, Denmark and Sweden are reaching rates of antidepressant use approaching that of the Unites States – that is, 8–10 % or more of adults taking antidepressant medications at any one time – with rates generally doubling over the past few years (OECD 2013). For example, during the period from 2000 to 2011, rates of antidepressant use grew by 150 % in Germany and by over 100 % in many other OECD countries, including Italy, Australia, Spain, Portugal, Denmark, and the United Kingdom (OECD 2013). France, already one the highest users of antidepressants in the OECD in 2000, nonetheless saw its rate of use grow by about another 20 % between 2000 and 2011 (OECD 2013), with approximately 10 % of the country's population reimbursed for at least one antidepressant at any one time, mostly prescribed by general medical practitioners (Mercier et al. 2011).

Of particular concern is an expansion internationally and in the United States of antidepressant use for milder forms of sadness that may not even carry a psychiatric diagnosis (Hollingworth et al. 2010; Mercier et al. 2011; Mitchell et al. 2009; Mojtabai 2013). Other factors hypothesized to account for increased use include guidelines that recommend increased duration of treatment to prevent relapse (Moore et al. 2009), extension of antidepressants to related anxiety conditions such as social phobia and generalized anxiety disorder (Hollingworth et al. 2010; Mercier et al. 2011), and even depressive reactions to the economic downturn (Gili et al. 2013), although data suggest that rates of antidepressant use were already rising rapidly before the downturn (OECD 2013). A recent study revealed that in Europe as a whole, 8 % of all individuals and 10 % of middle-aged adults took antidepressants in 2010, with about three-quarters of those taking them for over a month (Blanchflower and Oswald 2011). Moreover, under the influence of culturally sophisticated marketing campaigns, the upswing in depression diagnoses and antidepressant prescriptions in the United States and Europe over the past few decades is now being replicated in other countries that formerly had relatively few depression cases, such as Japan (see Kitanaka 2016, this volume; Watters 2010).

These increases in antidepressant use have occurred despite growing skepticism about the effectiveness of these medications. Evidence increasingly suggests that the improvement that occurs with antidepressant treatment is largely attributable to placebo effects (Kirsch et al. 2002, 2008; Moncrieff et al. 2004; Pigott et al. 2010). Other evidence suggests that most patients do not benefit, but that possibly there is a beneficial effect for a small subgroup, perhaps consisting of more severe depressions (Gueorguieva et al. 2011; Kirsch et al. 2008; Thase et al. 2011).

This upward trend in antidepressant use has also occurred despite increasing evidence that the negative side effects of antidepressants are considerably greater than generally thought (Read et al. 2014). Indeed, some researchers are finally attempting to explore the question of why human beings are biologically designed to experience sadness at all, and what the costs might be of interfering with this response (Andrews and Thomson 2009). There is also growing concern about the challenges of going off these drugs after prolonged treatment due to serious negative reactions, often labeled a "discontinuation syndrome" to avoid any connotations of dependence or addiction. Such difficulties are reported by a substantial percentage of patients, ranging between 20 and 75 % in various studies (Lane 2011). Disturbingly, difficulties going off of antidepressants, while related to length of time taking them, seems to affect some patients who are on antidepressants for as little as six weeks (Haddad 2001; Haddad and Anderson 2007; Schatzberg et al. 2006; Warner et al. 2006; Zajecka et al. 1997). Nonetheless, perhaps influenced by pharmaceutical advertising and by a perception of beneficial effects on patients, general medical practitioners tend to see antidepressants as a safe and effective treatment for depressed mood (Mercier et al. 2011). The entire area remains actively controversial in both scholarly and popular publications (Angell 2011a, b; Horgan 2011; Kirsch 2010; Kramer 2011; Melander et al. 2008; Oldham et al. 2011; Stewart et al. 2012; Sunday Dialogue 2011).

## Medicalization of Treatment

Trends in treatment, and specifically shifts in who treats depression and how it is treated, reflect a growing view of sadness as a medical disorder that is a "brain disease" best treated by physicians and with medication. A combination of factors, including the rise of novel antidepressant medications, the perception that there is an epidemic of untreated depressive disorder based on epidemiologic surveys applying DSM diagnostic criteria to community samples, and the current popularity of a brain-disease model of depression, have been influential in changing treatment patters. In the United States, there has been a documented shift towards treatment of depression by general physicians and towards medication rather than psychotherapy.

The most authoritative treatment and provider data concerning recent outpatient depression treatment in the U.S. comes from Marcus and Olfson's (2010) analysis that compares the 1998 and 2007 Medical Expenditure Panel Surveys, which are surveys sponsored by the Agency for Healthcare Research and Quality to provide estimates of the use of health care services in a nationally representative sample of the US civilian non-institutionalized population (in 2007, N = 29,370). Each survey consists of three rounds of in-person interviews during the study year, as well as a medical events diary kept by the respondent. By comparing two successive surveys, Marcus and Olfson are able to identify trends across a decade of growth and change in depression treatment.

One of Marcus and Olfson's (2010) major findings was that the use of psychotherapy in outpatient treatment of depression is decreasing, with the percentage receiving psychotherapy going from 54 % in 1998 to 43 % in 2007 (Marcus and Olfson 2010). This continues a trend documented in an earlier study of a drop from 71 to 60 % getting psychotherapy between 1987 and 1997, the period during which SSRI antidepressants became available (Olfson et al. 2002). Marcus and Olfson also report that about 35 % of outpatient depression patients received both psychotherapy and medication in 2007, implying that the percentage receiving psychotherapy alone was very small, perhaps about 8 % of depression outpatients.

As to providers, as one might expect, the vast majority of 2007 depression outpatients saw physicians, of which about half were psychiatrists. The figure for how many outpatients saw physicians closely tracks the figure for medication use, with 85 % seeing a physician (including psychiatrists and other physicians) and 82 % receiving medication in 2007. Of the prescriptions written for antidepressants in recent years, 80 % were written by general physicians, and of those, about three-quarters were written with no accompanying formal psychiatric diagnosis (Mojtabai and Olfson 2011). Seeing a physician is obviously a necessary condition for receiving a prescription for medication, but these data also tell us that seeing a physician with any hint of depression is virtually a sufficient condition for receiving medication. A striking finding is the limited involvement of non-physician mental health professionals in the overall provision of outpatient depression treatment. The previous decade had seen a major increase in the physician portion of outpatient treatment from 69 to 87 % of all depression outpatients, and a drop in the psychologist share from 30 to 19 % (Olfson et al. 2002). In 2007, both psychologists (21 %) and social workers (7 %) served rather small percentages of the outpatient depression group. The very low figure for social workers, which has stayed about the same since 1998, is particularly striking since they constitute by far the largest segment of the mental health profession in the United States. It would appear that the medicalization of depression has generally worked to direct these cases to physicians.

## LoS and the DSM-5's Bereavement Exclusion

LoS used a wide range of evidence to show that the fundamental flaw of the MDD diagnosis was its use of symptoms without consideration of the contexts in which they developed. It surveyed thousands of years of medical history, which routinely separated normal sadness that arises and persists in the context of some loss from depressive disorders that are unrelated to their contexts. Reviewing the evolutionary, social, and psychological literatures on sadness, we described normal sadness as having three basic qualities. First, it was inherently context specific in the sense that it is biologically designed to emerge in response to a specific range of the "right" stimuli consisting of losses and stresses and not to occur in response to events outside that range. The second component was that the emotional and symptomatic severity of the response was of roughly proportionate intensity to the magnitude of the loss that generated it, with the understanding that there is great individual variability as well as cultural shaping of the intensity of response. The third and final component of nondisordered sadness was that symptoms not only emerge but also persist in accordance with external contexts, but then naturally remit when the context changes for the better or as people reconstruct their lives and their meaning systems to adapt to their losses. Depressive disorders, according to us, always lack at least one of these qualities of nondisordered reactions.

One particular aspect of the MDD diagnosis was of special interest. MDD's symptom-based definition contained one exception – diagnoses were not given to bereaved people unless their symptoms were still present after two months or were especially severe. This exception was known as the "bereavement exclusion" (BE), and was stated, somewhat confusingly, as follows:

> The symptoms are not better accounted for by Bereavement, i.e., after the loss of a loved one, the symptoms persist for longer than 2 months or are characterized by marked functional impairment, morbid preoccupation with worthlessness, suicidal ideation, psychotic symptoms, or psychomotor retardation. (American Psychiatric Association 2000, 356)

In other words, patients are exempt from a diagnosis of depression if their symptoms are better explainable as part of normal grief following the loss of a loved one. It is well known that grief can occasionally trigger a genuine mental disorder (Parkes 1964), so the BE could not simply exclude all depressive feelings after loss from diagnosis. Instead, based on classic studies of normal grief (Clayton et al. 1968), the BE distinguished the kinds of depressive feelings that are common in normal general-stress reactions (e.g., sadness, crying, difficulty sleeping, lessened appetite, loss of interest in or lack of pleasure from usual activities, difficulty concentrating, fatigue) and thus would indicate a likely normal response to loss from those more severe symptoms (e.g., psychotic ideation, suicidal ideation, psychomotor retardation, sense of worthlessness, marked impairment in functioning, prolonged duration) that possibly indicated that the reaction had become pathological. Thus, to be excluded from MDD diagnosis, depressive feelings after a loss had to pass six tests; they had to be of normal-range duration (the DSM-IV defined a normal period of depressive feelings during bereavement after the death of a loved one as lasting no more than 2 months) and they had to include none of the five other especially serious symptoms. An episode that would otherwise have enough symptoms to qualify as MDD but occurred after loss and had only general distress symptoms and none of the six marks suggestive of pathology was called an "uncomplicated" bereavement-related depression and was excluded from MDD diagnosis.

## Wakefield et al.'s (2007) Study Showing that the BE Should Be Extended to Other Stressors

The BE was especially important because it was the sole exception to the symptom-based nature of the MDD diagnosis. In contrast to the DSM, we believe that bereavement was not a unique exemption to the depression criteria but was a model for all kinds of loss situations. Remarkably, the distinction between uncomplicated versus complicated depressive episodes that the DSM applied to bereavement-related depression to distinguish normal from abnormal depressive responses to loss had never been applied to depressive reactions to other stressors to see whether it worked there as well, despite the fact that accumulating evidence suggested that transient normal depressive responses to other stressors are common.

With colleagues Michael First and Mark Schmitz, we conducted a study to examine whether depressive reactions to other stressors, such as loss of a valued job, marital dissolution, financial ruin, loss of possessions in a natural disaster, and negative medical diagnosis in oneself or a loved one, also fell into the same pattern of milder uncomplicated responses and more severe complicated and possibly disordered responses (Wakefield et al. 2007). The study, published soon after LoS, examined whether depressive-like feelings after other stress-related losses that did not feature especially severe symptoms or extended duration – and thus were also "uncomplicated" according to the DSM's definition in the BE – were similar to uncomplicated bereavement-related depressions in other respects, and thus presumably also normal-range responses that should be excluded from diagnosis. Follow-up studies addressed some weaknesses in the initial study and confirmed the results (Wakefield and Schmitz 2013a, b).

We found that all kinds of loss-triggered episodes of depression that were not especially severe or prolonged and met the requirements for being "uncomplicated" (i.e., included only general-distress-type depressive feelings and not any of the six features suggesting pathology) had similar symptoms, durations, treatment histories, and degree of impairment as uncomplicated bereavement (Wakefield et al. 2007; Wakefield and Schmitz 2013a, b). Moreover, all loss-related uncomplicated MDD conditions differed greatly from other MDD conditions in a variety of ways indicating lower levels of pathology indicators, suggesting normal emotional conditions (Wakefield and Schmitz 2012a).

Our empirical research thus convincingly showed that the depression criteria mistakenly singled out bereavement as the single exclusion to the MDD diagnosis. The mental health consequences of uncomplicated bereavement were similar to depressions that stemmed from any kind of loss whether the death of a loved one, divorce, unemployment, and the like and were distinct from complicated depressive conditions. The critical distinction was not between bereavement and other losses but between uncomplicated conditions following loss and conditions with especially severe patho-suggestive symptoms such as suicidal thoughts, marked functional impairment, morbid preoccupation with worthlessness, or psychotic symptoms, or prolonged duration. These findings seemed to indicate that the bereavement exclusion should be extended to cover all kinds of losses that weren't particularly intense or lengthy. We proposed this narrowing of the domain of MDD as a target for DSM-5 revision, and a first step towards reigning in the excessive diagnosis of MDD in cases of intense normal sadness. We estimated that correcting this one problem alone, by excluding from MDD diagnosis uncomplicated depressive reactions to recent losses, would reduce the prevalence of community cases of DSM-diagnosable depressive illness by about 25 %.

## DSM-5's Reaction: Elimination of the Bereavement Exclusion

Researchers connected to the development of the DSM-5 reacted with alarm to these findings. One prominent member of the DSM-5 depression task force, psychiatrist Kenneth Kendler, used his own data set to test our contention. His findings, however, replicated our own: depression that developed after bereavement was identical to that following other stressful life events, and fell into the same two classes of uncomplicated and complicated reactions with overall similar features (Kendler et al. 2008). All parties were in agreement on this point. However, there was a vast difference in how they interpreted its implications. For Wakefield et al., given that the BE's excluded cases are not disorders, the similarity to analogous reactions to other stressors meant that those reactions to other stressors are not disorders either. We therefore argued that the DSM criteria should be revised to expand the BE to apply to uncomplicated reactions to all major stressors. However, to Kendler and others working on DSM-5, the similarity just showed that it was wrong to single out bereavement for exclusion, so something had to change. "The DSM-IV position is not logically defensible," Kendler wrote in a subsequent piece (2010). A later analysis suggested that it was Kendler's many claims in support of eliminating the BE that were indefensible (Wakefield 2011).

Rather than agreeing that the BE should be extended, Kendler and others reasoned in the opposite direction. They agreed that given the similarity bereavement could not be singled out, but argued that this likeness only implied that "either the grief exclusion criterion needs to be eliminated or extended" (Kendler 2010). Either option would resolve the inconsistency. Those who supported eliminating the exclusion altogether argued that since the uncomplicated other-stressor responses are now considered disorders by the DSM, the similarity result simply meant that we had been wrong all along about the bereavement cases. However, the fact is that the pathological versus normal status of depressive reactions to stressors other than grief had not been empirically studied at the time of DSM-III in the way that grief had been studied, and the issue of whether other reactions should be excluded simply never came up. The question of how such reactions should be understood has never been considered seriously or empirically evaluated by any DSM work group in any revision of the manual, and remains an unresolved issue. In any event, proponents of elimination of the BE strongly resisted extending the BE to other stressors, which would have lowered the number of conditions diagnosable with MDD and thereby potentially missed some genuine cases.

The president of the American Psychiatric Association in 2011–12, John Oldham, similarly reacted to this research by emphasizing the lack of justification for a unique bereavement exclusion, and embracing the implication that therefore the BE should be eliminated, not extended, because all such reactions should be considered disorders:

> (The bereavement exclusion is) very limited; it only applies to a death of a spouse or a loved one. Why is that different from a very strong reaction after you have had your entire home and possessions wiped out by a tsunami, or earthquake, or tornado; or what if you are in financial trouble, or laid off from work out of the blue? In any of these situations, the exclusion doesn't apply. What we know is that any major stress can activate significant depression in people who are at risk for it. It doesn't make sense to differentiate the loss of a loved one as understandable grief from equally severe stress and sadness after other kinds of loss. (Brooks 2012)

Oldham and many others argued, as had Kendler et al. (2008), that because uncomplicated depressive reactions during grief look similar to uncomplicated reactions to other stressors, and because the DSM considers the reactions to other stressors to be disorders, therefore the bereavement exclusion should be eliminated in DSM-5. However, the DSM-IV equally considered the uncomplicated bereavement-related depressive reactions to be normal, so once the uncomplicated depressive reactions to various stressors were discovered to be equivalent, the argument could be run in either direction with equal appeal to the authority of the DSM. Thus, citing the DSM became irrelevant. Once the bereavement-related depressive feelings and depressive feelings related to other stressors and losses were shown to look the same, this created a real dilemma for the DSM-5 that could not be resolved by appealing to features of the DSM-IV, because the DSM-IV was inconsistent on the very point at issue. The question then became whether all of the uncomplicated depressive reactions to loss or stress – that is, all of the reactions to bereavement and to other stressors that had none of the six patho-suggestive features and thus could potentially be best explained as part of a normal reaction – should all be excluded from or included in major depression diagnosis. None of those arguing for the elimination of the BE ever directly addressed this question on empirical grounds.

Other proponents of abandoning the BE argued that the presence of the DSM's depressive symptoms themselves, regardless of context or type, constituted a disorder. "When someone has a myocardial infarction (MI), physicians regard it as an instantiation of cardiac disease, regardless of its 'context'," psychiatrist Ronald Pies claimed. "The MI may have occurred in the context of the patient's poor diet, smoking, and high levels of psychic stress – but it is still an expression of disease" (Pies 2008). For Pies, depression is depression, just as a heart attack is a heart attack. For all of these psychiatrists, the clinical symptomatic similarity of uncomplicated depression during grief to uncomplicated depression after other stressors indicated that the BE should be abandoned, not extended.

Pies and other proponents of eliminating the BE claimed that physicians don't fail to diagnose serious diseases such as heart attacks, cancer, or tuberculosis that had environmental precipitants. Likewise, they argued, all depressive conditions should be diagnosed, regardless of their cause. Yet, unlike a heart attack, grief is a naturally designed and self-limited response, not a failure of natural functioning like a heart attack. Moreover, physicians do take context into account in deciding whether, for example, heightened pulse or blood pressure likely signify a disorder or a reaction to circumstances in the individual's life. However, there is a difference between psychiatric and other medical diagnosis in this regard simply because psychological functions are biologically designed to be highly sensitive to environmental context, and in fact it is this context-dependence that makes them adaptive and useful. Fear, for example, would not be very useful if it was happening all the time or randomly; it is useful because it is selectively triggered by perceived danger. Sadness similarly is highly sensitive to context, so that context must be taken into account when evaluating whether a disorder exists. In any event, the BE in DSM-IV already classified most depression during grief as MDD based on the presence of even one of the six features that were prohibited from exclusion. The notion that depression was depression just as a heart attack was a heart attack was both false and could not justify changing the previous criteria that considered especially severe grief as a disorder.

An important form of evidence in a consideration of diagnostic validity is predictive validity, whether over time the sequelae of a condition suggest it was a disorder or not. The BE debate was transformed when studies of the predictive validity of the BE began emerging. Several studies showed that at either one- or three-year follow-up periods after an episode of uncomplicated bereavement-related depression, people were no more likely than the non-depressed to have subsequent depressive episodes or various forms of anxiety (Gilman et al. 2012; Mojtabai 2011; Wakefield and Schmitz 2012a).

These results were soon generalized to all stressors; uncomplicated depressive reactions to stressors in general turned out to be much lower on pathology indicators than other forms of depression (Wakefield and Schmitz 2013b). To address the critique that grief was not unique and so there was no justification for the BE, Wakefield and his collaborators went on to conduct studies that showed an even more striking finding: people who developed uncomplicated depressions after all kinds of losses were more similar to those who were *never depressed* than to those who had complicated depressive conditions. Using data gathered at two points of time, they found that individuals with uncomplicated cases have similar recurrence rates (3.4 %) to people with no history of depression (1.7 %) during a one-year follow-up period; both groups had far lower rates than those with complicated cases (14.6 %) (Wakefield and Schmitz 2013c). The analysis was replicated in another data set and also applied to other possible sequelae of depression, such as anxiety disorders and suicide attempts (Wakefield and Schmitz 2014a, b). Not only were those with uncomplicated stress-related depressive conditions similar to one another, but they were far more comparable to people who had never been depressed than ones with serious or enduring symptoms.

These findings posed a stark choice for the DSM-5 mood disorders work group. On the one hand, they could expand the bereavement exclusion to cover all uncomplicated responses to loss-related stressors. On the other hand, they could abolish the BE so that all symptoms meeting the two-week MDD criteria were mental disorders. This was an especially consequential decision because MDD had been psychiatry's central diagnosis for the past 30 years. Extending the bereavement exclusion threatened both the symptom-based principles that were foundational for psychiatric diagnosis since 1980 and a substantial portion of the potential clientele of mental health professionals.

Given the international influence of the DSM, it was not only in the United States that concern was expressed about the proposed elimination of the BE. Given the limited ability of most nations' mental health systems to meet the treatment needs of the enormous numbers of genuinely psychiatrically disordered individuals, some European clinicians reacted to the proposed elimination of the BE by questioning whether it made sense to encompass a large number of false positive diagnoses to avoid the small chance that a case might be missed. For example, an article in the German national newspaper *Suddeutche Zeitung* described a report issued by the German Society for Psychiatry and Psychotherapy, Psychosomatics and Neurology (DGPPN) on the DSM-5 changes, and reported on an interview with Wolfgang Maier, President of the Society and Director of the Psychiatric Clinic of the University of Bonn (Weber 2013). Here is a translation of part of the article:

> The specialist organisation DGPPN advises against overdiagnosis in the DSM-5. There is the 'danger of pathologising ordinary states of suffering as well as natural adaptation and aging processes', says the president of the DGPPN and director of the psychiatric clinic of the University of Bonn, Wolfgang Maier, in a statement on Monday.
>
> The statement names a number of examples, where the new catalogue shifts the boundaries between health and sickness in an inadmissible way according to the DGPPN. Thus, in the DSM-5 a sadness of over two weeks after a death shall be diagnosed as depression if it shows its usual symptoms: cheerlessness, lack of drive/energy, indifference, sleeping problems, lack of appetite.
>
> "Such an overdiagnosis constitutes a threat, which is put up with by the APA authors with open eyes," says DGPPN president Maier: "Their premise is, we prefer false positive diagnoses rather than we fail to see a real sick person." But this is, according to Maier, a calculation that doesn't work, alone for economical reasons, at least not in Germany. One should always take into consideration that a diagnosis entitles the person affected to a provision of medical care through the system, whose resources are limited. The consequence could be that for the psychically truly sick there will be less possibilities for treatment. (Frances 2013a)

An additional generally unstated issue in the European response to DSM-5 is that in many European countries with generous disability benefits there are large numbers of individuals classified as disabled based on depression diagnoses that may not in all cases represent a genuine disorder. Further broadening the scope of depression to include what seem to be normal reactions seemed to open the floodgates to increased public expenditures for psychiatric claims that may not be warranted. However, this issue played a small role in the debate, which was focused on whether the change was indeed a diagnostically valid one.

## The Death of the Bereavement Exclusion

The symptoms and two-week duration criteria for Major Depressive Disorder (MDD) that appeared in the DSM-5 replicated the criteria of the earlier DSM-IV-TR (2000). The one major change to MDD criteria in the new edition of the manual was that it eliminated the bereavement exclusion from the category's diagnostic criteria. The DSM-5 mood disorders work group insisted that all conditions that met MDD symptom and duration criteria should be liable to a diagnosis of depression. William Coryell, a work group member, explained this decision in a DSM-5 website posting defending the decision after some negative commentary appeared in the New York Times, explaining that bereavement-related depression is similar to other depression. He quoted the work group's own earlier posting and a review article by Kendler et al.: "The DSM-5 Mood Disorders Work-group has recommended the elimination of the bereavement exclusion criteria from major depressive episodes in light of evidence that 'the similarities between bereavement related depression and depression related to other stressful life events substantially outweigh their differences' (Kendler et al. 2008)" (Coryell 2012).

This rationale begged the crucial question of whether all uncomplicated depressive reactions to stress (whether caused by bereavement or other losses and stress) were different from other MDD in a way that suggested they are normal emotional responses. The implicit assumption that the excluded depressions were similar to other depressions was based on three reviews of the literature by overlapping authors all of which claimed that the excluded depressions were in fact quite similar to all other MDD (Lamb et al. 2010; Zisook and Kendler 2007; Zisook et al. 2007). These reviews were later shown in a "review of the reviews" to be spurious because they cited no studies that were directly relevant to the question at issue (Wakefield and First 2012a). Such evidence was just starting to be generated. Two more recent reviews focus on the empirical evidence generated out of the debate and its interpretation and provide strong support for extending the BE to all major stressors rather than eliminating it (Wakefield and Schmitz 2012b; Wakefield 2013a).

Despite going ahead with the elimination of the BE, in response to intense criticism the DSM-5 added a note to the MDD diagnostic criteria that states:

> Responses to a significant loss (e.g. bereavement, financial ruin, losses from a natural disaster, a serious medical illness or disability) may include the feelings of intense sadness, rumination about the loss, insomnia, poor appetite, and weight loss noted in [the symptom criteria], which may resemble a depressive episode. Although such symptoms may be understandable or considered appropriate to the loss, the presence of a major depressive episode in addition to the normal response to a significant loss should also be carefully considered. This decision inevitably requires the exercise of clinical judgment based on the individual's history and the cultural norms for the expression of distress in the context of loss. (American Psychiatric Association 2013, 161)

It is of interest that the note, by referring to several stressors and neglecting to mention any durational limit, in effect recognizes two of the points we made in LoS and subsequent publications. First, uncomplicated normal depressive reactions can occur in response to any stressor, not just bereavement. Second, the two-month durational limit for uncomplicated bereavement-relate depression in DSM-IV is unrealistically brief and without any scientific foundation – a conclusion supported by recent research that suggests that 6 months or 1 year would be a more valid cut-point (Wakefield and Schmitz 2012a, b, 2013a, b; Wakefield et al. 2011a, b).

This note, however, is not part of the formal diagnosis and does not contain any diagnostic criteria. The MDD criteria themselves encompass all uncomplicated normal sadness reactions as well as depressive disorder, and then the note suggests that it is up to the clinician to make a further judgment about the suitability of the diagnosis. The interpretation of the note is itself a matter of contention. Most DSM-5 work group members believe this note to be largely superfluous, perhaps applying to the rare case or to subthreshold conditions, but not actually changing the fact that virtually all conditions satisfying MDD symptom and duration criteria are now considered MDD whether or not they follow loss of a loved one or any other stressor; most members of the work group believe that the work group completely eliminated the BE, and this is how it is being represented in the revisions of major instruments used for diagnosis and research (Michael First, personal communication). On the other hand, one prominent member of the work group, Mario Maj (2013), argues that the note leaves MDD diagnosis after a stressor entirely open to clinical judgment that can override the formal criteria, and thus in effect opens the door to the kind of subjective clinical judgment about MDD diagnosis that was problematic prior to DSM-III and was the reason for creating descriptive criteria in the first place. In any event, experience suggests that a note like this one will not be used by researchers and thus will have little or no impact on thinking in psychiatry. Such notes without criteria are inevitably ignored by researchers as well as by most clinicians, thus do not change the fact that DSM-5 eliminated the BE and, in so doing, created the likelihood of millions of additional incorrect diagnoses among a vulnerable population.

The DSM-5 criteria without the BE in effect modify the earlier definition in two major ways. First, any grieving person with depressive feelings is liable to a depressive diagnosis after a two-week period, rather than a two-month period, which many experts believed was already far too short (Kleinman 2012). Second, the criteria no longer require the presence of especially severe depressive symptoms during bereavement to be included as having MDD. Anyone who has suffered the loss of an intimate and has normal symptoms of grief such as sadness, a loss of pleasure, sleeping and eating problems, and fatigue that last for a two-week period following the death would meet the new criteria. Not only did the DSM-5 newly pathologize millions of people who are not currently diagnosed, but it missed the opportunity to correct the criteria and depathologize even larger numbers of people with normal depressive feelings who are currently liable to diagnosis.

Each of the committee's arguments for eliminating the BE was seriously deficient. Consider the DSM-5's own definition of mental disorder:

A mental disorder is a syndrome characterized by clinically significant disturbance in an individual's cognition, emotion regulation, or behavior that reflects a dysfunction in the psychological, biological, or developmental processes underlying mental functioning. Mental disorders are usually associated with significant distress or disability in social, occupational, or other important activities. An expectable or culturally approved response to a common stressor or loss, such as the death of a loved one, is not a mental disorder. (American Psychiatric Association 2013, 20)

This definition of mental disorder uses "the death of a loved one" to illustrate the *difference* between a painful but normal emotion and a mental disorder. Surely after the loss of a loved one it is not only within expectable range but a "culturally approved response" to experience general distress symptoms such as sadness, lack of sleep, lessened appetite, loss of interest in usual activities, and difficulty concentrating on usual tasks. The MDD definition as explicitly stated thus appears to be in tension with the DSM'5 own sensible requirement that "An expectable ... response to a common stressor or loss, such as the death of a loved one, is not a mental disorder."

The removal of the BE also undermines the central logic behind psychiatric diagnosis itself. The point of distinguishing one diagnosis from another is that distinctions help specify the causes, courses, outcomes, and treatments of the condition. Yet, combining uncomplicated depressive symptoms that stem from grief, unemployment, divorce, and the like with those that are disproportionate to their contexts does the opposite: it blurs conditions with environmental causes with those stemming from some dysfunction within the individual, those that are transient and unlikely to recur with ones that are more enduring; and those that are likely to improve enduringly on their own from those that may require professional interventions. The decision to remove the BE from the MDD criteria also challenges the as-yet-unrealized assumption that mental disorders will ultimately be found to stem from abnormal brain functioning (Greenberg 2013, 240). As diagnosticians have long recognized, *normal* brains (or minds) naturally respond to losses with periods of sadness. Neuroscientific research that relies on the DSM-5 criteria will hopelessly confound brains that are operating normally with those that are dysfunctional.

The DSM-5 work group also argued that the bereavement exclusion could prevent grieving people from getting treatment that can help them. The Chair of the work group, Jan Fawcett, cited the effectiveness of medication in helping the BE-excluded cases as the primary reason for eliminating the exclusion (Fawcett 2010). Reviews supporting elimination of the BE (Zisook and Kendler 2007; Zisook et al. 2007) cited as the only or primary evidence of medication benefit psychiatrist Sidney Zisook et al.'s one study of 22 recently bereaved people, in which they reported that over half of those were treated with the anti-depressant buproprion improved after two months (Zisook et al. 2001). Yet, this study had no placebo group and its claimed success rate of a little more than half (13 of 22) did not exceed placebo recovery rates in other studies. Early bereavement is, after all, a period in which it is well documented that symptoms plummet without medication (Clayton et al. 1968). The claims of drug benefit made on the basis of this uncontrolled study would not be taken seriously in any scientific branch of medicine.

Proponents of removing the BE exclusion also cited the possibility of untreated grief leading to suicide in the absence of treatment. They urged diagnosis of the bereaved on the grounds that the benefits of treating people who have "suicidal ideation, major role impairment or a substantial clinical worsening" far outweigh the costs of eliminating the exclusion (Kendler 2010). "I'd rather make the mistake of calling someone depressed who may not be depressed," Zisook stated, "than missing the diagnosis of depression, not treating it, and having that person kill themselves" (Zisook 2010). This was a disingenuous argument: the preexisting DSM-IV bereavement criteria *already* considered grieving persons with especially severe or impairing symptoms such as suicidal risk as not meeting the exclusion criteria. Recent studies have confirmed that the reference to possible suicide attempts was sheer scaremongering and that the evidence shows uncomplicated depressive reactions to stressors, which exclude suicidal ideation, do not involve elevated suicide attempt rates, as one would expect given the screening for suicidal ideation (Wakefield and Schmitz 2014a, b).

Finally, the abandonment of the bereavement exclusion in the DSM-5 risks an enormous pathologization that can occur when the MDD criteria consider bereaved people as disordered. Given that about 40 % of grieving people meet these criteria a month after their loss, it is likely that a majority of the bereaved could be diagnosed with MDD after the two-week period the diagnosis specifies (Clayton et al. 1972; Clayton 1982). In the U.S. alone, some 8 to 10 million people suffer the loss of an intimate every year and about half of these would meet the new criteria for bereavement. Because nearly everyone will suffer the loss of an intimate, abandoning the bereavement exclusion renders a majority of the population liable to a diagnosis of depressive disorder at some point in their lives.

The elimination of the bereavement exclusion in the DSM-5 thus has no good conceptual, empirical, or treatment-related grounds. "There is no scientific basis," Wakefield and First concluded after reviewing the evidence, "for removing the bereavement exclusion from the DSM-5" (2012a, 9). Moreover, as one critic noted, the BE "was necessary: without it the DSM loses its credibility" (Greenberg 2013, 114). Another leading critic, Allen Frances, asserted: "This was a stubbornly misguided decision in the face of universal opposition from clinicians, professional associations and journals, the press, and hundreds of thousands of grievers from all around the world" (Frances 2013b, 186). Remarkably, even psychiatrists' colleagues in general medicine questioned the DSM-5's elimination of the BE, with editorials appearing in leading medical journals largely siding with the critics (Editorial 2012; Friedman 2012).

In the course of the debate, two legitimate empirically supported points were made by those arguing for elimination of the BE. The first point was that the BE was stated in DSM-IV in a confusing way, so that without proper training a clinician could easily get confused as to how to apply the exclusion (Corruble et al. 2009). The appropriate way to address this problem is by rephrasing the exclusion, not by eliminating it. If we eliminated every frequently misapplied but scientifically valid diagnostic criteria set in the DSM, then MDD itself would have to be eliminated because it is known that general practitioners, who do the majority of treatment of MDD, misdiagnose more cases than they correctly diagnose.

The second legitimate empirically supported point is that the exclusion's validity is dramatically reduced when individuals already have a history of depressive disorder before the loss occurs (Wakefield and First 2012a). In such cases, there is a high likelihood not only of a depressive reaction to the loss, but of later recurrences or a chronic episode that in the long run reverses the exclusion (which requires limited duration). When one looks at those who have clinically problematic depressive reactions to loss, a large percentage consist of those who have experienced depressive disorder before the loss. In fact, this caveat was already implicitly taken into account in the DSM-IV BE's initial instruction that an episode should be diagnosed as MDD only if it is not better explained by normal bereavement. A depressive reaction to loss in an individual who has experienced recurrent depression in the past that was not itself explainable as a normal reaction to loss cannot be best explained as normal, but rather is most likely a recurrence (or at very high risk of becoming a recurrence) of the long-term depressive vulnerability. In such cases, the power of the "normal response to loss" explanation is weakened considerably, and a diagnosis of MDD becomes appropriate. However, this reasoning is not made explicit and so there is the real danger of the BE being applied automatically to recurrent cases. Although such recurrent cases are only a very small fraction of BE candidate cases, they account for a large percentage of later recurrences and should be more clearly and explicitly excluded from the exclusion.

To address both the clarity of the exclusion and the need to avoid applying the exclusion to recurrent cases, Wakefield and First (2012a) drafted a revised statement of the exclusion. However, their draft applied only to the bereavement case and not to other stressors, and it did not take into account the increasingly strong empirical evidence that a longer durational threshold than the DSM's 2 months is more valid. With these two additional corrections, an alternative statement of a "major stressor exclusion" might look as follows:

> If the episode occurs in the context of a major loss or stressor, it is not diagnosed as major depression if it is better explained as a normal distress reaction. If the episode includes any one or more of the following features that are suggestive of major depression, then it is disqualified form being considered normal distress and should be diagnosed as major depression: duration greater than 6 months; suicidal ideation; morbid preoccupation with worthlessness; marked psychomotor retardation; prolonged and marked global functional impairment; psychotic symptoms; or a history of major depressive disorder in the past. Stressor-related depressive episodes that have none of these features should be given a diagnosis of "normal bereavement-related depression, provisional."

What led the DSM-5 to alter the MDD diagnosis in the face of such powerful opposition? The charitable way of viewing the arguments of the proponents of the new DSM-5 criteria is that they are genuinely interested in alleviating the suffering that accompanies grief. Yet, drugs and psychotherapy are not known to be more effective for uncomplicated grief than simply letting the condition run its natural course. A more cynical explanation it that the removal of the BE can expand the clientele of mental health professionals. Because drugs are by far the most common response to grieving people who seek treatment, the DSM-5 changes could also produce a bonanza of new clients for pharmaceutical companies. Eight of the eleven members of the APA committee that recommended the new criteria had financial connections to the drug industry (Whoriskey 2012), and the consultant to the work group, Sidney Zisook, who provided most of the public defense of eliminating the BE, had been the lead author on the one study of using medication during early bereavement-related depression that was cited by the work group to justify the BE's elimination. The chairman of the work group, Jan Fawcett, enthusiastically pro-pounds drug treatments for depression: "I'm still working at 78 because I love to watch patients who have been depressed for years come to life again. You need those medicines to do that" (Whoriskey 2012). While drugs can help some people overcome grief, the new MDD criteria will mostly encompass people whose natural suffering will heal without interference from powerful medications. In any case, the criteria they replaced provided ample protection that grieving people with espe-cially severe or prolonged conditions would receive depressive diagnosis.

Perhaps the best explanation for the DSM-5's decision stems from the nature of professional legitimacy. Psychiatry is primarily a legitimate source of treatment for pathological conditions. The BE recognized that one form of common loss was not pathological but extending this logic would have also excluded many others from diagnosis and treatment. Expanding the BE could have had led to a major contrac-tion in the number of people who meet diagnostic criteria for depression. The evi-dence forced the DSM-5 committee to accept that bereavement was equivalent to other losses but it then had no choice but to abandon the exclusion in order to main-tain psychiatry's range of authority.

## DSM-5's Expansion of the Categories of Depressive and Grief Disorders

We have focused thus far on DSM-5's elimination of the bereavement exclusion because this is the DSM-5 change that is most relevant to the argument of LoS, which focused on MDD as the primary locus of psychiatry's confusion of normal sadness with mental disorder. However, the overall changes to the category of depressive disorders went well beyond this change. Indeed, DSM-5 dramatically altered – and in a variety of ways greatly expanded – the domain of diagnosable depressive illness, compounding the problem of potential overdiagnosis and the use of psychiatry to control normal human variation.

Three of the other changes are particularly notable, because they introduce new categories of disorders. Two of the new categories are depressive disorders intro-duced into the main list of depressive disorders, and the other is a new disorder of grief that is listed as a target of further study.

First, DSM-5 depressive disorders include a controversial new child depressive disorder category, *Disruptive Mood Dysregulation Disorder* (DMDD). DMDD diagnostic criteria include temper outbursts on average at least 3 times a week with generally irritable or dysphoric mood between outbursts, lasting for a year. Diagnosis of DMDD precludes diagnosis of oppositional defiant disorder (ODD), although most DMDD cases qualify for ODD diagnosis. This largely unstudied diagnosis was introduced to address an embarrassing problem for psychiatry – the excessive diagnosis of child bipolar disorder, and the consequent overtreatment of children with heavy-duty medications such as mood stabilizers and antipsychotics. DMDD is aimed at providing an alternative category for the diagnosis of such children.

Difficult children often present with chronic irritability and dysphoria punctuated by frequent tantrums, and this is often interpreted as indicating bipolar disorder. However, research suggests that such children are in fact generally neither experiencing an early form of bipolar disorder nor a stable mood disorder. Many children with these symptoms are brought to treatment by desperate parents, but the children seem to outgrow these behaviors and almost all are alternatively classifiable as having oppositional defiant disorder (Axelson et al. 2012). Consequently, the new DMDD diagnosis means that children whose defiance and tantrums are causing distress to parents may now come to be illegitimately diagnosed as having a mood disorder and receive antidepressant medication. Many children with various problems present with these symptoms, so the potential for overdiagnosis is substantial. Admittedly, if one is going to overdiagnose, depressive disorders have somewhat more benign medication implications than bipolar disorders, but it remains uncertain that this category will be used to shift the bipolar diagnoses into depression rather than simply opening up a new way to diagnose a large number of normal children as depressively disordered.

A second new category of disorder, Premenstrual Dysphoric Disorder (PMDD), has been added to DSM-5. This category was extremely controversial when first suggested for earlier DSM editions, and was listed in the appendix of DSM-IV as a category requiring further study. It has now been "promoted" to a full, regularly listed depressive disorder. PMDD has long been controversial due to concerns that the category would inevitably pathologize a common and natural female response that varies in intensity but is not a mental disorder except under very rare circumstances. The diagnostic criteria require that during the week before onset of menses and subsiding in the week following menses the patient experience at least five symptoms with marked severity, including depressive symptoms (e.g., mood swings, increased sensitivity, tearfulness, irritability or increased conflict, depressed mood, anxiety, decreased interest in usual activities, difficulty concentrating, fatigue). It is claimed that only a modest percentage of women, perhaps 8 % (European Medicines Agency 2011), would qualify for diagnosis, but there is the potential for extending this vaguely defined diagnosis to many more women given that as many as 90 % of women report significant premenstrual symptoms (Halbreich 2004; Halbreich et al. 2003). Since the Food and Drug Administration has already approved antidepressants for the treatment of PMDD, the inclusion of this category in DSM-5 was a foregone conclusion.

Finally, there is a new grief disorder, *Persistent Complex Bereavement-Related Disorder (PCBD)*, listed for further study. Although also concerned with grief, this category is not related to the elimination of the bereavement exclusion. The BE specifically concerned depressive symptoms during grief, and specified when such depressive symptoms should be diagnosed as disordered versus considered part of normal grief. PCBD is concerned with the non-depressive symptoms of grief, which before DSM-5 have never been subject to disorder diagnosis in the DSM. These non-depressive grief feelings include, for example, yearning for the lost person, being pained by or avoiding reminders of the person, feeling disbelief that the person is gone, preoccupation with the deceased or with the circumstances of the death, bitterness or anger over the loss, blame oneself or feeling guilty that one did not do enough to save the person, wanting to join the deceased, loneliness or detachment, and a sense of meaninglessness or emptiness. The proposed diagnostic criteria specify that if several of such symptoms continue for over a year after the loss at an intense level, then the grief reaction is to be considered pathological. Grief researchers themselves continue to argue for a six-month threshold for disorder rather than one year (Prigerson et al. 2009; Shear et al. 2011), claiming that grief that lasts that long has become interminable and has gone off track. However, these proposals have little relation to what research studies actually show, which is that many people, especially those who have lost a close dependent relationship, continue to progress in their mourning process and to further adapt to the loss long after 6 months or even a year (Wakefield 2012, 2013b). Thus, there is the potential for massively pathologizing intense normal grief, even when no depressive symptoms are involved.

Note that although PCBD is listed as a category requiring further study that has no official diagnostic code, it is explicitly mentioned as a diagnostic option under the coded main-list category of "other specified trauma- and stress-related disorders" (the DSM-5 version of DSM-IV's "not otherwise specified" disorders). Thus, this disorder can in fact be diagnosed immediately within the DSM-5 system.

In sum, the DSM-5 made dramatic changes to the diagnosis of depressive and grief conditions quite aside from the elimination of the bereavement exclusion and the consequent expansion of MDD. DSM-5 also added three new categories of disorder addressing the experiences of children, women, and the grief-stricken, respectively. Each of these categories might well encompass some genuine disorders, but they are all drawn in broad terms and defined in terms of symptoms common among normal individuals. They each, therefore, make the problem of false positive diagnosis potentially worse and provide a foundation for a possible new epidemic of overdiagnosis. They clearly reveal psychiatry's ongoing refusal to take seriously the problem of distinguishing normal intense emotion from psychiatric disorder.

## Conclusions

When DSM-5 finally emerged, it went in the direction opposite to that we had suggested in LoS and in subsequent research articles. Rather than more carefully drawing the distinction between intense normal sadness and MDD to make diagnosis and research more valid, DSM-5 expanded MDD diagnosis as well as diagnosis of depressive disorder in general into ever more areas, accelerating the trends we observed in LoS. The pathologization of sadness is thus proceeding more rapidly and more boldly, and with more blatant disregard of the scientific evidence, than we ever imagined possible. In this chapter, we have provided some perspective on these developments by offering an overview of how psychiatry, more than ever, is confusing the normal with the disordered and encompassing normal sadness within the category of major depressive disorder.

As *The Loss of Sadness* showed, the distinction between normal sadness and depressive disorder has been part of Western science, philosophy, and literature since the earliest recorded documents. Only since 1980 has this distinction been greatly eroded and become in danger of being substantially lost. The change to decontextualized symptom-based criteria for depressive illness was instrumental in triggering the Age of Depression that we now inhabit, because psychological functions are by their nature contextually sensitive, so that symptoms that are normal responses versus disorders cannot be generally discriminated without context (Wakefield and First 2012b). Our book posed a choice for psychiatric diagnosticians: they should either recognize the distinction between normal, albeit painful, emotions and mental disorders or risk pathologizing all forms of suffering. The DSM-5 chose the path towards the latter option. However, in abandoning the bereavement exclusion and greatly expanding the categories of depressive disorder, DSM-5 might have overreached. Time will tell if this affront to common sense, empirical evidence, and intellectual coherence will destroy the profession's credibility as the official social arbiter of normality and abnormality.

# References

American Psychiatric Association. (1980). *Diagnostic and statistical manual of mental disorders* (3rd ed.: DSM-III). Washington, DC: American Psychiatric Association.

American Psychiatric Association. (2000). *Diagnostic and statistical manual of mental disorders: DSM-IV-TR* (4th ed., text revision; DSM-IV-TR). Washington, DC: American Psychiatric Association.

American Psychiatric Association. (2013). *Diagnostic and statistical manual of mental disorders* (5th ed.: DSM-5). Arlington: American Psychiatric Association.

Andrews, P. W., & Thomson, J. A., Jr. (2009). The bright side of being blue: Depression as an adaptation for analyzing complex problems. *Psychological Review, 116*(3), 620–654.

Angell, M. (2011a). The epidemic of mental illness: Why? *New York Review of Books*, June 23, 2011. http://www.nybooks.com/articles/archives/2011/jun/23/epidemic-mental-illness-why. Accessed 6 April 2014.

Angell, M. (2011b). The illusions of psychiatry. *New York Review of Books*, July 14, 2011. http://www.nybooks.com/articles/archives/2011/jul/14/illusions-of-psychiatry. Accessed 6 April 2014.

Axelson, D., Findling, R. L., Fristad, M. A., Kowatch, R. A., Youngstrom, E. A., Horwitz, S. M., et al. (2012). Examining the proposed disruptive mood dysregulation disorder diagnosis in children in the Longitudinal Assessment of Manic Symptoms Study. *Journal of Clinical Psychiatry, 73*(10), 1342–1350.

Blanchflower, D. G., & Oswald, A. J. (2011). *Antidepressants and age*. Institute for the Study of Labor (IZA), Bonn. http://ftp.iza.org/dp5785.pdf. Accessed 6 April 2014.

Brooks, M. (2012, February 16). Lancet weighs in on DSM-5 Bereavement exclusion. *Medscape.* http://www.medscape.com/viewarticle/758788. Accessed 6 April 2014.

Clayton, P. J. (1982). Bereavement. In E. S. Paykel (Ed.), *Handbook of affective disorders* (pp. 15–46). London: Churchill Livingstone.

Clayton, P. J., Desmarais, L., & Winokur, G. (1968). A study of normal bereavement. *American Journal of Psychiatry, 125,* 168–178.

Clayton, P. J., Halikas, J. A., & Maurice, W. L. (1972). The depression of widowhood. *British Journal of Psychiatry, 120,* 71–78.

Corruble, E., Chouinard, V. A., Letierce, A., et al. (2009). Is DSM-IV bereavement exclusion for major depressive episode relevant to severity and pattern of symptoms? A case control, cross-sectional study. *Journal of Clinical Psychiatry, 70,* 1091–1097.

Coryell, W. (2012, April 17). Proposal to eliminate bereavement exclusion criteria from major depressive episode in DSM-5. *DSM5ORG, Major depressive Episode, Rationale.* http://www.dsm5.org/ProposedRevisions/Pages/proposedrevision.aspx?rid=427. Accessed 5 May 2012.

Eaton, W. W., Badawi, M., & Melton, B. (1995). Prodromes and precursors: Epidemiologic data for primary prevention of disorders with slow onset. *American Journal of Psychiatry, 152,* 967–972.

Editorial. (2012). Living with grief. *Lancet, 379,* 589.

European Medicines Agency. (2011). *Guideline on the treatment of premenstrual dysphoric disorder (PMDD).* http://www.ema.europa.eu/docs/en_GB/document_library/Scientific_guide-line/2011/08/WC500110103.pdf. Accessed 4 May 2013.

Fawcett, J. (2010). An overview of mood disorders in the DSM-5. *Current Psychiatry Report, 12,* 531–538.

First, M. B., & Wakefield, J. C. (2013). Diagnostic criteria as dysfunction indicators: Bridging the chasm between the definition of mental disorder and diagnostic criteria for specific disorders. *Canadian Journal of Psychiatry, 58*(12), 663–669.

Frances, A. (2013a, April 25). The international reaction to DSM 5. *Psychology Today Blog.* http://www.psychologytoday.com/blog/saving-normal/201304/the-international-reaction-dsm-5. Accessed 5 April 2014.

Frances, A. (2013b). *Saving normal.* New York: William Morrow.

Friedman, R. A. (2012). Grief, depression, and the DSM-5. *New England Journal of Medicine, 366,* 1855–1857.

Gili, M., Roca, M., Stuckler, D., Basu, S., & McKee, M. (2013). 2255-The mental health risks of economic crisis in Spain: Evidence from primary care centres, 2006 and 2010. *European Psychiatry, 28*(Suppl 1), 1.

Gilman, S. E., Breslau, J., Trinh, N. H., Fava, M., Murphy, J. M., & Smoller, J. W. (2012). Bereavement and the diagnosis of major depressive episode in the National Epidemiologic Survey on Alcohol and Related Conditions. *Journal of Clinical Psychiatry, 73,* 208–215.

Goldberg, D. (2011). The heterogeneity of "major depression". *World Psychiatry, 10,* 226–228.

Greenberg, G. (2013). *The book of Woe: The DSM and the unmaking of psychiatry.* New York: Blue Rider Press.

Gueorguieva, R., Mallinckrodt, C., & Krystal, J. H. (2011). Trajectories of depression severity in clinical trials of duloxetine: Insights into antidepressant and placebo responses. *Archives of General Psychiatry, 68*(12), 1227–1237.

Haddad, P. M. (2001). Antidepressant discontinuation syndromes. *Drug Safety, 24*(3), 183–197.

Haddad, P. M., & Anderson, I. M. (2007). Recognising and managing antidepressant discontinuation symptoms. *Advances in Psychiatric Treatment, 13,* 447–457.

Halbreich, U. (2004). The diagnosis of premenstrual syndromes and premenstrual dysphoric disorder–clinical procedures and research perspectives. *Gynecological Endocrinology, 19*(6), 320–334.

Halbreich, U., Borenstein, J., Pearlstein, T., & Kahn, L. S. (2003). The prevalence, impairment, impact, and burden of premenstrual dysphoric disorder (PMS/PMDD). *Psychoneuroendocrinology, 28*(3), 1–23.

Hasin, D. S., Goodwin, R. D., Stinson, F. S., & Grant, B. F. (2005). The epidemiology of major depressive disorder: Results from the National Epidemiologic Survey on Alcohol and Related Conditions. *Archives of General Psychiatry, 62*, 1097–1106.

Hollingworth, S., et al. (2010). Affective and anxiety disorders: Prevalence, treatment and antidepressant medication use. *Australian and New Zealand Journal of Psychiatry, 44*, 513–519.

Horgan, J. (2011, July 12). *Are Antidepressants Just Placebos with Side Effects?* CrossCheck, Scientific American Blog Network. http://blogs.scientificamerican.com/crosscheck/2011/07/12/are-antidepressants-just-placebos-with-side-effects/. Accessed 6 April 2014.

Horwitz, A. V., & Wakefield, J. C. (2007). *The loss of sadness: How psychiatry transformed normal sorrow into depressive disorder*. New York: Oxford University Press.

Horwitz, A. V., & Wakefield, J. C. (2010). *Tristesse ou depression? Comment la psychiatrie a medicalise nos tristesses*. Traduit de l'anglais par Francoise Parot. Wavre: Edition Mardaga.

Kendler, K. S. (2010). *Statement on the proposal to eliminate the grief exclusion criterion from major depression*. http://www.dsm5.org/. Accessed 16 October 2010.

Kendler, K. S., Myers, J., & Zisook, S. (2008). Does bereavement related major depression differ from major depression associated with other stressful life events? *American Journal of Psychiatry, 165*, 1449–1455.

Kessler, R. C., McGonagle, K. A., Zhao, S., Nelson, C. B., Eshelman, S., Wittchen, H. U., et al. (1994). Lifetime and 12-month prevalence of DSM-III-R psychiatric disorders in the United States: Results from the National Comorbidity Survey. *Archives of General Psychiatry, 51*, 8–19.

Kessler, R. C., Nelson, C. B., McGonagle, K. A., Liu, J., Swartz, M. S., & Blazer, D. G. (1996). Comorbidity of DSM-III-R major depressive disorder in the general population: Results from the US National Comorbidity Survey. *British Journal of Psychiatry, 168*(suppl. 30), 17–30.

Kessler, R. C., Beglund, P., Demler, O., Jin, R., Koretz, D., Merikangas, K. R., et al. (2003). The epidemiology of major depressive disorder: Results from the National Comorbidity Survey replication. *Journal of the American Medical Association, 289*, 3095–3105.

Kessler, R. C., Berglund, P., Demler, O., Jin, R., Merikangas, K. R., & Walters, E. E. (2005). Lifetime prevalence and age-of-onset distributions of *DSM-IV* disorders in the National Comorbidity Survey Replication. *Arch Gen Psychiatry, 62*, 593–602.

Kirsch, I. (2010). *The emperor's new drugs: Exploding the antidepressant myth*. New York: Basic Books.

Kirsch, I., Moore, T. J., Scoboria, A., & Nicholls, S. S. (2002). The emperor's new drugs: An analysis of antidepressant medication data. *Prevention and Treatment, 5*, 23. doi:10.1037/1522-3736.5.1.523a.

Kirsch, I., Deacon, B. J., Huedo-Medina, T. B., Scoboria, A., Moore, T. J., & Johnson, B. (2008). Initial severity and antidepressant benefits: A meta-analysis of data submitted to the Food and Drug Administration. *PLoS Medicine, 5*(2), e45. doi:10.1371/journal.pmed.0050045.

Kitanaka, J. (2016). Depression as a problem of labor: Japanese debates about work, stress, and a new therapeutic ethos. In J. C. Wakefield & S. Demazeux (Eds.), *Sadness or depression? International perspectives on the depression epidemic and its meaning*. Dordrecht: Springer.

Klein, D. F., & Thase, M. (1997). Medication versus psychotherapy for depression: Progress notes. *American Society of Clinical Psychopharmacology, 8*, 41–47.

Kleinman, A. (2012). Culture, bereavement and psychiatry. *Lancet, 379*, 608–609.

Kramer, P. D. (2011, July 9). In defense of antidepressants. *New York Times Sunday Review*. http://www.nytimes.com/2011/07/10/opinion/sunday/10antidepressants.html?pagewanted=all. Accessed 25 July 2011.

Kruijshaar, M. E., Barendregt, J., Vos, T., de Graaf, R., Spijker, J., & Andrews, G. (2005). Lifetime prevalence estimates of major depression: An indirect estimate and a quantification of recall bias. *European Journal of Epidemiology, 20*, 103–111.

Lamb, K., Pies, R., & Zisook, S. (2010). The bereavement exclusion for the diagnosis of major depression: To be or not to be. *Psychiatry, 7*, 19–25.

Lane, C. 2011. Antidepressant withdrawal syndrome: Why SSRI antidepressants often produce a withdrawal syndrome. *Psychology Today Blog*. http://www.psychologytoday.com/blog/side-effects/201107/antidepressant-withdrawal-syndrome. Accessed 20 March 2014.

Maj, M. (2011a). When does depression become a mental disorder? *British Journal of Psychiatry, 199*, 85–86.

Maj, M. (2011b). Refining the diagnostic criteria for major depression on the basis of empirical evidence. *Acta Psychiatrica Scandinavica, 123*, 317.

Maj, M. (2013). "Clinical judgment" and the DSM-5 diagnosis of major depression. *World Psychiatry, 12*(2), 89–91.

Marcus, S. C., & Olfson, M. (2010). National trends in the treatment for depression from 1998 to 2007. *Archives of General Psychiatry, 67*(12), 1265–1273.

Mathers, C. D., & Loncar, D. (2006). Projections of global mortality and burden of disease from 2002 to 2030. *PLoS Medicine, 3*, e442. doi:10.1371/journal.pmed.0030442.

Melander, H., et al. (2008). A regulatory Apologia – A review of placebo-controlled studies in regulatory submissions of new-generation antidepressants. *European Neuropsychopharmacology, 18*(9), 623–627.

Mercier, A., Auger-Aubin, I., Lebeau, J.-P., Van Royen, P., & Peremans, L. (2011). Understanding the prescription of antidepressants: A qualitative study among French GPs. *BMC Family Practice, 12*(99), 1–9. http://www.biomedcentral.com/1471-2296/12/99.

Mitchell, A. J., Vaze, S., & Rao, S. (2009). Clinical diagnosis of depression in primary care: A metaanalysis. *Lancet, 374*, 609–619.

Moffitt, T. E., Harrington, H. L., Caspi, A., Kim-Cohen, J., Goldberg, D., Gregory, A. M., & Poulton, R. (2007). Depression and generalized anxiety disorder: Cumulative and sequential comorbidity in a birth cohort followed prospectively to age 32 years. *Archives of General Psychiatry, 64*, 651–660.

Moffitt, T. E., Caspi, A., Taylor, A., Kokaua, J., Milne, B., Polanczyk, G., & Poulton, R. (2010). How common are common mental disorders? Evidence that lifetime prevalence rates are doubled by prospective versus retrospective ascertainment. *Psychological Medicine, 40*(6), 899–909.

Mojtabai, R. (2008). Increase in antidepressant medication in the US adult population between 1990 and 2003. *Psychotherapy and Psychosomatics, 77*(2), 83–92.

Mojtabai, R. (2011). Bereavement-related depressive episodes: Characteristics, 3-year course, and implications for DSM-5. *Archives of General Psychiatry, 68*, 920–928.

Mojtabai, R. (2013). Clinician-identified depression in community settings: Concordance with structured-interview diagnoses. *Psychotherapy and Psychosomatics, 82*, 161–169.

Mojtabai, R., & Olfson, M. (2011). Proportion of antidepressants prescribed without a psychiatric diagnosis is growing. *Health Affairs, 30*(8), 1434–1442. doi:10.1377/hlthaff.2010.1024.

Moncrieff, J., Wessely, S. & Hardy, R. (2004). Active placebos versus antidepressants for depression. *Cochrane Database of Systematic Reviews, 2004*(1):CD003012.

Moore, M., Yuen, H. M., Dunn, N., Mullee, M. A., Maskell, J., & Kendrick, T. (2009). Explaining the rise in antidepressant prescribing: A descriptive study using the general practice research database. *British Medical Journal, 339*, 1–7. doi:10.1136/bmj.b3999.

Narrow, W. E., Rae, D. S., Robin, L. N., & Regier, D. A. (2002). Revised prevalence estimates of mental disorder in the United States: Using a clinical significance criterion to reconcile 2 survey's estimates. *Archives of General Psychiatry, 59*, 115–123.

OECD. (2013). *Health at a glance 2013: OECD indicators*. OECD Publishing. http://dx.doi.org/10.1787/health_glance-2013-en

Oldham, J., Carlat, D., Friedman, R., et al. (2011, August 18). 'The illusions of psychiatry': An exchange. *New York Review of Books*. http://www.nybooks.com/articles/archives/2011/aug/18/illusions-psychiatry-exchange. Accessed 6 April 2014.

Olfson, M., Marcus, S. C., Druss, B., & Pincus, H. A. (2002). National trends in the use of outpatient psychotherapy. *American Journal of Psychiatry, 159*, 1914–1920.

Parker, G. (1979). Sex differences in non-clinical depression. *Australian and New Zealand Journal of Psychiatry, 13*, 127–132.

Parker, G. (2007). Is depression overdiagnosed? Yes. *BMJ, 335*(7615), 328. doi:10.1136/bmj.39268.475799.AD.

Parker, G. (2011). Classifying clinical depression: An operational proposal. *Acta Psychiatrica Scandinavica, 123*, 314–316.

Parkes, C. (1964). Recent bereavement as a cause of mental illness. *British Journal of Psychiatry, 110*, 198–204.

Pies, R. (2008, December 12). Major depression after recent loss is major depression – Until proved otherwise. *Psychiatric Times*, p. 12.

Pigott, H. E., Leventhal, A. M., Alter, G. S., & Boren, J. J. (2010). Efficacy and effectiveness of antidepressants: Current status of research. *Psychotherapy and Psychosomatics, 79*(5), 267–279. doi:10.1159/000318293. Epub 2010 Jul 9.

Pratt, L. A., Brody, D. J., & Gu, Q. (2011). *Antidepressant use in persons aged 12 and over: United States, 2005–2008* (NCHS data brief, no 76). Hyattsville: National Center for Health Statistics.

Prigerson, H. G., Horowitz, M. J., Jacobs, S. C., Parkes, C. M., Aslan, M., Goodkin, K., et al. (2009). Prolonged grief disorder: Psychometric validation of criteria proposed for DSM-V and ICD-11. *PLoS Medicine, 6*, e1000121.

Read, J., Cartwright, C., & Gibson, K. (2014). Adverse emotional and interpersonal effects reported by 1829 New Zealanders while taking antidepressants. *Psychiatry Research, 216*, 67–73.

Regier, D. A., Kaelber, C. T., Rae, D. S., Farmer, M. E., Knauper, B., Kessler, R. C., et al. (1998). Limitations of diagnostic criteria and assessment instruments for mental disorders: Implications for research and policy. *Archives of General Psychiatry, 55*, 109–115.

Robins, L. N., & Regier, D. A. (1991). *Psychiatric disorders in America*. New York: Free Press.

Rohde, P., Lewinsohn, P. M., Klein, D. N., Seeley, J. R., & Gau, J. M. (2013). Key characteristics of major depressive disorder occurring in childhood, adolescence, emerging adulthood, and adulthood. *Clinical Psychological Science, 1*(1), 41–53.

Schatzberg, A. F., Blier, P., Delgado, P. L., Fava, M., Haddad, P. M., & Shelton, R. C. (2006). Antidepressant discontinuation syndrome: Consensus panel recommendations for clinical management and additional research. *Journal of Clinical Psychiatry, 67*(Suppl 4), 27–30.

Shear, M., Katherine, N., Simon, M., Wall, S., Zisook, R., Neimeyer, N. D., et al. (2011). Complicated grief and related bereavement issues for DSM-5. *Depression and Anxiety, 28*, 103–117.

Spitzer, R. L., & Wakefield, J. C. (1999). DSM-IV diagnostic criterion for clinical significance: Does it help solve the false positives problem? *American Journal of Psychiatry, 156*, 1856–1864.

Stewart, J. A., Deliyannides, D. A., Hellerstein, D. J., McGrath, P. J., & Stewart, J. W. (2012). Can people with nonsevere major depression benefit from antidepressant medication? *Journal of Clinical Psychiatry, 73*(4), 518–525.

Sunday dialogue: seeking a path through depression's landscape. (2011, July 16). *New York Times Sunday Review.* http://www.nytimes.com/2011/07/17/opinion/sunday/l17dialogue.html?pagewanted=all. Accessed 5 August 2011.

Thase, M. E., Larsen, K. G., & Kennedy, S. H. (2011). Assessing the 'true' effect of active antidepressant therapy v. placebo in major depressive disorder: Use of a mixture model. *British Journal of Psychiatry, 199*, 501–507.

Tyrer, P. (2009). Are general practitioners really unable to diagnose depression? *Lancet, 374*, 589–590.

Ustun, T. B., Yuso-Mateos, J. L., Chatterji, S., Mathers, C., & Murray, C. J. L. (2004). Global burden of depressive disorders in the year 2000. *British Journal of Psychiatry, 184*, 386–392.

Wakefield, J. C. (1992). The concept of mental disorder: On the boundary between biological facts and social values. *American Psychologist, 4*, 373–388.

Wakefield, J. C. (2006). The concept of mental disorder: Diagnostic implications of the harmful dysfunction analysis. *World Psychiatry, 6*, 149–156.

Wakefield, J. C. (2009). Disability and diagnosis: Should role impairment be eliminated from DSM/ICD diagnostic criteria? *World Psychiatry, 8*, 87–88.

Wakefield, J. C. (2011). Should uncomplicated bereavement-related depression be reclassified as a disorder in DSM-5? Response to Kenneth S. Kendler's statement defending the proposal to eliminate the bereavement exclusion. *Journal of Nervous and Mental Disease, 199*, 203–208.

Wakefield, J. C. (2012). Should prolonged grief be reclassified as a mental disorder in DSM-5? Reconsidering the empirical and conceptual arguments for proposed grief disorders. *Journal of Nervous and Mental Disease, 200*, 499–511.

Wakefield, J. C. (2013a). The DSM-5 debate over the bereavement exclusion: Psychiatric diagnosis and the future of empirically supported practice. *Clinical Psychology Review, 33*, 825–845.

Wakefield, J. C. (2013b). Is complicated/prolonged grief a disorder? Why the proposal to add "complicated grief disorder" to the DSM-5 is conceptually and empirically unsound. In M. Stroebe, H. Schut, & J. van den Bout (Eds.), *Complicated grief: Scientific foundations for health care professionals* (pp. 99–114). New York: Routledge.

Wakefield, J. C., & First, M. B. (2012a). Does the empirical evidence support the proposal to eliminate the major depression "bereavement exclusion" in DSM-5? *World Psychiatry, 11*, 3–10.

Wakefield, J. C., & First, M. B. (2012b). Placing symptoms in context: The role of contextual criteria in reducing false positives in DSM diagnosis. *Comprehensive Psychiatry, 53*, 130–139.

Wakefield, J. C., & First, M. B. (2013). The importance and limits of harm in identifying mental disorder. *Canadian Journal of Psychiatry, 58*(11), 618–621.

Wakefield, J. C., & Schmitz, M. F. (2012a). Recurrence of depression after bereavement-related depression: Evidence for the validity of the DSM-IV bereavement exclusion from the Epidemiologic Catchment Area Study. *Journal of Nervous and Mental Disease, 200*, 480–485.

Wakefield, J. C., & Schmitz, M. F. (2012b). Beyond reactive versus endogenous: Should uncomplicated stress-triggered depression be excluded from major depression diagnosis? A review of the evidence. *Minerva Psichiatrica, 53*, 251–276.

Wakefield, J. C., & Schmitz, M. F. (2013a). Normal vs. disordered bereavement-related depression: Are the differences real or tautological? *Acta Psychiatrica Scandinavica, 127*, 159–168.

Wakefield, J. C., & Schmitz, M. F. (2013b). Can the DSM's major depression bereavement exclusion be validly extended to other stressors?: Evidence from the NCS. *Acta Psychiatrica Scandinavica, 128*, 294–305.

Wakefield, J. C., & Schmitz, M. F. (2013c). When does depression become a disorder? Using recurrence rates to evaluate the validity of proposed changes in major depression diagnostic thresholds. *World Psychiatry, 12*, 44–52.

Wakefield, J. C., & Schmitz, M. F. (2014a). Uncomplicated depression, suicide attempt, and the DSM-5 bereavement-exclusion debate: An empirical evaluation. *Research on Social Work Practice, 24*(1), 37–49.

Wakefield, J. C., & Schmitz, M. F. (2014b). Predictive validation of single episode uncomplicated depression as a benign subtype of unipolar major depression. *Acta Psychiatrica Scandinavica, 129*, 445–457.

Wakefield, J. C., & Spitzer, R. L. (2002). Lowered estimates – But of what? *Archives of General Psychiatry, 59*, 129–130.

Wakefield, J. C., Schmitz, M. F., First, M. B., & Horwitz, A. V. (2007). Should the bereavement exclusion for major depression be extended to other losses? Evidence from the National Comorbidity Survey. *Archives of General Psychiatry, 64*, 433–440.

Wakefield, J. C., Schmitz, M. F., & Baer, J. C. (2010). Does the DSM-IV clinical significance criterion for major depression reduce false positives?: Evidence from the NCS-R. *The American Journal of Psychiatry, 167*, 298–304.

Wakefield, J. C., Schmitz, M. F., & Baer, J. C. (2011a). Relation between duration and severity in bereavement-related depression. *Acta Psychiatrica Scandinavica, 124*, 487–494.

Wakefield, J. C., Schmitz, M. F., & Baer, J. C. (2011b). Did narrowing the major depression bereavement exclusion from DSM-III-R to DSM-IV increase validity? Evidence from the National Comorbidity Survey. *Journal of Nervous and Mental Disease, 199*, 66–73.

Warner, C. H., Bobo, W., Warner, C., Reid, S., & Rachal, J. (2006). Antidepressant discontinuation syndrome. *American Family Physician, 74*(3), 449–456.

Watters, E. (2010). *Crazy like us: The globalization of the American psyche.* New York: The Free Press.

Weber, C. (2013). Wenn Trauer zur Krankheit wird. *Suddeutche Zeitung.* http://www.sueddeutsche.de/gesundheit/neue-diagnosekriterien-in-der-psychiatrie-wenn-trauer-zur-krankheit-wird-1.1649873. Accessed 5 April 2014.

Wells, J. E., & Horwood, L. J. (2004). How accurate is recall of key symptoms of depression? A comparison of recall and longitudinal reports. *Psychological Medicine, 34*, 1001–1011.

Whoriskey, P. (2012, December 26). Antidepressants to treat grief? Psychiatry panelists with ties to drug industry say yes. *The Washington Post.* http://www.washingtonpost.com/business/economy/antidepressants-to-treat-grief-psychiatry-panelists-with-ties-to-drug-industry-say-yes/2012/12/26/ca09cde6-3d60-11e2-ae43-cf491b837f7b_story.html. Accessed 6 April 2014.

Wilhelm, K., Parker, G., & Hadzi-Pavlovic, D. (1996). Fifteen years on: Evolving ideas in researching sex differences in depression. *Psychological Medicine, 27*, 875–883.

Wilhelm, K., Mitchell, P. B., Niven, H., Finch, A., Wedgwood, L., Scimone, A., Blair, I. P., Parker, G., & Schofield, P. R. (2006). Life events, first depression onset and the serotonin transporter gene. *British Journal of Psychiatry, 188*, 210–215.

World Health Organization. (1992). *ICD-10: International statistical classification of diseases and related health problems, tenth revision.* Geneva: World Health Organization.

Zajecka, J., Tracy, K. A., & Mitchell, S. (1997). Discontinuation symptoms after treatment with serotonin reuptake inhibitors: A literature review. *Journal of Clinical Psychiatry, 58*, 291–297.

Zisook, S.. (2010, August 2). Today in your health: Bereavement. *National Public Radio, Morning Edition.*

Zisook, S., & Kendler, K. S. (2007). Is bereavement-related depression different than nonbereavement-related depression? *Psychological Medicine, 37*, 779–794.

Zisook, S., Shuchter, S. R., Pedrelli, P., Sable, J., & Deaciuc, S. C. (2001). Bupropion sustained release for bereavement: Results of an open trial. *Journal of Clinical Psychiatry, 62*, 227–230.

Zisook, S., Shear, K., & Kendler, K. S. (2007). Validity of the bereavement exclusion criterion for the diagnosis of major depressive episode. *World Psychiatry, 6*, 102–107.

# Index

© Springer Science+Business Media Dordrecht 2016
J.C. Wakefield, S. Demazeux (eds.), *Sadness or Depression?*
History, Philosophy and Theory of the Life Sciences 15,
DOI 10.1007/978-94-017-7423-9

CPSIA information can be obtained
at www.ICGtesting.com
Printed in the USA
LVHW080411180521
687657LV00002B/205